Critical Rehabilitation for Partial and Total Knee Arthroplasty

Frank R. Noyes • Sue Barber-Westin
Editors

Critical Rehabilitation for Partial and Total Knee Arthroplasty

Guidelines and Objective Testing to Allow Return to Physical Function, Recreational and Sports Activities

Springer

Editors
Frank R. Noyes
Cincinnati Sportsmedicine and Orthopedic Center
Noyes Knee Institute
Cincinnati, OH
USA

Sue Barber-Westin
Noyes Knee Institute
Cincinnati, OH
USA

ISBN 978-3-030-87002-7 ISBN 978-3-030-87003-4 (eBook)
https://doi.org/10.1007/978-3-030-87003-4

This Springer imprint is published by the registered company Springer Nature Switzerland AG
The registered company address is: Gewerbestrasse 11, 6330 Cham, Switzerland

Preface

The successful treatment of patients undergoing partial and total knee replacements has multiple facets that require careful planning and strict compliance of issues that span the entire program. These include preoperative assessments, understanding patient goals and individual issues, and technical operative details. Most important, and the major topic of this book, is the postoperative rehabilitation program that successfully restores knee motion, function, strength, and return to daily and recreational activities.

Many younger, athletic patients that undergo knee replacement have a strong desire to resume an active lifestyle after surgery. This places a sometimes daunting responsibility on the clinical team to design and implement rehabilitation protocols that allow a higher level of activities postoperatively. The task of setting realistic patient goals and expectations in younger patients who expect to have nearly normal knee function may be difficult, even with the best of operative outcomes.

Complicating matters is the fact that these individuals commonly delay surgery for a few years due to arthritis-induced symptoms. They typically present with muscle atrophy and altered limb function encompassing all muscle groups of the hip and lower extremity. Preoperative rehabilitation may be required to improve muscle strength and function, and evidence of the effectiveness of such programs is described in this book.

It is interesting to note from a historical standpoint that published knee replacement rehabilitation programs commonly failed to provide parameters for return to athletic activities. They lacked an emphasis on individual assessments, objective methods to determine function and strength, and outcome instruments that specifically detailed the return to recreational and athletic pursuits. A similar observation existed for rehabilitation and return to sports protocols after athletic knee injuries that underwent extensive changes in the past decade [1]. At our Knee Institute, there is very little difference in the entire rehabilitation program for treatment of both sports injuries and knee replacements. Our extensive clinical experience has shown that patients who desire to return to recreational sports after knee replacement need more robust and advanced programs.

The majority of published knee replacement rehabilitation protocols often discharge all patients 12 weeks after surgery. This book emphasizes the need for extended rehabilitation to completely restore lower limb function, strength, and coordination parameters for patient who desire to resume recreational and athletic activities. Individualized programs to match patient goals and recreational pursuits, detailed in several chapters, may require up to 12 months to achieve a high degree of success and patient satisfaction. Gone are the days when patients are discharged from therapy just a few months postoperatively who are barely recovered and still harbor extensive muscle disuse and poor function due to surgery and prior inactivity.

We wish to thank all of the authors of *Critical Rehabilitation for Partial and Total Knee Replacement* whose contributions provide the successful aspects they have implemented in the monitoring and structure of rehabilitation programs. This knowledge base should assist patient clinics worldwide in implementing these strategies into their own postoperative programs. The advanced rehabilitation concepts detailed in this book will help achieve a high level of patient satisfaction for the achievement of an active lifestyle following knee replacement surgery.

Cincinnati, OH, USA Frank R. Noyes
Cincinnati, OH, USA Sue Barber-Westin

Reference

1. Noyes FR, Barber-Westin Sue. Return to sport after ACL reconstruction and other knee operations. Limiting the risk of reinjury and maximizing athletic performance. Springer ISBN 978-3-030-22360-1.

Contents

Contributors

Albert T. Anastasio Department of Orthopaedic Surgery, Duke University Medical Center, Durham, NC, USA

Sue Barber-Westin Noyes Knee Institute, Cincinnati, OH, USA

Lefko T. Charalambous Department of Orthopaedic Surgery, Duke University Medical Center, Durham, NC, USA

Niall H. Cochrane Department of Orthopaedic Surgery, Duke University Medical Center, Durham, NC, USA

Timothy Heckmann Noyes Knee Institute, Cincinnati, OH, USA

David L. Kerr Department of Orthopaedic Surgery, Duke University Medical Center, Durham, NC, USA

A. J. Kievit Department of Orthopedic Surgery, Amsterdam Movement Sciences, Amsterdam Centre for European Studies, Amsterdam University Medical Centers, Amsterdam, Netherlands

P. P. F. M. Kuijer Department of Public and Occupational Health, Amsterdam Public Health Research Institute, Amsterdam Movement Sciences, Amsterdam University Medical Centers, Amsterdam, Netherlands

Frank R. Noyes Cincinnati SportsMedicine and Orthopaedic Center, The Noyes Knee Institute, Cincinnati, OH, USA

M. U. Schafroth Department of Orthopedic Surgery, Amsterdam Movement Sciences, Amsterdam Centre for European Studies, Amsterdam University Medical Centers, Amsterdam, Netherlands

Thorsten M. Seyler Department of Orthopaedic Surgery, Duke University Medical Center, Durham, NC, USA

Mark Wu Department of Orthopaedic Surgery, Duke University Medical Center, Durham, NC, USA

Introduction: Epidemiology of Knee Arthroplasty in a Younger Patient Population

1

Sue Barber-Westin and Frank R. Noyes

1.1 Introduction

Total knee arthroplasty (TKA) is one of the most commonly performed elective surgical procedures in the USA, with an exponential growth in volume noted in the past few decades [1–7]. In 2011–2012, an estimated 14–15 million individuals in the USA had symptomatic knee osteoarthritis (OA), of whom more than half had sufficient progression of the disease to warrant consideration for TKA [8]. In 2012, over 700,000 TKAs were performed, for a rate of 223 per 100,000 individuals [9]. This was the highest rate of TKAs among 24 OECD (Organisation for Economic Co-operation and Development) countries studied that year. Other countries with high incidence rates included Austria (218 per 100,000 inhabitants), Germany (206 per 100,000 inhabitants), and Switzerland (205 per 100,000 inhabitants) [10]. Globally, from 2005 to 2011, the highest annual TKA growth rate occurred in patients <65 years of age, and significant associations were noted between increased TKA utilization rates and higher gross national product ($r = 0.53$, $P < 0.01$), greater health expenditures ($r = 0.68$, $P < 0.001$), and obesity ($r = 0.46$–0.72, $P < 0.05$).

Many studies have provided estimated future projections of TKA volume and incidence rates using different epidemiological models [6, 11–15]. Incidence rates are typically calculated as the number of TKAs during a specified time period divided by the size of the US population (using US Census Bureau data) during the same time period. This chapter assesses the most current data available as of May 2020 and discusses factors that affect models and projections for future TKA numbers in the USA. Factors such as age and gender are taken into account when

S. Barber-Westin (✉)
Noyes Knee Institute, Cincinnati, OH, USA
e-mail: sbwestin@csmref.org

F. R. Noyes
Cincinnati SportsMedicine and Orthopaedic Center, The Noyes Knee Institute, Cincinnati, OH, USA

F. R. Noyes, S. Barber-Westin (eds.), *Critical Rehabilitation for Partial and Total Knee Arthroplasty*, https://doi.org/10.1007/978-3-030-87003-4_1

available. The effect of long-term participation in athletics and sports injuries on the future development of knee osteoarthritis (OA) and potentially TKA is reviewed.

1.2 Historic Annual Numbers and Incidence Rates of Primary TKA in the USA

The number and incidence rates of primary TKA performed in the USA according to various studies are shown in Table 1.1 [3, 6, 7, 9, 12]. Although all of the studies except one [10] used the same databases – the National Inpatient Sample (NIS) taken from the US Healthcare Cost and Utilization Project (HCUP) and the US Census Bureau – the volume and incidence rates varied among the investigations. The NIS is an annual national survey of discharge information from approximately 1000 hospitals and is considered statistically valid because it represents 95% of the US population [12, 15].

In a published report from HCUP, Fingar et al. [9] reported that 421,700 TKAs were performed in 2003, which increased to 700,100 in 2012, representing an overall 66% increase in volume. This study included patients of all ages. Sloan et al. [6] reported fewer procedures (in patients of all ages): 369,405 TKAs in 2012 and 630,509 TKAs in 2013, for an overall 71% increase in volume from 2000. Interestingly, these authors found that the mean annual increase in TKA volume significantly decreased from 2008 to 2014 compared with the time period of 2000–2008 (3.6% and 10.2%, respectively, $P = 0.015$). Inacio et al. [12] reported numbers in patients >40 years of age that were very similar to those of Sloan et al.; however, the incidence rates were more than twice as those of Sloan's for unknown reasons.

Gender comparisons of TKA incidence rates have been conducted in two studies [6, 7], both of which found higher incidence rates in women compared with men (Table 1.2). Williams et al. [7] in a report from the US Department of Health and Human Services found similar increases in the rate of TKA for men and women from 2000 through 2010 (86% and 99%, respectively). However, the rate of TKA for women was higher compared with men in 2000 (33.0 and 24.3 per 10,000, respectively) and in 2010 (65.5 and 45.3 per 10,000, respectively). The difference in rates is most notable in patients aged 45 to 64. Sloan et al. [6] reported large differences in incidence rates between men and women in 2000 and again in 2014. This study also reported large increases in incidence rates according to patient age in 2014 compared with 2000. For instance, the incidence rate in patients aged 65–69 was 498.3 per 100,000 individuals in 2000 and 909.2 per 100,000 individuals in 2014.

As of the time of writing, only two studies estimated prevalence rates of TKA in the USA [16, 17]. Prevalence rates represent the proportion of patients who are alive on a certain date who had TKA, regardless of what year the procedure was performed. One study [16] estimated that in 2010, approximately 4.55% of the entire US population ≥50 years of age, or 4.7 million individuals, had a TKA. The rates increased with each decade of age until ≥90 years and were 1.48% for ages 50–59,

Table 1.1 Historic volume and incidence rates of primary total knee arthroplasty in the USA

Year TKA volume reported	Study	Patient ages studied (year)	Volume TKA	Incidence rate per 100,000 individuals
2000	Sloan et al. [6]	All	274,025	97
	Inacio et al. [12]	≥40	274,463	229
	Kim et al. [3]	All	281,534	Not done
2001	Sloan et al. [6]	All	305,108	107
	Inacio et al. [12]	≥40	305,572	249
	Kim et al. [3]	All	313,618	Not done
2002	Sloan et al. [6]	All	339,225	118
	Inacio et al. [12]	≥40	339,681	272
	Kim et al. [3]	All	350,122	All
2003	Sloan et al. [6]	All	369,405	127
	Inacio et al. [12]	≥40	369,985	290
	Kim et al. [3]	All	379,719	Not done
	Fingar et al. [9]	All	421,700	145.4
2004	Sloan et al. [6]	All	431,852	147
	Inacio et al. [12]	≥40	419,774	323
	Kim et al. [3]	All	431,485	Not done
2005	Sloan et al. [6]	All	482,369	163
	Inacio et al. [12]	≥40	483,067	365
	Kurtz et al. [15]	All	471,088	Not done
	Pabinger et al. [10]	All	Not done	185
2006	Sloan et al. [6]	All	481,941	161
	Inacio et al. [12]	≥40	482,689	358
	Pabinger et al. [10]	All	Not done	175
	Kurtz et al. [13]	All	524,600	Not done
		<45	9900	Not done
		45–54	59,100	Not done
		55–64	147,100	Not done
2007	Sloan et al. [6]	All	532,883	177
	Inacio et al. [12]	≥40	533,602	390
	Pabinger et al. [10]	All	Not done	172
2008	Sloan et al. [6]	All	591,564	194
	Inacio et al. [12]	≥40	592,323	427
	Losina et al. [41]	All	615,050	Not done
	Pabinger et al. [10]	All	Not done	201
2009	Sloan et al. [6]	All	596,939	194
	Inacio et al. [12]	≥40	597,541	424
	Pabinger et al. [10]	All	Not done	213
2010	Sloan et al. [6]	All	632,091	204
	Inacio et al. [12]	≥40	632,862	442
	Williams et al. [7]	≥45	693,400	Not done
	Pabinger et al. [10]	All	Not done	226
2011	Sloan et al. [6]	All	617,945	198
	Inacio et al. [12]	≥40	618,604	426
	Pabinger et al. [10]	All	Not done	235
2012	Sloan et al. [6]	All	630,509	201
	Inacio et al. [12]	≥40	631,214	429
	Fingar et al. [9]	All	700,100	223
2013	Sloan et al. [6]	All	661,695	209
2014	Sloan et al. [6]	All	680,150	213

Table 1.2 Historic annual incidence rates of primary total knee arthroplasty according to gender and age in the USA

Year TKA incidence rate reported	Study	Age (year): incidence rate	Gender: incidence rate	Age (year) and gender: incidence rate
2000	Sloan et al. [6]	<45: 3.0/100,000 45–54: 66.7/100,000 55–64: 249.6/100,000 65–69: 498.3/100,000 70–74: 614.7/100,000 75–79: 635/100,000 80–84: 501.8/100,000 ≥85: 209.9/100,000	Female: 120.7/100,000 Male: 73.1/100,000	Not done
	Williams et al. [7]	Not done	Female: 33.0/10,000 Male: 24.3/10,000	Female 45–64: 16.4/10,000 Male 45–64: 8.7/10,000 Female ≥65: 58.8/10,000 Male >65: 57.0/10,000
2005	Pabinger et al. [10]	≤64: 36/100,000 ≥65: 149/100,000	Not done	Not done
2006	Pabinger et al. [10]	≤64: 35/100,000 ≥65: 140/100,000	Not done	Not done
2007	Pabinger et al. [10]	≤64: 35/100,000 ≥65: 137/100,000	Not done	Not done
2008	Pabinger et al. [10]	≤64: 44/100,000 ≥65: 157/100,000	Not done	Not done
2009	Pabinger et al. [10]	≤64: 48/100,000 ≥65: 165/100,000	Not done	Not done
2010	Pabinger et al. [10]	≤64: 53/100,000 ≥65: 173/100,000	Not done	Not done
2011	Pabinger et al. [10]	≤64: 58/100,000 ≥65: 177/100,000	Not done	Not done
2014	Sloan et al. [6]	<45: 5.8/100,000 45–54: 168.3/100,000 55–64: 525.3/100,000 65–69: 909.2/100,000 70–74: 1016.6/100,000 75–79: 966.6/100,000 80–84: 716.7/100,000 ≥ 85: 259.2/100,000	Female: 259.8/100,000 Male: 165.3/100,000	Not done

Table 1.2 (continued)

Year TKA incidence rate reported	Study	Age (year): incidence rate	Gender: incidence rate	Age (year) and gender: incidence rate
2015	Williams et al. [7]	Not done	Female: 65.5/10,000 Male: 45.3/10,000	Female 45–64: 46.6/10,000 Male 45–64: 828.6/10,000 Female ≥65: 99.3/10,000 Male >65: 82.6/10,000

4.59% for ages 60–69, 8.80% for ages 70–79, 10.13% for ages 80–89, and 7.40% for ages >90. Women had higher prevalence rates than men for all ages except the ≥90 category (7.39% and 7.41%, respectively). An earlier study [17] published rates that were approximately 20% lower due to differing statistical methods and inclusion of older data. Even so, that study found prevalence rates higher among females than males and increasing rates with each decade of age.

1.3 Projected Volume of TKA

Investigations have used various models, including linear, Poisson, and logistic, to estimate or project future TKA volume and incidence rates [3, 6, 11–15]. Factors entered into the models typically include US Census Bureau data and historic TKA volume calculated from the NIS database, which provides an approximate 20% sample of patients discharged from 1000 hospitals in 44 states, which is 95% representative of the US population [12]. US population growth is projected, and other factors such as age, gender, ethnicity, obesity, and US census region that produce different incidence rates [6, 11, 14, 15] may be included. Poisson and linear regression models assume an exponential or continuous increase in demand for TKA throughout the study time period and have been used most frequently in recent literature [6, 11–14]. A logistic model uses an upper limit (estimated maximum incidence) in the number of TKAs as one of several parameters and produces a more conservative projection [12].

A comparison of projected volume and incidence rates from the most recent studies for the years 2025 to 2050 is shown in Table 1.3. Tremendous variability exists, even in studies that used the same model. For instance, the Poisson model estimates for the total number of TKA for the year 2030 ranged from 1,678,200 to 4,344,900. Two studies conducted analyses according to patient age [6, 13]. The projected volume for patients <45 years of age in 2030 ranged from 9800 to 95,200; for patients aged 45 to 54, from 51,500 to 994,600; and for patients aged 55 to 64, from 162,300 to 1,300,200. These models use historic data to predict data typically at least 10 years ahead, and authors acknowledge there are several limitations in projection methodology. These include the inability to account for future population

Table 1.3 Projected volume and incidence rates of primary total knee arthroplasty in the USA

Year TKA projected	Study/regression model	Age (year)/ gender studied	Volume TKA	Incidence rate per 100,000 individuals
2025	Bashinskaya et al. [11]/ linear	All	2,428,810	NA
	Inacio et al. [12]/ logistic/Poisson	>40	1,027,494/1,446,387	603/849
2030	Bashinskaya et al. [11]/ linear	All	3,008,718	NA
	Sloan et al. [6]/linear/ Poisson	All	1,252,900/1,678,200	NA
		<45 years	17,900/25,600	NA
		45–54 years	123,500/158,600	NA
		55–64 years	334,800/452,800	NA
		65–69 years	284,400/400,500	NA
		70–74 years	278,200/410,600	NA
		75–79 years	209,400/310,500	NA
		80–84 years	104,600/163,800	NA
		≥85 years	28,600/49,800	NA
		All men	491,100/643,900	NA
		All women	761,800/1,026,100	NA
	Inacio et al. [12]/ logistic/Poisson	>40	1,163,697/1,950,967	645/1082
	Kurtz et al. [14]/Poisson	All	3,480,000	NA
	Kurtz et al. [13]/Poisson/ constant	All	4,344,900/792,200	NA
		<45 years	95,200/9800	NA
		45–54 years	994,100/51,500	NA
		55–64 years	1,300,200/162,300	NA
2035	Bashinskaya et al. [11]/ linear	All	3,394,921	NA
	Inacio et al. [12]/ logistic/Poisson	>40	1,286,531/2,621,920	676/1379
2040	Bashinskaya et al. [11]/ linear	All	3,656,712	NA
	Inacio et al. [12]/ logistic/Poisson	>40	1,383,809/3,479,536	699/1757
2045	Bashinskaya et al. [11]/ linear	All	3,884,707	NA
	Inacio et al. [12]/ logistic/Poisson	>40	1,463,313/4,587,552	714/2239
2050	Bashinskaya et al. [11]/ linear	All	4,174,554	NA
	Inacio et al. [12]/ logistic/Poisson	>40	1,531,566/6,030,029	725/2854

numbers, unexpected changes in healthcare systems, politics, surgeon availability, more sports injuries, changes in life expectancy, increasing incidence of obesity, economic resources, recessions, and potential national disasters that limit accessibility to elective surgery (such as the recent COVID-19 pandemic). It is also difficult to project the prevalence of severe symptomatic knee OA, which is increasing rapidly [8, 18]. In addition, these models do not take into account the impact of new technologies – such as cartilage restoration, tissue engineering, and drug therapies – that could lessen the need for TKA. Longer-term projections, such as those 30 years in advance, are expected to be more unreliable [12].

1.4 Impact of Athletic Knee Injuries on Future Osteoarthritis and TKA

Serious knee injuries are a strong risk factor for the development of OA [19–26]. These include anterior cruciate ligament (ACL) ruptures [25, 27, 28], especially those combined with complex meniscus tears requiring meniscectomy [20, 25, 29–31], as well as patellar dislocations [32–34] and complete knee dislocations [35–37]. Recent data suggests that ACL and meniscus injuries significantly increase the risk of a subsequent TKA. In a matched case-control study of 49,723 TKA patients and 104,353 controls in the UK, Khan et al. [38] reported that a history of an ACL injury increased the odds of a subsequent TKA by nearly sevenfold (odds ratio [OR], 6.96; 95% confidence interval [CI] 4.73 to 10.31) and a meniscus injury increased the odds by 15-fold (OR, 15.24; 95% CI 13.88–16.69). The study was based on 20-year longitudinal data, and unfortunately, the investigators were unable to determine the treatment of the ACL and meniscus injuries. However, the findings were similar to those reported by Leroux et al. [39] in a study from Canada that reported that the cumulative incidence of TKA following cruciate ligament reconstruction (ACL or posterior cruciate ligament) was seven times greater than that of a matched control group from the general population (OR, 7.26; 95% CI 5.79–9.11). This study involved 30,277 patients who had undergone cruciate ligament reconstruction and 151,362 individuals from the general population. The majority of patients followed were <50 years of age and had undergone TKA in a mean of 11 years after the knee ligament reconstruction.

A study from Australia found that a history of a sports knee injury more than doubled the odds of a TKA compared with injuries to other areas of the body (OR, 2.41; 95% CI 1.73–3.37), after adjusting for potential confounding factors including age, gender, insurance type, and length of hospital stay for the injury [40]. This study included 64,038 patients who sustained a sports injury between 2000 and 2005 and were followed until 2015. There were 357 patients (0.6%) that required TKA. Suter et al. [21] used the Osteoarthritis Policy Model to project the cumulative incidence of TKA in four patient cohorts: no knee injury, isolated ACL rupture treated conservatively, isolated ACL reconstruction, and ACL reconstruction and medial meniscus tear treated either conservatively or operatively (Table 1.4). Patients who sustained an ACL and meniscus tear by age 25 had a nearly fourfold increase in the estimated lifetime risk of TKA compared with individuals who had no injury (22.3%; 95% CI 16.8–27.9).

Table 1.4 Risk of symptomatic knee osteoarthritis and TKA[a]

Outcome	No injury	Isolated ACL reconstruction[b]	Isolated ACL tear treated conservatively[b]	ACL reconstruction with meniscus tear[b, c]
Lifetime risk of symptomatic knee osteoarthritis	13.5%	16.2%	17.3%	34.2%
Lifetime risk of TKA	6.0%	8.0%	8.9%	22.3%

[a]From Suter et al. [21]
[b]Injured by age 25
[c]Treated in any manner

1.5 Conclusions

In conclusion, the most recent data at the time of writing shows marked increases in the incidence of TKA by 60–70% over the last 15 years. Prior athletic injuries are an important aspect of TKA prevalence. Granted, over the past decade there have been many improved treatment options for common knee ligament injuries and meniscus tears which may be repaired instead of removed that likely will decrease the effect of athletic injuries on knee arthritis in the future. Still, a prior injury (whether athletic or other trauma) increases the odds for subsequent knee replacement surgery in younger and active patients. In addition, there have been major advances in TKA surgery including pre-emptive programs for patient optimization and prehabilitation before surgery, surgical advances of decreasing blood loss and need for transfusion, improved instrumentation for predictable results, and better understanding by patients that the risks of TKA are in fact very small. Patient-reported outcome measures (PROMs) after TKA show major improvements in symptoms and quality of life that have led to more patients requesting the surgery rather than living with advancing knee osteoarthritis. This is a dynamic issue with knee osteoarthritis affecting millions of patients worldwide, and this book is dedicated to showing the major advances that clinics and institutions have implemented that are important to acknowledge and disseminate.

References

1. Cram P, Lu X, Kates SL, Singh JA, Li Y, Wolf BR. Total knee arthroplasty volume, utilization, and outcomes among Medicare beneficiaries, 1991–2010. JAMA. 2012;308(12):1227–36. https://doi.org/10.1001/2012.jama.11153.
2. Jain NB, Higgins LD, Ozumba D, Guller U, Cronin M, Pietrobon R, Katz JN. Trends in epidemiology of knee arthroplasty in the United States, 1990–2000. Arthritis Rheum. 2005;52(12):3928–33. https://doi.org/10.1002/art.21420.
3. Kim S. Changes in surgical loads and economic burden of hip and knee replacements in the US: 1997–2004. Arthritis Rheum. 2008;59(4):481–8. https://doi.org/10.1002/art.23525.
4. Kurtz SM, Ong KL, Schmier J, Zhao K, Mowat F, Lau E. Primary and revision arthroplasty surgery caseloads in the United States from 1990 to 2004. J Arthroplasty. 2009;24(2):195–203. https://doi.org/10.1016/j.arth.2007.11.015.

5. Mehrotra C, Remington PL, Naimi TS, Washington W, Miller R. Trends in total knee replacement surgeries and implications for public health, 1990–2000. Public Health Rep. 2005;120(3):278–82.
6. Sloan M, Premkumar A, Sheth NP. Projected volume of primary total joint arthroplasty in the U.S., 2014 to 2030. J Bone Joint Surg Am. 2018;100(17):1455–60. https://doi.org/10.2106/JBJS.17.01617.
7. Williams SN, Wolford ML, Bercovitz A. Hospitalization for total knee replacement among inpatients aged 45 and over: United States, 2000–2010. NCHS Data Brief. 2015;210:1–8.
8. Deshpande BR, Katz JN, Solomon DH, Yelin EH, Hunter DJ, Messier SP, Suter LG, Losina E. Number of persons with symptomatic knee osteoarthritis in the US: impact of race and ethnicity, age, sex, and obesity. Arthritis Care Res. 2016;68(12):1743–50. https://doi.org/10.1002/acr.22897.
9. Fingar KR, Stocks C, Weiss AJ, Steiner CA. Most frequent operating room procedures performed in US hospitals, 2003–2012: statistical brief# 186. Healthcare Cost and Utilization Project (HCUP) Statistical Briefs. Rockville: Agency for Health Care Policy and Research (US); 2014.
10. Pabinger C, Lothaller H, Geissler A. Utilization rates of knee-arthroplasty in OECD countries. Osteoarthr Cartil. 2015;23(10):1664–73. https://doi.org/10.1016/j.joca.2015.05.008.
11. Bashinskaya B, Zimmerman RM, Walcott BP, Antoci V. arthroplasty utilization in the United States is predicted by age-specific population groups. ISRN Orthop. 2012. https://doi.org/10.5402/2012/185938.
12. Inacio MCS, Paxton EW, Graves SE, Namba RS, Nemes S. Projected increase in total knee arthroplasty in the United States - an alternative projection model. Osteoarthr Cartil. 2017;25(11):1797–803. https://doi.org/10.1016/j.joca.2017.07.022.
13. Kurtz SM, Lau E, Ong K, Zhao K, Kelly M, Bozic KJ. Future young patient demand for primary and revision joint replacement: national projections from 2010 to 2030. Clin Orthop Relat Res. 2009;467(10):2606–12. https://doi.org/10.1007/s11999-009-0834-6.
14. Kurtz S, Ong K, Lau E, Mowat F, Halpern M. Projections of primary and revision hip and knee arthroplasty in the United States from 2005 to 2030. J Bone Joint Surg Am. 2007;89(4):780–5. https://doi.org/10.2106/JBJS.F.00222.
15. Kurtz SM, Ong KL, Lau E, Bozic KJ. Impact of the economic downturn on total joint replacement demand in the United States: updated projections to 2021. J Bone Joint Surg Am. 2014;96(8):624–30. https://doi.org/10.2106/JBJS.M.00285.
16. Maradit Kremers H, Larson DR, Crowson CS, Kremers WK, Washington RE, Steiner CA, Jiranek WA, Berry DJ. Prevalence of total hip and knee replacement in the United States. J Bone Joint Surg Am. 2015;97(17):1386–97. https://doi.org/10.2106/JBJS.N.01141.
17. Weinstein AM, Rome BN, Reichmann WM, Collins JE, Burbine SA, Thornhill TS, Wright J, Katz JN, Losina E. Estimating the burden of total knee replacement in the United States. J Bone Joint Surg Am. 2013;95(5):385–92. https://doi.org/10.2106/JBJS.L.00206.
18. Sebbag E, Felten R, Sagez F, Sibilia J, Devilliers H, Arnaud L. The world-wide burden of musculoskeletal diseases: a systematic analysis of the World Health Organization Burden of Diseases Database. Ann Rheum Dis. 2019;78(6):844–8.
19. Oiestad BE, Engebretsen L, Storheim K, Risberg MA. Knee osteoarthritis after anterior cruciate ligament injury: a systematic review. Am J Sports Med. 2009;37(7):1434–43. https://doi.org/10.1177/0363546509338827.
20. van Meer BL, Meuffels DE, van Eijsden WA, Verhaar JA, Bierma-Zeinstra SM, Reijman M. Which determinants predict tibiofemoral and patellofemoral osteoarthritis after anterior cruciate ligament injury? A systematic review. Br J Sports Med. 2015;49(15):975–83. https://doi.org/10.1136/bjsports-2013-093258.
21. Suter LG, Smith SR, Katz JN, Englund M, Hunter DJ, Frobell R, Losina E. Projecting lifetime risk of symptomatic knee osteoarthritis and total knee replacement in individuals sustaining a complete anterior cruciate ligament tear in early adulthood. Arthritis Care Res. 2017;69(2):201–8. https://doi.org/10.1002/acr.22940.

22. Prien A, Boudabous S, Junge A, Verhagen E, Delattre BMA, Tscholl PM. Every second retired elite female football player has MRI evidence of knee osteoarthritis before age 50 years: a cross-sectional study of clinical and MRI outcomes. Knee Surg Sports Traumatol Arthrosc. 2020;28(2):353–62. https://doi.org/10.1007/s00167-019-05560-w.
23. Poulsen E, Goncalves GH, Bricca A, Roos EM, Thorlund JB, Juhl CB. Knee osteoarthritis risk is increased 4–6 fold after knee injury - a systematic review and meta-analysis. Br J Sports Med. 2019;53(23):1454–63. https://doi.org/10.1136/bjsports-2018-100022.
24. Silverwood V, Blagojevic-Bucknall M, Jinks C, Jordan JL, Protheroe J, Jordan KP. Current evidence on risk factors for knee osteoarthritis in older adults: a systematic review and meta-analysis. Osteoarthr Cartil. 2015;23(4):507–15. https://doi.org/10.1016/j.joca.2014.11.019.
25. Sanders TL, Pareek A, Kremers HM, Bryan AJ, Levy BA, Stuart MJ, Dahm DL, Krych AJ. Long-term follow-up of isolated ACL tears treated without ligament reconstruction. Knee Surg Sports Traumatol Arthrosc. 2017;25(2):493–500. https://doi.org/10.1007/s00167-016-4172-4.
26. Noyes FR, Barber-Westin S. Advantages and potential consequences of return to sport after ACL reconstruction: quality of life, reinjury rates, and knee osteoarthritis. In: Noyes FR, Barber-Westin S, editors. Return to sport after ACL reconstruction and other knee operations: limiting the risk of reinjury and maximizing athletic performance. Cham: Springer International Publishing; 2019. p. 3–23. https://doi.org/10.1007/978-3-030-22361-8_1.
27. Chalmers PN, Mall NA, Moric M, Sherman SL, Paletta GP, Cole BJ, Bach BR Jr. Does ACL reconstruction alter natural history?: a systematic literature review of long-term outcomes. J Bone Joint Surg Am. 2014;96(4):292–300. https://doi.org/10.2106/JBJS.L.01713.
28. Nordenvall R, Bahmanyar S, Adami J, Mattila VM, Fellander-Tsai L. Cruciate ligament reconstruction and risk of knee osteoarthritis: the association between cruciate ligament injury and post-traumatic osteoarthritis. A population based nationwide study in Sweden, 1987–2009. PLoS One. 2014;9(8):e104681. https://doi.org/10.1371/journal.pone.0104681.
29. van Yperen DT, Reijman M, van Es EM, Bierma-Zeinstra SMA, Meuffels DE. Twenty-year follow-up study comparing operative versus nonoperative treatment of anterior cruciate ligament ruptures in high-level athletes. Am J Sports Med. 2018;46(5):1129–36. https://doi.org/10.1177/0363546517751683.
30. Claes S, Hermie L, Verdonk R, Bellemans J, Verdonk P. Is osteoarthritis an inevitable consequence of anterior cruciate ligament reconstruction? A meta-analysis. Knee Surg Sports Traumatol Arthrosc. 2013;21(9):1967–76. https://doi.org/10.1007/s00167-012-2251-8.
31. Barenius B, Ponzer S, Shalabi A, Bujak R, Norlen L, Eriksson K. Increased risk of osteoarthritis after anterior cruciate ligament reconstruction: a 14-year follow-up study of a randomized controlled trial. Am J Sports Med. 2014;42(5):1049–57. https://doi.org/10.1177/0363546514526139.
32. Sanders TL, Pareek A, Johnson NR, Stuart MJ, Dahm DL, Krych AJ. Patellofemoral arthritis after lateral patellar dislocation: a matched population-based analysis. Am J Sports Med. 2017;45(5):1012–7.
33. Sanders TL, Pareek A, Hewett TE, Stuart MJ, Dahm DL, Krych AJ. High rate of recurrent patellar dislocation in skeletally immature patients: a long-term population-based study. Knee Surg Sports Traumatol Arthrosc. 2018;26(4):1037–43. https://doi.org/10.1007/s00167-017-4505-y.
34. Conchie H, Clark D, Metcalfe A, Eldridge J, Whitehouse M. Adolescent knee pain and patellar dislocations are associated with patellofemoral osteoarthritis in adulthood: a case control study. Knee. 2016;23(4):708–11.
35. Moatshe G, Dornan GJ, Ludvigsen T, Løken S, LaPrade RF, Engebretsen L. High prevalence of knee osteoarthritis at a minimum 10-year follow-up after knee dislocation surgery. Knee Surg Sports Traumatol Arthrosc. 2017;25(12):3914–22.
36. Engebretsen L, Risberg MA, Robertson B, Ludvigsen TC, Johansen S. Outcome after knee dislocations: a 2-9 years follow-up of 85 consecutive patients. Knee Surg Sports Traumatol Arthrosc. 2009;17(9):1013–26. https://doi.org/10.1007/s00167-009-0869-y.

37. Hantes M, Fyllos A, Papageorgiou F, Alexiou K, Antoniou I. Long-term clinical and radiological outcomes after multiligament knee injury using a delayed ligament reconstruction approach: a single-center experience. Knee. 2019;26(6):1271–7.
38. Khan T, Alvand A, Prieto-Alhambra D, Culliford DJ, Judge A, Jackson WF, Scammell BE, Arden NK, Price AJ. ACL and meniscal injuries increase the risk of primary total knee replacement for osteoarthritis: a matched case-control study using the Clinical Practice Research Datalink (CPRD). Br J Sports Med. 2019;53(15):965–8. https://doi.org/10.1136/bjsports-2017-097762.
39. Leroux T, Ogilvie-Harris D, Dwyer T, Chahal J, Gandhi R, Mahomed N, Wasserstein D. The risk of knee arthroplasty following cruciate ligament reconstruction: a population-based matched cohort study. J Bone Joint Surg Am. 2014;96(1):2–10. https://doi.org/10.2106/JBJS.M.00393.
40. Ackerman IN, Bohensky MA, Kemp JL, de Steiger R. Likelihood of knee replacement surgery up to 15 years after sports injury: a population-level data linkage study. J Sci Med Sport. 2019;22(6):629–34. https://doi.org/10.1016/j.jsams.2018.12.010.
41. Losina E, Thornhill TS, Rome BN, Wright J, Katz JN. The dramatic increase in total knee replacement utilization rates in the United States cannot be fully explained by growth in population size and the obesity epidemic. J Bone Joint Surg Am. 2012;94(3):201–7. https://doi.org/10.2106/JBJS.J.01958.

2 Preoperative Nutrition and General Health Concerns, Patient Indications, and Selection Criteria

Frank R. Noyes and Sue Barber-Westin

2.1 Preoperative Nutrition: Effect of Malnutrition on Total Joint Arthroplasty Outcomes

Malnutrition is a state of altered body composition and function resulting from a lack of nutritional uptake or intake [1] that has been identified from 6% [2] to 26% of total joint arthroplasty patients [3]. Before total knee arthroplasty (TKA), malnutrition is typically defined by serum protein values of albumin (<3.5 g/dL), prealbumin (<16 mg/dL), transferrin (<200 mg/dL), and total lymphocyte count (<1500 cells/mm^3). Albumin is the most widely used marker in orthopedic surgery [4]. It is one of the most abundant proteins that transports fatty acids, steroids, and hormones and is an essential component of serum that plays a crucial role in wound healing and immune function. Patients with low albumin are likely to also lack other important vitamins that are essential for wound healing and proper immune function. They are also more likely to have comorbidities such as liver disease, cardiac disease, and renal malfunction that are associated with higher post-TKA complication rates [5, 6] and hospital charges [7]. Many investigations have reported strong correlations between a low albumin level (<3.5 dg/L) and postoperative total joint arthroplasty complications [5, 6, 8–13].

Prealbumin is a protein synthesized in the liver that is used to formulate other proteins and is also important to assay prior to surgery to determine the nutritional status of the patient. A low level (<16 mg/dL) is indicative of a number of medical conditions including malnutrition, liver disease, digestive disorders, low diet zinc, and hyperthyroidism. Prealbumin reflects short-term changes in nutritional status

F. R. Noyes
Cincinnati SportsMedicine and Orthopaedic Center, The Noyes Knee Institute, Cincinnati, OH, USA

S. Barber-Westin (✉)
Noyes Knee Institute, Cincinnati, OH, USA
e-mail: sbwestin@csmref.org

F. R. Noyes, S. Barber-Westin (eds.), *Critical Rehabilitation for Partial and Total Knee Arthroplasty*, https://doi.org/10.1007/978-3-030-87003-4_2

and is a more reliable test than serum albumin levels that provides a longer-term assessment. This test has become a standard at joint replacement centers. A serum globulin test may be ordered to assay a patient's overall nutrition and more specifically to diagnose any medical conditions related to the immune system. The normal range for serum globulin is 2.0–3.5 g/dL. Other factors that play a role in immune system function identified in arthroplasty patients include vitamin D, serum zinc, and adiposity [14]. Obesity, low body mass index (BMI), prior gastric bypass, malabsorption states, and hypermetabolic states may also increase the risk of malnutrition.

A systematic review of 20 studies concluded that serologic preoperative malnutrition led to deteriorated postoperative outcomes and increased complications after joint arthroplasty, including increased rates of infection and wound healing problems [10]. Albumin levels were reported in all 20 studies; ninety percent showed a correlation between low albumin content and poorer outcomes, and the authors' meta-analysis indicated that a level <3.5 dg/L had increased odds of developing a postoperative wound complication (odds ratio [OR], 2.18; 95% confidence interval [CI] 1.92–2.47). Roche et al. [13] in a study of 161,625 TKAs reported that patients with low preoperative levels of albumin (<3.5 g/dL), prealbumin (<16 mg/dL), and transferrin (<200 mg/dL) had increased odds of sustaining postoperative complications compared with patients with normal serum protein values (Table 2.1).

Bohl et al. [6] in a study of 49,603 total joint arthroplasty patients reported that compared with patients with normal preoperative albumin concentration, patients with levels <3.5 g/dL had an increased risk for any complication (7.3% vs. 4.0%; relative risk [RR], 1.5; 95% CI 1.2–1.7, $P < 0.001$), for a serious complication (2.1% vs. 1.2%; RR, 1.4; 95% CI 1.0–1.9, $P < 0.05$), for surgical site infection (2.29% vs. 0.96%; RR, 2.0; 95% CI 1.5–2.8, $P < 0.001$), and for pneumonia (1.27% vs 0.30%; RR, 2.5; 95% CI 1.6–4.0, $P < 0.001$). Nelson et al. [12] analyzed 37,143 TKAs and reported multiple statistically significant associations between low albumin and postoperative complications (Table 2.2).

In a study of 1911 total joint arthroplasty patients, Huang et al. [11] reported that malnourished patients (low albumin <3.5 mg/dl or transferrin <200 mg/dl) had a significantly higher risk of any complication compared with normal nourished individuals (12.0% and 2.9%, respectively, $P < 0.001$), as well as a significantly longer

Table 2.1 Odds of sustaining postoperative complications in patients with preoperative malnutrition compared with patients with normal serum protein values (n = 161,625 TKAs)[a]

Preoperative abnormal serum protein value	Infection OR	Wound complication OR	Concomitant infection with wound complication OR	Infection after wound complication OR
Albumin <3.5 g/dL	2.20	2.30	2.90	2.87
Prealbumin <16 mg/dL	1.87	1.90	2.27	2.22
Transferrin <200 mg/dL	1.87	1.90	1.79	1.78

OR odds ratio

[a]From Roche et al. [13]. Note: 95% confidence intervals not provided

Table 2.2 Postoperative complications related to low albumin values <3.5 g/dL ($N = 37,143$ TKAs)[a]

Complication	% Preoperative abnormal albumin	% Preoperative normal albumin	OR, 95% CI	*P* value
Any infection	5.0	2.4	2.0; 1.53–2.61	<0.001
Any major complication	2.4	1.3	1.41; 1.00–1.97	0.05
Blood transfusion	17.8	12.4	1.56; 1.35–1.81	<0.001
Pneumonia	1.21	0.29	3.55; 2.14–5.89	<0.001
Superficial surgical site infection	1.27	0.64	1.27; 1.09–2.75	0.02
Deep surgical site infection	0.38	0.12	3.64; 1.54–8.63	0.003
Unplanned intubation	0.51	0.17	2.24; 1.07–4.69	0.03
Progressive renal insufficiency	0.45	0.12	2.71; 1.21–6.07	0.01
Acute renal failure	0.32	0.06	5.19; 1.96–13.73	0.001
Cardiac arrest requiring resuscitation	0.19	0.12	3.74; 1.50–9.28	0.005
Septic shock	0.38	0.08	4.4; 1.74–11.09	0.002
Mortality	0.64	0.015	3.17; 1.58–6.35	0.001

CI confidence intervals, *OR* odds ratio
[a]From Nelson et al. [12]

length of hospital stay (>3 days, 45% and 16%, respectively, $P < 0.001$). Compared with normal nourished individuals, malnourished patients had significant increases in complications related to cardiovascular (0% and 0.5%, respectively, $P = 0.001$), neurovascular (0% and 2.7%, respectively, $P < 0.001$), renal (0.8% and 5.4%, respectively, $P < 0.001$), irrigation and debridement (0.6% and 2.7%, respectively, $P = 0.002$), hematoma (0.7% and 3.8%, respectively, $P < 0.001$), and infection within 3 months of surgery (0.4% and 2.7%, respectively, $P < 0.001$).

Blevins et al. [5] reported that low albumin was the most specific marker and had the highest positive predictive value compared with other markers (platelets, hemoglobin, and platelet-to-white blood cell ratio) in predicting infection within 2 years of total joint arthroplasty in a study of 30,863 patients. In a multivariate regression model, low albumin increased the odds of development of infection (OR, 4.69; 95% CI 2.43–9.08, $P < 0.0001$). Low hemoglobin (anemia) also significantly increased the odds of infection (OR, 1.73; 95% CI 1.10–2.72, $P = 0.02$). A study of 78 total joint replacements reported that preoperative albumin level was a significant predictor for surgical site infection ($P = 0.01$) [8]. Preoperative and postoperative total lymphocyte count and postoperative albumin were not significant predictors.

Interestingly, the most recent guidelines based on recommendations from the World Health Organization and the Center for Disease Control and Prevention for the prevention of surgical site infection at the time of writing failed to mention preoperative malnutrition issues [15, 16]. A systematic review by Alamanda and Springer [17] on studies that investigated modifiable risk factors for reducing infection recommended albumin or transferrin preoperative testing, as well as advice from a dietitian in the presence of malnutrition. Other methods to detect undernutrition include anthropometric measurements such as calf circumference (<31 cm), arm muscle circumference (<22), and triceps skinfold [4]. However, there are no standard values, and the use of these measurements is not as well supported as the use of serologic laboratory values.

There are also standardized malnutrition screening tools, including the Mini Nutritional Assessment (MNA) that has been shown to be reliable and valid in the geriatric population [18] (Table 2.3). Six questions are answered, and based on the score, 14 other items may then be required to determine nutritional status. Guigoz [18] conducted a review of the sensitivity and specificity of the MNA and concluded this instrument is accurate in identifying nutrition risk. Sensitivity compared with low albumin concentrations ranged from 72% to 100% in eight studies. In addition, receiver operating characteristic curves showed high accuracy of 0.916 for albumin levels <3.5 g/dL.

The subjective global assessment [19] and the Nutritional Risk Screening 2002 (NRS 2002, Table 2.4) [20] are two other commonly used screening tools for malnutrition. Ozkalkanli et al. [21] compared these two instruments in 223 patients scheduled for orthopedic surgery. Sensitivity, specificity, and positive and negative predictive values for the prediction of postoperative complications were calculated. The NRS 2002 had higher sensitivity (69% vs. 50%) and specificity (80% vs. 77%) values and higher OR for the association between malnutrition and occurrence of postoperative complications (4.1 vs. 3.5).

It is important to know all aspects of the dietary status of the patient before surgery including weight loss, change in dietary habits, and loss of appetite. In addition, the psychological status of the patient should be understood including bereavement, loss of a loved one, and home care status. In this regard, the importance of determining the home care that will be provided is paramount. This includes identification of individuals who will provide meals to maintain adequate nutrition, assist with bodily functions, and drive the patient to orthopedic and rehabilitation follow-up visits. The goal is to have the patient remain at home if possible; however, if a postoperative rehabilitation facility is required, the patient's status is closely monitored including diet, hydration, anemia from blood loss, and rehabilitation progress as there may exist quality differences in rehabilitation facilities.

2.2 Effects of Preoperative Obesity and Underweight States

In the USA, the prevalence of obesity (BMI $\geq$ 30 kg/m^2) among adults in 2017–2018 was 42.4%. The rates according to age were 40% in individuals aged 20–39, 44.8% in ages 40–59, and 42.8% in ages ≥60 [22]. Severe obesity (BMI $\geq$ 40 kg/m^2) was present in 9.2% of all adults. In comparison, prevalence rates in 1999–2000 were

Table 2.3 Mini Nutritional Assessment (MNA)[a]

Complete the screening (A–F); if the summed score is <11 points, continue with the remaining questions to derive a malnutrition indicator score		
Question	Responses	Points
A. Has food intake declined over the past 3 months due to loss of appetite, digestive problems, and chewing or swallowing difficulties?	Severe decrease in food intake	0
	Moderate decrease in food intake	1
	No decrease in food intake	2
B. Weight loss during the last 3 months	Does not know	0
	Between 1 and 3 kg (2.2–6.6 lbs)	1
	No weight loss	2
C. Mobility	Bed or chair bound	0
	Able to get out of bed/chair but does not go out	1
	Goes out	2
D. Has suffered psychological stress or acute disease in the past 3 months	Yes	0
	No	2
E. Neuropsychological problems	Severe dementia or depression	0
	Mild dementia	1
	No psychological problems	2
F. Body mass index	<19	0
	19–21	1
	21–23	2
	>23	3
Sum items A–F	*0–7 points: malnourished*	
	8–11 points: at risk of malnutrition	
	12 14 points: normal nutritional status	
G. Lives independently (not in nursing home or hospital)	No	0
	Yes	1
H. Takes more than 3 prescription drugs a day	No	1
	Yes	0
I. Pressure sores or skin ulcers	No	1
	Yes	0
J. How many full meals does the patient eat daily?	1 meal	0
	2 meals	1
	3 meals	2
K. Selected consumption markers for protein intake: 1. At least 1 serving of dairy products per day 2. Two or more servings of legumes or eggs per week 3. Meat, fish, or poultry every day	If 0 or 1 yes responses	0
	If 2 yes responses	0.5
	If 3 yes responses	1
L. Consumes 2 or more servings of fruit or vegetables per day	No	0
	Yes	1
M. How much water (water, juice, coffee, tea, milk) is consumed per day	<3 cups	0
	3–5 cups	0.5
	>5 cups	1

(continued)

Table 2.3 (continued)

Complete the screening (A–F); if the summed score is <11 points, continue with the remaining questions to derive a malnutrition indicator score		
Question	Responses	Points
N. Mode of feeding	Unable to eat without assistance	0
	Self-fed with some difficulty	1
	Self-fed without any problem	2
O. Self-view of nutritional state	Views self as malnourished	0
	Is uncertain of nutritional state	1
	Views self as having no nutritional problem	2
P. In comparison with other people of the same age, how does the patient consider his/her health status?	Not as good	0
	Does not know	0.5
	As good	1
	Better	2
Q. Midarm circumference in cm	<21	0
	21–22	0.5
	>22	1
R. Calf circumference in cm	<31	0
	≥31	1
Sum items A–F		
Sum items G–R		
Total score	*<17 points = malnourished*	
	17–23.5 points = at risk of malnutrition	
	24–30 points = normal nutritional status	

[a]From Guigoz et al. [18]

Table 2.4 Nutrition Risk Screening 2002 for patients >70 years of age[a]

Factor	Score
Nutrition score:	1
Weight loss >5% in 3 months or food intake below 50–75% in preceding week	
Weight loss >5% in 2 months, BMI 18.5–20.5 kg/m^2 and impaired general condition, or food intake 25–60% in preceding week	2
Weight loss >5% in 1 month or >15% in 3 months, BMI <18.5 kg/m^2 and impaired general condition, or food intake 0–25% in preceding week	3
Severity of disease score:	1
Hip fracture, chronic patient with acute complications	
Major abdominal surgery, stroke, severe pneumonia, hematologic malignancies	2
Head injury, bone marrow transplantation, intensive care patients with Acute Physiology and Chronic Health Evaluation >10	3
Overall score: Total ≥3 = nutritional risk; ≥5 high risk	

[a]From Kondrup et al. [20]

30.5% for obesity and 4.7% for severe obesity. A study from Norway that followed 225,908 individuals for 12 years reported that weight gain increased the risk for TKA in patients <40 years of age [23]. For men, an increase of 5 kg of weight resulted in a 26% increased risk of TKA in those aged 17–20 years at their first screening and a 13% increased risk in those aged 21–40. For women, an increase of 5 kg was associated with a 43% increased risk for TKA in those aged 17–20 years and a 24% increased risk for those aged 21–40.

Many investigations have reported that obesity is associated with increased rates of postoperative infection (Table 2.5) and other major complications following total joint arthroplasty [2, 7, 24–35]. One study [36] found an association between aseptic tibial component loosening and TKA failure and increased BMI. Patients with a BMI ≥35 kg/m^2 had an increased cumulative probability of revision at 15 years compared with those with BMI <35 kg/m^2 (4.27% and 1.23%, respectively; hazard ratio [HR], 2.3; 95% CI 1.3–3.9; $P < 0.01$). Boyer et al. [37] in a registry study of 28,483 TKAs reported no association between BMI and revision for any reason, septic loosening, or aseptic loosening.

D'Apuzzo et al. [25] compared postoperative complication rates between 90,143 morbidly obese (≥40 kg/m^2) patients and 90,442 nonobese (<30 kg/m^2) patients and reported significant increases in infection, anemia, wound dehiscence, genitourinary disease, peripheral vascular disease, respiratory disease, and death in the morbidly obese cohort (OR range 0.7–3.2; $P < 0.05$). In a study of 34,800 TKA patients, Fu et al. [2] found that morbid obesity (BMI ≥40 kg/m^2) significantly increased the odds of postoperative complications (OR, 1.31; $P = 0.005$), wound complications (OR, 1.99; $P = 0.001$), and return to the operating room within 30 days (OR, 1.59; $P = 0.01$). However, this study reported that a multivariable analysis that adjusted for BMI found that preoperative malnutrition (albumin <3.5 g/dL) was a stronger predictor for multiple complications (Table 2.6).

A study of 34,744 patients from the Danish nationwide registry [32] who underwent total joint replacement surgery found that patients with a BMI >35 kg/m^2 ($N = 3295$) had an increased risk of a major cardiovascular event within 30 days (HR, 1.2; 95% CI 0.67–2.1), mortality within 30 days (HR, 2.3; 95% CI 1.08–5.0), cardiovascular mortality within 30 days (HR, 2.4; 95% CI 0.94–6.2), mortality within 1 year (HR, 1.7; 95% CI 1.2–2.4), and cardiovascular mortality within 1 year (HR, 2.2; 95% CI 1.4–3.5). However, the highest risk group in this study was underweight patients ($n = 353$) with a BMI <18.5 kg/m^2 who had an increased risk (compared with patients with a BMI of 25–29 kg/m^2) of a major cardiovascular event within 30 days (HR, 2.0; 95% CI 0.7–5.4), mortality within 30 days (HR, 7.7; 95% CI 3.1–19.0), cardiovascular mortality within 30 days (HR, 4.1; 95% CI 0.9–18.0), mortality within 1 year (HR, 5.7; 95% CI 3.8–8.4), and cardiovascular mortality within 1 year (HR, 2.5; 95% CI 1.09–5.9).

Wallace et al. [34] followed 32,485 TKA patients and reported that increased BMI was associated with an increased risk of pulmonary embolism (PE) or deep venous thrombosis (DVT) and wound infection by 6 months postoperatively. The greatest increase was found in patients with BMI >35 kg/m^2 for PE/DVT (OR, 1.93; 95% CI 1.45–2.57; $P < 0.001$) and for wound infection (OR, 1.39; 95% CI 1.11–1.72;

Table 2.5 Association between obesity/body mass index and total joint arthroplasty infection

Study	Arthroplasty type	Infection type	Cohort (N)	BMI (kg/m²)	OR	95% CI
Kunutsor et al. [30]	TKA and THA	Periprosthetic joint	N/A (29 studies, meta-analysis)	≥30 vs. <30	1.60	1.29–1.99
				≥35 vs. <35	1.53	1.22–1.92
				≥40 vs. <40	3.68	2.25–6.01
Jamsen et al. [28]	TKA and THA	Periprosthetic joint	1105	≤25	(reference)	NA
			2461	25–29	1.24	0.39–3.89
			1635	30–34	2.38	0.78–7.24
			559	35–39	1.49	0.33–6.66
			193	≥40	13.46	4.10–44.17
Everhart et al. [26]	All primary and revision joint arthroplasties	Surgical site	1875	<18.5	1.90	0.26–13.7
				25–29.9	0.60	0.24–1.50
				30–39.9	0.84	0.51–1.41
				40–49.9	1.28	0.61–2.65
				≥50	15.69	5.97–41.21
Jung et al. [29]	TKA	Periprosthetic joint	983	<25	(reference)	NA
			2712	25–30	0.36	0.10–1.26
			2757	30–35	0.86	0.30–2.45
			1570	35–40	1.51	0.53–4.31
			923	>40	1.72	0.56–5.27
George et al. [27]	TKA	Periprosthetic joint	14,989	<25	(reference)	NA
			41,155	25–29.9	0.90	0.61–1.32
			71,709	30–39.9	1.14	0.80–1.62
			23,081	≥40	2.14	1.48–3.10
		Superficial	14,989	<25	(reference)	NA
			41,155	25–29.9	0.85	0.64–1.14
			71,709	30–39.9	1.24	0.95–1.61
			23,081	≥40	2.02	1.53–2.67
Alvi et al. [24]	TKA and THA	Deep incision	6016	<25	(reference)	NA
			13,289	25–30	0.73	0.23–2.27
			11,558	30–35	1.06	0.38–2.97
			6820	35–40	1.40	0.52–3.73
			5184	>40	3.22	1.34–7.22

		Superficial	6016	<25	(reference)	NA
			13,289	25–30	0.76	0.34–1.69
			11,558	30–35	1.37	0.71–2.66
			6820	35–40	1.68	0.83–3.40
			5184	>40	2.29	1.14–4.61
D'Apuzzo et al. [25]	TKA	In-hospital	90,045	≥40	1.3	1.1–1.7
Fu et al. [2]	TKA	Wound complication	34,800	≥40	1.99	1.33–2.98
Wallace et al. [34]	TKA	Wound infection	32,303	18.5–25	(reference)	NA
				25–30	1.41	1.13–1.75
				30–35	1.59	1.26–1.99
				>35	1.93	1.45–2.57
Werner et al. [35]	TKA	Infection	1,681,681	<30	(reference)	NA
				≥50	13.0	12.0–14.2

NA not applicable, *THA* total hip arthroplasty, *TKA* total knee arthroplasty

Table 2.6 Adjusted odds of developing postoperative complications by obesity classification and preoperative malnutrition[a]

Complication	Category	OR	95% CI	P value
Any	Obese III	1.31	1.08–1.58	0.005
	Malnutrition	1.37	1.11–1.68	0.003
Any major	Obese III	1.18	0.95–1.47	NS
	Malnutrition	1.32	1.04–1.68	0.02
Any wound	Obese III	1.99	1.33–2.98	0.001
	Malnutrition	1.78	1.20–2.64	0.005
Cardiac	Obese III	0.96	0.45–1.23	NS
	Malnutrition	2.23	1.21–4.12	0.01
Respiratory	Obese III	0.52	0.29–0.95	0.03
	Malnutrition	3.75	2.46–5.71	<0.001
Return to OR within 30 days	Obese III	1.59	1.11–2.27	0.01
	Malnutrition	1.10	0.71–1.71	NS
Death	Obese III	1.40	0.47–4.21	NS
	Malnutrition	3.17	1.46–6.90	0.004

[a]From Fu et al. [2]
Obese III (≥40 kg/m^2), preoperative malnutrition (albumin <3.5 g/dL), Note, no significant findings for obese class I or II

$P = 0.003$). This study found no increased risk of mortality within 6 months according to BMI. Tohidi et al. [33] followed a cohort of 9817 TKA patients for 10 years postoperatively and reported that morbidly obese patients (BMI ≥45 kg/m^2) had a 50% higher risk of mortality than nonmorbidly obese patients (risk ratio, 1.50; 95% CI 1.22–1.85).

The effects of super-obesity (BMI ≥ 50 kg/m^2) on postoperative complications were reported by Werner et al. [35] in a cohort of 1,681,681 primary TKA patients. Patients in this category had a higher overall rate of complications within 90 days postoperatively (24.7%) compared with non-obese (3.0%), obese (8.3%), and morbidly obese (13.1%) patients. For infection, ORs for super-obese patients were 13.0 compared with non-obese, 5.3 compared with obese, and 2.5 compared with morbidly obese ($P < 0.0001$ for all comparisons).

Several studies have compared functional outcomes between obese and non-obese patients with differing outcomes [38–45]. Xu et al. [44] followed 126 patients for 10 years postoperatively and compared results from 34 obese (BMI ≥ 30 kg/m^2) to those of 92 non-obese patients. After adjusting for age, gender, and Charlson Comorbidity Index, there was a distinct association between obesity and poorer outcome scores for American Knee Society (AKS) Function Score, Oxford Knee Score, and Physical and Mental Component score of the 36-Item Short-Form Health Survey (SF-36; $P < 0.01$). Liljensoe et al. [42] reported 3- to 5-year outcomes on 197 patients that underwent primary TKA. These authors found that after adjusting for age, gender, primary disease, and surgical approach, a difference in BMI of 1 was associated with an 8% increased risk of a poorer score in the SF-36 Physical Component Score, a 4–12% increased risk of a poorer score for eight of the SF-36 individual domains, and a 3–14% increased risk of a poorer result in AKS overall and function scores.

Yoo et al. [45] found no significant differences in AKS scores between obese patients (BMI ≥ 30 kg/m^2, n = 78) and non-obese patients (n = 114, BMI <25 kg/m^2 and n = 179, BMI 25–29 kg/m^2) 5 years postoperatively. Baker et al. [38] reported no effect of BMI on Oxford Knee Score, EuroQol 5D index, and EuroQol 5D visual analogue scale measures in 13,673 primary TKAs followed a mean of 7 months postoperatively. The authors concluded that patients with high BMIs experienced similar magnitude of improvements in these scores as those with normal BMI (<25 versus > 25 kg/m^2). In a separate report [39], these authors reported similar findings at 3 years postoperatively in Western Ontario and McMaster Universities Osteoarthritis Index (WOMAC) and SF-36 scores. Patients with a BMI of >35 kg/m^2 did have lower rates of patient satisfaction with pain relief compared to those with a BMI of 18.5–25.0 kg/m^2 (84.6% versus 93.3%, P = 0.01). Collins et al. [40] in a report of 445 primary TKAs followed 9 years postoperatively concluded that obesity had a small adverse effect on outcomes; however, substantial improvements were experienced in mildly and highly obese patients. There were no significant differences in complications, revisions, or implant survival between obese and non-obese patients.

Stevens-Laspely et al. [43] evaluated functional performance after TKA in 140 patients 6 months postoperatively. BMI did not account for variance in postoperative timed up-and-go test, stair-climbing test, 6-minute walk test, or SF-36 scores. This population had a mean BMI of 30.8 ± 5.2 kg/m^2 (range, 21.2–40.0 kg/m^2) and did not include severely obese patients. As of the time of writing, we were unable to find other studies in which objective function was determined according to BMI.

2.3 Effects of Preoperative Vitamin D Deficiency

Vitamin D plays an important role on the regulation of bone health and fracture healing, as well as soft tissue healing and function [46]. It is biologically synthesized using ultraviolet B (UVB) rays from the sun and is acquired from food such as liver, cod liver oil, fatty fish, and egg yolks. There remains debate regarding normal ranges according to the level of serum 25-hydroxyvitamin D_3 (25 OHD) [47]. The Vitamin D Council reported ≤30 ng/mL as deficient, 31–39 ng/mL as insufficient, and 40–80 ng/mL as sufficient [48]. The Endocrine Society reported ≤20 ng/mL as deficient, 21–29 ng/mL as insufficient, and 30–100 ng/mL as sufficient [49]. The Food and Nutrition Board Institute of Medicine reported 0–11 ng/mL as deficient, 12–20 ng/mL as insufficient, and >20 ng/Ml as sufficient [50]. Further complicating the matter was a report by Manson et al. [47] that stated that approximately 97.5% of the population require 20 ng/mL or less, and 50% requires 16 ng/mL or less, to maintain good bone health. It is understandable that a wide range of patients undergoing primary total joint arthroplasty (10–80%) have been identified as vitamin D deficient or insufficient [51].

A meta-analysis of the prevalence of preoperative vitamin D deficiency (hypovitaminosis D) and its association with total joint arthroplasty outcomes was recently conducted by Emara et al. [52]. Eighteen studies had a pooled prevalence for vitamin D insufficiency (20 to <30 ng/mL) of 53.4% and deficiency (<20 ng/mL) of 39.4%. Hypovitaminosis D was associated with higher complications rates ($P < 0.05$). Individual studies have reported that vitamin D deficiency resulted in increased hospital length of stay [53–55], higher perioperative complications rates [55–58], and poorer postoperative functional outcomes [53, 59–62]. Hegde et al. [56] reported that vitamin D deficiency (serum 25D <20 nm/mL) resulted in higher manipulation rates (OR, 1.69; $P < 0.001$), surgical site infection (OR, 1.76; $P = 0.001$), DVT (OR, 1.80; $P < 0.001$), and myocardial infarction (OR, 2.11; $P < 0.001$).

Maniar et al. [61] studied the effect of preoperative vitamin D deficiency and postoperative supplementation on functional outcomes in 120 TKA patients. Of the 120 patients, 64 (53%) were found to be deficient (<30 nm/mL), and the remaining were sufficient before surgery. Preoperatively, the deficient group had significantly worse WOMAC scores (48.3 versus 42.3, $P < 0.05$). Postoperatively, all patients took oral vitamin D supplements (5 μg/day) from the 14th postoperative day for 4 weeks. At 3 months postoperatively, there were no significant differences between the two groups in several patient-reported outcome measures.

Piuzzi et al. [63] studied prevalence and risk factors of preoperative vitamin D deficiency and insufficiency in 226 total joint arthroplasty patients in the North Midwest region of the USA. Vitamin D insufficiency was defined as <30 ng/mL and deficiency as <20 ng/mL. There were 137 patients (60.6%) in the insufficient group and 61 (26.9%) in the deficient group. On multivariate analysis, an American Society of Anesthesiologists (ASA) score ≥3 was an independent risk factor for vitamin D insufficiency (OR, 2.44; $P < 0.001$), while ACA ≥3 (OR, 3.57; $P < 0.001$) and younger age (OR, 0.96; $P = 0.002$) were independent risk factors for deficiency. There was no association in other factors such as BMI, gender, race, joint type, and comorbidities with deficiency or insufficiency. There were significantly quarterly seasonal changes, with the lowest mean levels of vitamin D found in the first quarter of the year (January, February, and March) and the highest found in the fourth quarter. The authors suggested the clinicians pay particular attention in patients with an ASA score ≥3 and surgery performed during the winter season.

In 2020, Arshi et al. [51] estimated that the implementation of widespread preoperative 25 OHD testing and repletion in deficient cases would result in cost savings (for reducing joint infection) of over $1,000,000 per 10,000 cases. The use of selective preoperative screening to detect vitamin D-deficient patients (<20 ng/mL) and the use of repletion with oral supplements to normal levels (>30 ng/mL) in these individuals were projected to result in $1,504,857 (range, $215,084–$4,256,388) in cost savings. The use of vitamin D supplementation preoperatively in all patients (without screening) was projected to result in $1,906,077 (range, $616,304–$4,657,608) in cost savings.

Accordingly, preoperative 25 OHD has become a routine screening test at our center for a number of years and should be assessed well before surgical planning in older adults to allow for optimization if a deficiency is present.

2.4 Indications for Bariatric Surgery Before TKA

It is important to develop a relationship with a nutritional and dietary center to assist patients who require preoperative optimization. There are many options available in this field, and patients are advised of specific programs available on the Internet, through commercial companies, or based in hospitals that may be effective. Frequently, when the surgeon states that surgery must be postponed due to increased complication rates already discussed, the patient and their family become more serious on obesity issues and will adopt a program, thereby delaying surgery for 3–6 months. Simple suggestions are often effective such as avoiding a high-carbohydrate diet including candy and soft drinks, decreasing portion sizes by one-half, use of protein supplements for one portion of meal, and avoiding snacking. An important part of weight loss is to initiate any type of physical activity including water therapy, stationary biking, flexibility, low intensity yoga or pilates, and upper body workouts. This represents a comprehensive program at our center involving the entire team to encourage and assist patients with weight loss to avoid bariatric surgery, which is considered the last resort in the treatment strategy.

It is unfortunate that weight loss strategies are frequently ineffective in morbidly obese patients (BMI $\geq$ 40 kg/m^2). Bariatric surgery (BS) may be considered when all conservative management programs fail, including lifestyle modification and pharmacotherapy, especially in patients with obesity-related comorbidities such as hypertension and diabetes [64]. The literature is conflicted on the impact of preoperative BS on outcomes and complications after total joint arthroplasty. A recent systematic review of 13 studies encompassing 11,770 patients found no consensus of the effect of previous BS on short-term outcomes of total hip or knee arthroplasty [65]. A prior systematic review of five studies that compared obese patients who had undergone BS to those who had not found no significant difference in outcomes including infection, DVT, readmission, revision surgery, or mortality [66].

A report published after the two systematic reviews just discussed used data from the Nationwide Inpatient Sample in the USA to compare complications between 9803 patients with morbid obesity who underwent BS to 9803 patients with morbid obesity who did not undergo this procedure [67]. The group that did not undergo BS had a significantly higher risk of postoperative complications and longer length of hospital stay (Table 2.7). However, incidences of blood transfusion and anemia were greater in the BS group. The authors believed this could have been secondary to malnutrition due to malabsorption after BS. The results of this study provided a general conclusion that BS may be of benefit for obese patients undergoing total joint arthroplasty but cautioned that not all complications will be reduced.

A study of 25,852 Medicare patients who underwent BS followed by TKA from 2004 to 2016 reported differences in complication rates according to the type of BS (Table 2.8) [68]. When compared with 2,675,575 TKA patients who had not undergone a BS, the BS group as a whole had higher risks of dislocation, implant failure, periprosthetic infection, pneumonia, and wound dehiscence (hazard ratios >2.0). The authors of this study concluded that BS did not normalize post-TKA risks. It is

Table 2.7 Effect of bariatric surgery on complications, length of stay, and costs of TKA[a]

Variable	Morbid obesity No preop BS (%)	Morbid obesity Preop BS (%)	OR (95% CI)	*P* value
Higher morbid obesity, no preop BS				
Pulmonary embolism	0.57	0.19	0.34 (0.20–0.57)	<0.0001
Respiratory complication	0.43	0.19	0.45 (0.26–0.78)	0.003
Death	0.15	0.01	0.07 (0.01–0.50)	0.0005
Length of stay, mean +/- SD	3.31 ± 1.84	3.12 ± 1.21		<0.0001
Cost, mean +/- SD	$18,162 ± 8265	$18,029 ± 8089		0.05
Higher preop BS				
Anemia	21.62	24.28	1.16 (1.09–1.24)	<0.0001
Blood transfusion	9.02	15.65	1.87 (1.71–2.04)	<0.0001

CI confidence interval, *OR* odds ratio
[a]From Wang et al. [67]

important to note that patients undergoing BS are at high risk for remaining nutritional and metabolic abnormalities already discussed that require optimization prior to surgery. Another study of 86,609 Medicare patients who underwent BS and then primary TKA from 1999 to 2012 reported that compared with controls, BS patients had increased risk of revision for any reason at 1 year (HR, 4.3; $P = 0.003$), 2 years (HR, 3.58; $P = 0.004$), and 5 years (HR, 3.37; $P = 0.003$) [69]. Patients who underwent BS were not at increased risk for postoperative infection.

McLawhorn et al. [70] compared complications and risk of revision between matched cohorts of 2636 patients who had BS and 2636 morbidly obese patients who did not before TKA. There were significantly increased odds of any in-hospital complications and 90-day postoperative complications in patients who did not undergo BS (OR, 0.69 and 0.61, respectively; $P < 0.05$). There was no difference between groups for revision. The authors concluded that preoperative discussions of referral for bariatric evaluation are appropriate for morbidly obese patients.

The experience of our center in regard to patients with morbid obesity and the problems in compliance with recommendations is entirely in agreement with a recent study. Springer [71] followed 289 patients who presented with BMI >40 kg/m^2 and were candidates for total hip or knee replacement. The patients were informed weight loss was required before total joint arthroplasty could be performed and were provided with referral information to bariatric practices for weight management. The patients were tracked for 2 years to determine what treatment occurred. One-third had no further contact with the office, 67 patients (23%) went for an appointment with a bariatric group, and just four (3%) had BS. Overall, 56 (19%) underwent total joint arthroplasty; not all lost weight but found another orthopedic surgeon who performed the procedure (BMI range at surgery, 27.5–53.0 kg/m^2). The author acknowledged that current methods failed to provide appropriate resources to patients and the majority do not lose weight.

Table 2.8 Hazard ratios comparing use of various Bariatric procedures and 90-day post-TKA complications in elderly Medicare patients, 2004–2016[a]

Complication	BS (reference: none)	HR (95% CI)	*P* value
Death	Gastric bypass	1.90 (1.00–3.64)	0.05
	Procedure NA	1.29 (1.00–1.65)	0.04
	Sleeve gastrectomy	1.18 (0.44–3.16)	NS
	Band gastroplasty	0.61 (0.20–1.88)	NS
Implant failure	Sleeve gastrectomy	2.54 (1.45–4.46)	0.001
	Procedure NA	1.71 (1.47–1.99)	<0.001
	Gastric bypass	1.57 (0.88–2.81)	NS
	Band gastroplasty	1.24 (0.70–2.18)	NS
Periprosthetic infection	Band gastroplasty	2.32 (1.54–3.50)	<0.001
	Procedure NA	1.96 (1.69–2.26)	<0.001
	Sleeve gastrectomy	1.76 (0.92–3.37)	NS
	Gastric bypass	0.82 (0.39–1.72)	NS
Pneumonia	Gastric bypass	2.08 (1.31–3.29)	0.002
	Band gastroplasty	1.44 (0.87–2.37)	NS
	Procedure NA	1.35 (1.14–1.59)	<0.001
	Sleeve gastrectomy	0.94 (0.42–2.09)	NS
Readmission	Procedure NA	1.44 (1.38–1.51)	<0.001
	Sleeve gastrectomy	1.37 (1.12–1.68)	0.002
	Band gastroplasty	1.34 (1.16–1.55)	<0.001
	Gastric bypass	1.24 (1.06–1.46)	0.007
Renal failure	Sleeve gastrectomy	1.63 (1.06–2.51)	0.03
	Procedure NA	1.47 (1.31–1.64)	<0.001
	Band gastroplasty	1.39 (0.96–2.01)	NS
	Gastric bypass	1.13 (0.72–1.77)	NS
Revision	Band gastroplasty	1.90 (1.22–2.94)	0.004
	Procedure NA	1.68 (1.44–1.96)	<0.001
	Sleeve gastrectomy	1.45 (0.73–2.89)	NS
	Gastric bypass	0.79 (0.38–1.66)	NS
Wound dehiscence	Band gastroplasty	2.54 (1.59–4.05)	<0.001
	Procedure NA	2.11 (1.78–2.52)	<0.001
	Sleeve gastrectomy	1.98 (0.95–4.13)	NS
	Gastric bypass	1.58 (0.82–3.04)s	NS

CI confidence interval, *HR* hazard ratio, *NA* not available, *NS* not significant
[a]From Meller et al. [68]

Recommendation was made for collaboration to occur between the American Association of Hip and Knee Surgeons and the American Society of Metabolic and Bariatric Surgeons in order to define optimal care and develop national programs.

2.5 Strategies to Improve Nutritional Status

The importance of adequate albumin levels has been discussed previously. Patients with low albumin are likely to also lack other important vitamins that are essential for wound healing and proper immune function. All of our patients undergo preoperative protein testing to ensure either adequate levels exist or if supplementation is required. We recommend adding proteins and amino acids to patients' diets 4 weeks preoperatively and 8 weeks postoperatively. Many good liquid preparations are available online and at major retail or pharmacy stores that are high in protein but low in carbohydrates and calories. Patients who are lactose intolerant are encouraged to use plant-based products. Yogurt or probiotic products are recommended 4 weeks before surgery to help prevent gastrointestinal problems postoperatively. A daily multivitamin including vitamins D and C is recommended 8 weeks before and after surgery. Vitamin D levels are tested on all patients and deficiencies expected in patients not routinely exposed to sunlight. Calcium supplementation is recommended for patients with decreased bone density as determined with a DEXA scan. Iron deficiency anemia should be excluded with appropriate hemoglobin and hematocrit testing, and if present, referral is required for determination of the causes including necessity for appropriate colon screening tests.

Few studies have determined the effect of preoperative nutritional supplementation on outcomes in TKA patients [72]. In one study [73], 19 patients who received essential amino acid supplementation (1 week before and 6 weeks after TKA) had reduced muscle volume atrophy 6 weeks postoperatively compared with 20 patients who received a placebo. Quadriceps atrophy in the involved side was significantly greater in the placebo group compared with the supplementation group ($-13.4\% \pm 1.9\%$ and $-8.5\% \pm 2.5\%$, $P < 0.05$), as was hamstrings atrophy ($-12.2\% \pm 1.4\%$ and $-7.4\% \pm 2.0\%$, $P < 0.05$). However, there was no significant difference in isometric muscle strength or functional measures such as the timed up-and-go and stair-climb tests between groups. In a double-blind randomized controlled trial (RCT) [74], 30 patients received essential amino acid supplementation and 30 a placebo 1 week before to 2 weeks after TKA. Four weeks postoperatively, the supplementation group demonstrated superior relative changes in rectus femoris muscle area and quadriceps muscle diameter ($P < 0.05$) and better visual analogue scores for knee pain ($P < 0.05$). There was no significant difference between groups for quadriceps isometric strength or 6-m timed walk.

Schroer et al. [1] studied the effect of a high-protein, anti-inflammatory diet administered in patients with malnutrition on post-TKA length of stay, readmission rates, and costs. All TKA patients attended a mandatory preoperative education class and received instruction regarding the benefits of the diet (Table 2.9), which was to be followed for 1 month before surgery. Patients with a preoperative serum albumin levels ≤3.4 g/l were called and specifically encouraged to follow the diet. After surgery, these patients were seen by an inpatient dietitian during their hospital stay who reinforced maintenance of the diet postoperatively. There was a significant difference in the length of hospital stay, readmissions, and mean charges for

Table 2.9 Anti-inflammatory, high-protein diet for malnourished patients[a]

Anti-inflammatory diet goals
Limit or omit red meat, sugar, saturated fats, and simple carbohydrates
Increase fish, nuts, seeds, fruits, vegetables, and whole grains
Increase protein to 100 g per day unless medically contraindicated (i.e., renal disease)
Liquid protein supplements only when goals not met through food

[a]From Schroer et al. [1]

primary hospitalization, readmissions, and 90 days of care in the malnourished patients who received the nutritional intervention compared with those who did not ($P < 0.05$). The authors concluded that their program was effective and recommendable but remarked that there is no consensus regarding the length of time patients should optimize their nutrition before TKA. One limitation of this study was that patients did not receive a second albumin test after participation in the diet program and were not tracked postoperatively to determine if the diet was maintained.

Weight loss programs such as Weight Watchers and physician or dietitian-based exercise and diet treatment plans should be recommended in obese patients as already discussed. However, few studies have evaluated their overall efficacy in TKA patients, and more well-designed research is required. As discussed, the effects of preoperative BS are conflicting with regard to postoperative outcomes and complications. Caution is warranted and further research required to determine the optimal TKA candidates for these procedures.

2.6 Patient Indications and Selection Criteria

Criteria for TKA include failure of all nonoperative treatment measures (physical therapy, medications, weight control, injection therapeutic options, lifestyle modifications) and other surgical procedures to alleviate pain with daily activities. Bi- and tricompartmental severe loss of radiographic joint space and articular cartilage are indications, whereas single compartmental severe arthritis may be treated with a unicompartmental knee arthroplasty.

Women over 50 years of age or with any family history of low bone density or bone mass require a DEXA scan to rule out osteoporosis. There should be no gum infection or major dental problems. Any urinary risk factors such as recurrent infection or difficulty voiding require treatment before surgery. Iron deficiency anemia must be excluded. Diabetics is an added risk factor for surgery, and it is highly important that the patient's A1C test be normal (<5.7%) and not elevated. Patients with peripheral vascular disease risk factors should undergo assessment of current symptoms, history of vasculopathy, assessment of pulses, and ankle brachial pressure test [75, 76]. An index of <0.9 requires referral for vascular assessment before TKA.

Smoking increases the risk of complications and mortality after TKA [75, 77–80]. In a study of 56,212 TKAs, Matharu et al. [79] found that smokers had increased risk of lower respiratory tract infection (4.2% versus 2.7% non-smoker), increased usage of analgesics (7.4% versus 5.2%), and higher 1-year mortality rates (1.1% versus 0.9%) compared with non-smokers. Bedard et al. [77] conducted a meta-analysis of 14 studies encompassing 227,289 primary total hip and joint arthroplasty patients to determine the relationship between tobacco use and risk of postoperative complications. Tobacco use was associated with increased risk of wound complications (OR, 1.78; 95% CI 1.32–2.39) and periprosthetic joint infection (OR, 2.02; 95% CI 1.47–2.77). There was a significantly increased risk of wound complication and periprosthetic joint infection for current tobacco users compared with former users, suggesting that smoking cessation preoperatively could have a positive impact. Smoking should be stopped at least 1 month before surgery [81, 82].

Appropriateness criteria, a method that combines available scientific evidence with expert opinion, for TKA have been described by various authors (Table 2.10) [83–87]. The RAND approach, developed in the 1980s [88], was used in two studies that subsequently determined that 31% [85] to 49% [83] of TKA cases were "inappropriate" according to the RAND criteria. One of these investigations reported no significant difference in clinical outcome measures between patients classified as inappropriate and those classified as appropriate or inconclusive at 1 and 2 years postoperatively [85]. The American Academy of Orthopaedic Surgeons published appropriateness criteria for the management of knee osteoarthritis in 2016 that addressed the use of TKA, unicompartmental arthroplasty, and realignment osteotomy [89]. Katz et al. [90] described the limitations of appropriateness criteria and recommended constant reevaluation and updating of these systems. In addition, several studies have published recommended guidelines for TKA. Gademan et al. [91]

Table 2.10 Appropriateness criteria for TKA

Variable	AAOS system[a]	Modified Escobar (RAND) system[b]
Function: limiting pain	1 = moderate to long distance (walking >1/4 mile) 2 = short distance (walking 2 city blocks, length of a shopping mall) 3 = pain at rest or night	1 = slight; combined WOMAC pain and function score of 0–11 2 = moderate; combined WOMAC pain and function score of 12–22 3 = intense; combined WOMAC pain and function score of 23–33 4 = severe; combined WOMAC pain and function score ≥ 34
Range of motion	1 = full 2 = >5° flexion contracture and/or flexion <110° 3 = >10° flexion contracture and/or flexion <90°	1 = preserved mobility and stability (extension loss <5° and normal or mild medial or lateral gapping in 20° of flexion) 2 = extension loss ≥5° or moderate or severe medial or lateral gapping in 20° of flexion
Functional instability	1 = none 2 = functional instability	None
Pattern of arthritic involvement	1 = predominately 1 compartment 2 = >1 compartment	1 = unicompartmental tibiofemoral osteoarthritis 2 = bicompartmental osteoarthritis 3 = tricompartmental osteoarthritis
Imaging	1 = mild to moderate 2 = severe	1 = Kellgren-Lawrence grade ≤ 2 2 = Kellgren-Lawrence grade 3 3 = Kellgren-Lawrence grade 4
Limb alignment	1 = normal 2 = varus or valgus	None
Mechanical symptoms	1 = no 2 = yes	None
Age	1 = young 2 = middle-aged 3 = elderly	1 = <55 2 = 55–65 3 = >65

[a]From the American Academy of Orthopaedic Surgeons [92]
[b]From Riddle et al. [87]

systematically reviewed the literature and found that the quality of evidence for TKA guidelines was generally low and specific cut-off values or ranges for specific criteria (such as pain and function) were frequently not provided. Future work in this area should consider the constant evolution of TKA procedures, changes in demographic features of patient candidates, influence of reimbursement requirements, and the need to include cut-off values using validated symptom and function rating systems.

References

1. Schroer WC, LeMarr AR, Mills K, Childress AL, Morton DJ, Reedy ME. 2019 Chitranjan S. Ranawat Award: elective joint arthroplasty outcomes improve in malnourished patients with nutritional intervention: a prospective population analysis demonstrates a modifiable risk factor. Bone Joint J. 2019;101-B(7_Supple_C):17–21. https://doi.org/10.1302/0301-620X.101B7.BJJ-2018-1510.R1.
2. Fu MC, McLawhorn AS, Padgett DE, Cross MB. Hypoalbuminemia is a better predictor than obesity of complications after total knee arthroplasty: a propensity score-adjusted observational analysis. HSS J. 2017;13(1):66–74. https://doi.org/10.1007/s11420-016-9518-4.
3. Pruzansky JS, Bronson MJ, Grelsamer RP, Strauss E, Moucha CS. Prevalence of modifiable surgical site infection risk factors in hip and knee joint arthroplasty patients at an urban academic hospital. J Arthroplasty. 2014;29(2):272–6. https://doi.org/10.1016/j.arth.2013.06.019.
4. Cross MB, Yi PH, Thomas CF, Garcia J, Della Valle CJ. Evaluation of malnutrition in orthopaedic surgery. J Am Acad Orthop Surg. 2014;22(3):193–9. https://doi.org/10.5435/JAAOS-22-03-193.
5. Blevins K, Aalirezaie A, Shohat N, Parvizi J. Malnutrition and the development of periprosthetic joint infection in patients undergoing primary elective total joint arthroplasty. J Arthroplasty. 2018;33(9):2971–5. https://doi.org/10.1016/j.arth.2018.04.027.
6. Bohl DD, Shen MR, Kayupov E, Della Valle CJ. Hypoalbuminemia independently predicts surgical site infection, pneumonia, length of stay, and readmission after total joint arthroplasty. J Arthroplasty. 2016;31(1):15–21. https://doi.org/10.1016/j.arth.2015.08.028.
7. Schroer WC, Diesfeld PJ, LeMarr AR, Morton DJ, Reedy ME. Modifiable risk factors in primary joint arthroplasty increase 90-day cost of care. J Arthroplasty. 2018;33(9):2740–4. https://doi.org/10.1016/j.arth.2018.04.018.
8. Alfargieny R, Bodalal Z, Bendardaf R, El-Fadli M, Langhi S. Nutritional status as a predictive marker for surgical site infection in total joint arthroplasty. Avicenna J Med. 2015;5(4):117–22. https://doi.org/10.4103/2231-0770.165122.
9. Courtney PM, Rozell JC, Melnic CM, Sheth NP, Nelson CL. Effect of malnutrition and morbid obesity on complication rates following primary total joint arthroplasty. J Surg Orthop Adv. 2016;25(2):99–104.
10. Gu A, Malahias MA, Strigelli V, Nocon AA, Sculco TP, Sculco PK. Preoperative malnutrition negatively correlates with postoperative wound complications and infection after total joint arthroplasty: a systematic review and meta-analysis. J Arthroplasty. 2019;34(5):1013–24. https://doi.org/10.1016/j.arth.2019.01.005.
11. Huang R, Greenky M, Kerr GJ, Austin MS, Parvizi J. The effect of malnutrition on patients undergoing elective joint arthroplasty. J Arthroplasty. 2013;28(8 Suppl):21–4. https://doi.org/10.1016/j.arth.2013.05.038.
12. Nelson CL, Elkassabany NM, Kamath AF, Liu J. Low albumin levels, more than morbid obesity, are associated with complications after TKA. Clin Orthop Relat Res. 2015;473(10):3163–72. https://doi.org/10.1007/s11999-015-4333-7.
13. Roche M, Law TY, Kurowicki J, Sodhi N, Rosas S, Elson L, Summers S, Sabeh K, Mont MA. Albumin, prealbumin, and transferrin may be predictive of wound

complications following total knee arthroplasty. J Knee Surg. 2018;31(10):946–51. https://doi.org/10.1055/s-0038-1672122.
14. Golladay GJ, Satpathy J, Jiranek WA. Patient optimization-strategies that work: malnutrition. J Arthroplasty. 2016;31(8):1631–4. https://doi.org/10.1016/j.arth.2016.03.027.
15. Parvizi J, Shohat N, Gehrke T. Prevention of periprosthetic joint infection: new guidelines. Bone Joint J. 2017;99-B(4 Supple B):3–10. https://doi.org/10.1302/0301-620X.99B4.BJJ-2016-1212.R1.
16. Shohat N, Parvizi J. Prevention of periprosthetic joint infection: examining the recent guidelines. J Arthroplasty. 2017;32(7):2040–6. https://doi.org/10.1016/j.arth.2017.02.072.
17. Alamanda VK, Springer BD. The prevention of infection: 12 modifiable risk factors. Bone Joint J. 2019;101-b(1_Supple_A):3–9. https://doi.org/10.1302/0301-620x.101b1.Bjj-2018-0233.R1.
18. Guigoz Y. The Mini Nutritional Assessment (MNA) review of the literature--what does it tell us? J Nutr Health Aging. 2006;10(6):466–85; discussion 485-467.
19. Detsky AS, McLaughlin JR, Baker JP, Johnston N, Whittaker S, Mendelson RA, Jeejeebhoy KN. What is subjective global assessment of nutritional status? JPEN J Parenter Enteral Nutr. 1987;11(1):8–13. https://doi.org/10.1177/014860718701100108.
20. Kondrup J, Rasmussen HH, Hamberg O, Stanga Z, Ad Hoc EWG. Nutritional risk screening (NRS 2002): a new method based on an analysis of controlled clinical trials. Clin Nutr. 2003;22(3):321–36. https://doi.org/10.1016/s0261-5614(02)00214-5.
21. Ozkalkanli MY, Ozkalkanli DT, Katircioglu K, Savaci S. Comparison of tools for nutrition assessment and screening for predicting the development of complications in orthopedic surgery. Nutr Clin Pract. 2009;24(2):274–80. https://doi.org/10.1177/0884533609332087.
22. Hales CM, Carroll MD, Fryar CD, Ogden CL. Prevalence of obesity and severe obesity among adults: United States, 2017–2018;2020.
23. Apold H, Meyer HE, Nordsletten L, Furnes O, Baste V, Flugsrud GB. Weight gain and the risk of knee replacement due to primary osteoarthritis: a population based, prospective cohort study of 225,908 individuals. Osteoarthr Cartil. 2014;22(5):652–8. https://doi.org/10.1016/j.joca.2014.03.002.
24. Alvi HM, Mednick RE, Krishnan V, Kwasny MJ, Beal MD, Manning DW. The effect of BMI on 30 day outcomes following total joint arthroplasty. J Arthroplasty. 2015;30(7):1113–7. https://doi.org/10.1016/j.arth.2015.01.049.
25. D'Apuzzo MR, Novicoff WM, Browne JA. The John Insall Award: morbid obesity independently impacts complications, mortality, and resource use after TKA. Clin Orthop Relat Res. 2015;473(1):57–63. https://doi.org/10.1007/s11999-014-3668-9.
26. Everhart JS, Altneu E, Calhoun JH. Medical comorbidities are independent preoperative risk factors for surgical infection after total joint arthroplasty. Clin Orthop Relat Res. 2013;471(10):3112–9. https://doi.org/10.1007/s11999-013-2923-9.
27. George J, Piuzzi NS, Ng M, Sodhi N, Khlopas AA, Mont MA. Association between body mass index and thirty-day complications after total knee arthroplasty. J Arthroplasty. 2018;33(3):865–71. https://doi.org/10.1016/j.arth.2017.09.038.
28. Jamsen E, Nevalainen P, Eskelinen A, Huotari K, Kalliovalkama J, Moilanen T. Obesity, diabetes, and preoperative hyperglycemia as predictors of periprosthetic joint infection: a single-center analysis of 7181 primary hip and knee replacements for osteoarthritis. J Bone Joint Surg Am. 2012;94(14):e101. https://doi.org/10.2106/JBJS.J.01935.
29. Jung P, Morris AJ, Zhu M, Roberts SA, Frampton C, Young SW. BMI is a key risk factor for early periprosthetic joint infection following total hip and knee arthroplasty. N Z Med J. 2017;130(1461):24–34.
30. Kunutsor SK, Whitehouse MR, Blom AW, Beswick AD, Team I. Patient-related risk factors for periprosthetic joint infection after total joint arthroplasty: a systematic review and meta-analysis. PLoS One. 2016;11(3):e0150866. https://doi.org/10.1371/journal.pone.0150866.
31. Sayeed Z, Anoushiravani AA, Chambers MC, Gilbert TJ, Scaife SL, El-Othmani MM, Saleh KJ. Comparing in-hospital total joint arthroplasty outcomes and resource consumption among

underweight and morbidly obese patients. J Arthroplasty. 2016;31(10):2085–90. https://doi.org/10.1016/j.arth.2016.03.015.
32. Thornqvist C, Gislason GH, Kober L, Jensen PF, Torp-Pedersen C, Andersson C. Body mass index and risk of perioperative cardiovascular adverse events and mortality in 34,744 Danish patients undergoing hip or knee replacement. Acta Orthop. 2014;85(5):456–62. https://doi.org/10.3109/17453674.2014.934184.
33. Tohidi M, Brogly SB, Lajkosz K, Grant HJ, VanDenKerkhof EG, Campbell AR. Ten-year mortality and revision after total knee arthroplasty in morbidly obese patients. J Arthroplasty. 2018;33(8):2518–23. https://doi.org/10.1016/j.arth.2018.03.049.
34. Wallace G, Judge A, Prieto-Alhambra D, de Vries F, Arden NK, Cooper C. The effect of body mass index on the risk of post-operative complications during the 6 months following total hip replacement or total knee replacement surgery. Osteoarthr Cartil. 2014;22(7):918–27. https://doi.org/10.1016/j.joca.2014.04.013.
35. Werner BC, Cancienne JM, Miller MD, Gwathmey FW. Incidence of manipulation under anesthesia or lysis of adhesions after arthroscopic knee surgery. Am J Sports Med. 2015;43(7):1656–61. https://doi.org/10.1177/0363546515578660.
36. Abdel MP, Bonadurer GF 3rd, Jennings MT, Hanssen AD. Increased aseptic tibial failures in patients with a BMI >/=35 and well-aligned total knee arthroplasties. J Arthroplasty. 2015;30(12):2181–4. https://doi.org/10.1016/j.arth.2015.06.057.
37. Boyer B, Bordini B, Caputo D, Neri T, Stea S, Toni A. What are the influencing factors on hip and knee arthroplasty survival? Prospective cohort study on 63619 arthroplasties. Orthop Traumatol Surg Res. 2019;105(7):1251–6. https://doi.org/10.1016/j.otsr.2019.07.020.
38. Baker P, Petheram T, Jameson S, Reed M, Gregg P, Deehan D. The association between body mass index and the outcomes of total knee arthroplasty. J Bone Joint Surg Am. 2012;94(16):1501–8. https://doi.org/10.2106/JBJS.K.01180.
39. Baker P, Muthumayandi K, Gerrand C, Kleim B, Bettinson K, Deehan D. Influence of body mass index (BMI) on functional improvements at 3 years following total knee replacement: a retrospective cohort study. PLoS One. 2013;8(3):e59079. https://doi.org/10.1371/journal.pone.0059079.
40. Collins RA, Walmsley PJ, Amin AK, Brenkel IJ, Clayton RA. Does obesity influence clinical outcome at nine years following total knee replacement? J Bone Joint Surg. 2012;94(10):1351–5. https://doi.org/10.1302/0301-620X.94B10.28894.
41. Daniilidis K, Yao D, Gosheger G, Berssen C, Budny T, Dieckmann R, Holl S. Does BMI influence clinical outcomes after total knee arthroplasty? Technol Health Care. 2016;24(3):367–75. https://doi.org/10.3233/THC-151128.
42. Liljensoe A, Lauersen JO, Soballe K, Mechlenburg I. Overweight preoperatively impairs clinical outcome after knee arthroplasty: a cohort study of 197 patients 3–5 years after surgery. Acta Orthop. 2013;84(4):392–7. https://doi.org/10.3109/17453674.2013.799419.
43. Stevens-Lapsley JE, Petterson SC, Mizner RL, Snyder-Mackler L. Impact of body mass index on functional performance after total knee arthroplasty. J Arthroplasty. 2010;25(7):1104–9. https://doi.org/10.1016/j.arth.2009.08.009.
44. Xu S, Chen JY, Lo NN, Chia SL, Tay DKJ, Pang HN, Hao Y, Yeo SJ. The influence of obesity on functional outcome and quality of life after total knee arthroplasty: a ten-year follow-up study. Bone Joint J. 2018;100-b(5):579–83. https://doi.org/10.1302/0301-620x.100b5.Bjj-2017-1263.R1.
45. Yoo JH, Oh HC, Park SH, Kim JK, Kim SH. Does obesity affect clinical and radiological outcomes in minimally invasive total knee arthroplasty? Minimum 5-year follow-up of minimally invasive TKA in obese patients. Clin Orthop Surg. 2018;10(3):315–21. https://doi.org/10.4055/cios.2018.10.3.315.
46. Moon AS, Boudreau S, Mussell E, He JK, Brabston EW, Ponce BA, Momaya AM. Current concepts in vitamin D and orthopaedic surgery. Orthop Traumatol Surg Res. 2019;105(2):375–82. https://doi.org/10.1016/j.otsr.2018.12.006.
47. Manson J, Brannon PM, Rosen CJ, Taylor CL. Vitamin D deficiency-is there really a pandemic. N Engl J Med. 2016;375(19):1817–20.

48. Neal S, Sykes J, Rigby M, Hess B. A review and clinical summary of vitamin D in regard to bone health and athletic performance. Phys Sportsmed. 2015;43(2):161–8. https://doi.org/10.1080/00913847.2015.1020248.
49. Holick MF, Binkley NC, Bischoff-Ferrari HA, Gordon CM, Hanley DA, Heaney RP, Murad MH, Weaver CM, Endocrine S. Evaluation, treatment, and prevention of vitamin D deficiency: an Endocrine Society clinical practice guideline. J Clin Endocrinol Metab. 2011;96(7):1911–30. https://doi.org/10.1210/jc.2011-0385.
50. Ross AC, Manson JE, Abrams SA, Aloia JF, Brannon PM, Clinton SK, Durazo-Arvizu RA, Gallagher JC, Gallo RL, Jones G, Kovacs CS, Mayne ST, Rosen CJ, Shapses SA. The 2011 report on dietary reference intakes for calcium and vitamin D from the Institute of Medicine: what clinicians need to know. J Clin Endocrinol Metab. 2011;96(1):53–8. https://doi.org/10.1210/jc.2010-2704.
51. Arshi A, Shieh A, Adams JS, Bernthal NM, Zeegen EN, Sassoon AA. Preoperative vitamin D repletion in total knee arthroplasty: a cost-effectiveness model. J Arthroplasty. 2020;35(5):1379–83. https://doi.org/10.1016/j.arth.2019.12.037.
52. Emara AK, Nageeb E, George J, Buttaro MA, Higuera C, Piuzzi NS. Hypovitaminosis D in lower extremity joint arthroplasty: a systematic review and meta-analysis. J Orthop. 2020;21:109–16. https://doi.org/10.1016/j.jor.2020.03.010.
53. Jansen J, Tahmassebi J, Haddad FS. Vitamin D deficiency is associated with longer hospital stay and lower functional outcome after total knee arthroplasty. Acta Orthop Belg. 2017;83(4):664–70.
54. Maier GS, Maus U, Lazovic D, Horas K, Roth KE, Kurth AA. Is there an association between low serum 25-OH-D levels and the length of hospital stay in orthopaedic patients after arthroplasty? J Orthop Traumatol. 2016;17(4):297–302. https://doi.org/10.1007/s10195-016-0414-y.
55. Traven SA, Chiaramonti AM, Barfield WR, Kirkland PA, Demos HA, Schutte HD, Drew JM. Fewer complications following revision hip and knee arthroplasty in patients with normal vitamin D levels. J Arthroplasty. 2017;32(9S):S193–6. https://doi.org/10.1016/j.arth.2017.02.038.
56. Hegde V, Arshi A, Wang C, Buser Z, Wang JC, Jensen AR, Adams JS, Zeegen EN, Bernthal NM. Preoperative vitamin D deficiency is associated with higher postoperative complication rates in total knee arthroplasty. Orthopedics. 2018;41(4):e489–95. https://doi.org/10.3928/01477447-20180424-04.
57. Maier GS, Horas K, Seeger JB, Roth KE, Kurth AA, Maus U. Is there an association between periprosthetic joint infection and low vitamin D levels? Int Orthop. 2014;38(7):1499–504. https://doi.org/10.1007/s00264-014-2338-6.
58. Zajonz D, Prager F, Edel M, Möbius R, Daikos A, Fakler JK, Josten C, Kratzsch J, Roth A. The significance of the vitamin D metabolism in the development of periprosthetic infections after THA and TKA: a prospective matched-pair analysis of 240 patients. Clin Interv Aging. 2018;13:1429–35. https://doi.org/10.2147/cia.S171307.
59. Allain TJ, Beresford PA, Newman JH, Swinkels A. Vitamin D levels in patients undergoing knee arthroplasty: does vitamin D status effect postoperative outcomes? e-SPEN Eur e-J Clin Nutr Metab. 2008;3(1):e17–21.
60. Lee A, Chan SK, Samy W, Chiu CH, Gin T. Effect of hypovitaminosis D on postoperative pain outcomes and short-term health-related quality of life after knee arthroplasty: a cohort study. Medicine. 2015;94(42):e1812. https://doi.org/10.1097/md.0000000000001812.
61. Maniar RN, Patil AM, Maniar AR, Gangaraju B, Singh J. Effect of preoperative vitamin D levels on functional performance after total knee arthroplasty. Clin Orthop Surg. 2016;8(2):153–6. https://doi.org/10.4055/cios.2016.8.2.153.
62. Shin KY, Park KK, Moon SH, Yang IH, Choi HJ, Lee WS. Vitamin D deficiency adversely affects early post-operative functional outcomes after total knee arthroplasty. Knee Surg Sports Traumatol Arthrosc. 2017;25(11):3424–30. https://doi.org/10.1007/s00167-016-4209-8.
63. Piuzzi NS, George J, Khlopas A, Klika AK, Mont MA, Muschler GF, Higuera CA. High prevalence and seasonal variation of hypovitaminosis D in patients scheduled for lower

extremity total joint arthroplasty. Ann Transl Med. 2018;6(16):321. https://doi.org/10.21037/atm.2018.08.21.
64. Mechanick JI, Youdim A, Jones DB, Garvey WT, Hurley DL, McMahon MM, Heinberg LJ, Kushner R, Adams TD, Shikora S, Dixon JB, Brethauer S, American Association of Clinical E, Obesity S, American Society for M, Bariatric S. Clinical practice guidelines for the perioperative nutritional, metabolic, and nonsurgical support of the bariatric surgery patient--2013 update: cosponsored by American Association of Clinical Endocrinologists, the Obesity Society, and American Society for Metabolic & Bariatric Surgery. Endocr Pract. 2013;19(2):337–72. https://doi.org/10.4158/EP12437.GL.
65. Gu A, Cohen JS, Malahias MA, Lee D, Sculco PK, McLawhorn AS. The effect of bariatric surgery prior to lower-extremity total joint arthroplasty: a systematic review. HSS J. 2019;15(2):190–200. https://doi.org/10.1007/s11420-019-09674-2.
66. Smith TO, Aboelmagd T, Hing CB, MacGregor A. Does bariatric surgery prior to total hip or knee arthroplasty reduce post-operative complications and improve clinical outcomes for obese patients? Systematic review and meta-analysis. Bone Joint J. 2016;98-b(9):1160–6. https://doi.org/10.1302/0301-620x.98b9.38024.
67. Wang Y, Deng Z, Meng J, Dai Q, Chen T, Bao N. Impact of bariatric surgery on inpatient complication, cost, and length of stay following total hip or knee arthroplasty. J Arthroplasty. 2019;34(12):2884–2889.e2884. https://doi.org/10.1016/j.arth.2019.07.012.
68. Meller MM, Goodman S, Gonzalez MH, Lau E Does bariatric surgery normalize risks after total knee arthroplasty? Administrative medicare data. J Am Acad Orthop Surg Glob Res Rev. 2019;3(12). https://doi.org/10.5435/JAAOSGlobal-D-19-00102.
69. Lee GC, Ong K, Baykal D, Lau E, Malkani AL. Does prior bariatric surgery affect implant survivorship and complications following primary total hip arthroplasty/total knee arthroplasty? J Arthroplasty. 2018;33(7):2070–2074.e2071. https://doi.org/10.1016/j.arth.2018.01.064.
70. McLawhorn AS, Levack AE, Lee YY, Ge Y, Do H, Dodwell ER. Bariatric surgery improves outcomes after lower extremity arthroplasty in the morbidly obese: a propensity score-matched analysis of a New York statewide database. J Arthroplasty. 2018;33(7):2062–2069.e2064. https://doi.org/10.1016/j.arth.2017.11.056.
71. Springer BD. Management of the bariatric patient. What are the implications of obesity and total joint arthroplasty: the orthopedic Surgeon's perspective? J Arthroplasty. 2019;34(7s):S30–s32. https://doi.org/10.1016/j.arth.2018.12.021.
72. Burgess LC, Phillips SM, Wainwright TW. What is the role of nutritional supplements in support of total hip replacement and total knee replacement surgeries? A systematic review. Nutrients. 2018;10(7). https://doi.org/10.3390/nu10070820.
73. Dreyer HC, Owen EC, Strycker LA, Smolkowski K, Muyskens JB, Kirkpatrick TK, Christie AD, Kuehl KS, Lantz BA, Shah SN, Mohler CG, Jewett BA. Essential amino acid supplementation mitigates muscle atrophy after total knee arthroplasty: a randomized, double-blind, placebo-controlled trial. JB JS Open Access. 2018;3(2):e0006. https://doi.org/10.2106/jbjs.Oa.18.00006.
74. Ueyama H, Kanemoto N, Minoda Y, Taniguchi Y, Nakamura H. 2020 Chitranjan S. Ranawat Award: perioperative essential amino acid supplementation suppresses rectus femoris muscle atrophy and accelerates early functional recovery following total knee arthroplasty. Bone Joint J. 2020;102-b(6_Supple_A):10–8. https://doi.org/10.1302/0301-620x.102b6.Bjj-2019-1370.R1.
75. Adie S, Harris I, Chuan A, Lewis P, Naylor JM. Selecting and optimising patients for total knee arthroplasty. Med J Aust. 2019;210(3):135–41. https://doi.org/10.5694/mja2.12109.
76. Abu Dakka M, Badri H, Al-Khaffaf H. Total knee arthroplasty in patients with peripheral vascular disease. Surgeon. 2009;7(6):362–5. https://doi.org/10.1016/s1479-666x(09)80111-x.
77. Bedard NA, DeMik DE, Owens JM, Glass NA, DeBerg J, Callaghan JJ. Tobacco use and risk of wound complications and periprosthetic joint infection: a systematic review and meta-analysis of primary total joint arthroplasty procedures. J Arthroplasty. 2019;34(2):385–396.e384. https://doi.org/10.1016/j.arth.2018.09.089.

78. Gonzalez AI, Luime JJ, Uçkay I, Hannouche D, Hoffmeyer P, Lübbeke A. Is there an association between smoking status and prosthetic joint infection after primary total joint arthroplasty? J Arthroplasty. 2018;33(7):2218–24. https://doi.org/10.1016/j.arth.2018.02.069.
79. Matharu GS, Mouchti S, Twigg S, Delmestri A, Murray DW, Judge A, Pandit HG. The effect of smoking on outcomes following primary total hip and knee arthroplasty: a population-based cohort study of 117,024 patients. Acta Orthop. 2019;90(6):559–67. https://doi.org/10.1080/17453674.2019.1649510.
80. Schiffner E, Latz D, Karbowski A, Grassmann JP, Thelen S, Gehrmann S, Windolf J, Schneppendahl J, Jungbluth P. Possible risk factors for acute and chronic deep periprosthetic joint infections in primary total knee arthroplasty. Do BMI, smoking, urinary tract infections, gender, and ASA classification have an impact? J Orthop. 2020;19:111–3. https://doi.org/10.1016/j.jor.2019.11.035.
81. Sorensen LT. Wound healing and infection in surgery. The clinical impact of smoking and smoking cessation: a systematic review and meta-analysis. Arch Surg. 2012;147(4):373–83. https://doi.org/10.1001/archsurg.2012.5.
82. Wong J, Lam DP, Abrishami A, Chan MT, Chung F. Short-term preoperative smoking cessation and postoperative complications: a systematic review and meta-analysis. Can J Anaesth. 2012;59(3):268–79. https://doi.org/10.1007/s12630-011-9652-x.
83. Escobar A, Quintana JM, Arostegui I, Azkarate J, Guenaga JI, Arenaza JC, Garai I. Development of explicit criteria for total knee replacement. Int J Technol Assess Health Care. 2003;19(1):57–70. https://doi.org/10.1017/s0266462303000060.
84. Frankel L, Sanmartin C, Hawker G, De Coster C, Dunbar M, Bohm E, Noseworthy T. Perspectives of orthopaedic surgeons on patients' appropriateness for total joint arthroplasty: a qualitative study. J Eval Clin Pract. 2016;22(2):164–70. https://doi.org/10.1111/jep.12449.
85. Riddle DL, Perera RA, Jiranek WA, Dumenci L. Using surgical appropriateness criteria to examine outcomes of total knee arthroplasty in a United States sample. Arthritis Care Res. 2015;67(3):349–57. https://doi.org/10.1002/acr.22428.
86. Riddle DL, Perera RA. Appropriateness and total knee arthroplasty: an examination of the American Academy of Orthopaedic Surgeons appropriateness rating system. Osteoarthr Cartil. 2017;25(12):1994–8. https://doi.org/10.1016/j.joca.2017.08.018.
87. Riddle DL, Ghomrawi H, Jiranek WA, Dumenci L, Perera RA, Escobar A. Appropriateness criteria for total knee arthroplasty: additional comments and considerations. J Bone Joint Surg Am. 2018;100(4):e22. https://doi.org/10.2106/jbjs.17.00405.
88. Brook RH, Chassin MR, Fink A, Solomon DH, Kosecoff J, Park RE. A method for the detailed assessment of the appropriateness of medical technologies. Int J Technol Assess Health Care. 1986;2(1):53–63. https://doi.org/10.1017/s0266462300002774.
89. Manner PA, Tubb CC, Levine BR. AAOS appropriate use criteria: surgical management of osteoarthritis of the knee. JAAOS J Am Acad Orthop Surg. 2018;26(9):e194–7.
90. Katz JN, Winter AR, Hawker G. Measures of the appropriateness of elective orthopaedic joint and spine procedures. J Bone Joint Surg Am. 2017;99(4):e15. https://doi.org/10.2106/JBJS.16.00473.
91. Gademan MG, Hofstede SN, Vliet Vlieland TP, Nelissen RG, Marang-van de Mheen PJ. Indication criteria for total hip or knee arthroplasty in osteoarthritis: a state-of-the-science overview. BMC Musculoskelet Disord. 2016;17(1):463. https://doi.org/10.1186/s12891-016-1325-z.
92. American Academy of Orthopaedic S. Appropriate Use Criteria for Surgical Management of Osteoarthritis of the Knee. 2016. http://www.aaos.org/smoakauc. Accessed 23 July 2020.

3 Advances in Surgical Techniques for Robotic Computer-Navigated Total and Unicompartmental Knee Arthroplasty

David L. Kerr, Niall H. Cochrane, Albert T. Anastasio, Lefko T. Charalambous, Mark Wu, and Thorsten M. Seyler

3.1 Evolution of Robotic Arthroplasty

Surgical technology has developed increasing capabilities over the past 30 years, and robotic-assisted arthroplasty is one of many areas that have attracted significant interest from both patients and surgeons alike. Historically, alignment in total knee arthroplasty (TKA) has been based on preoperative radiographs combined with intraoperative assessments of deformity and alignment jigs that utilize either the anatomic axis—provided by intramedullary guides—or extramedullary and anatomic bony landmarks. While practical, conventional jigs and alignment techniques may be limited by variation in patient anatomy secondary to natural changes or progressive deformity from osteoarthritis [1]. Since the implementation of ROBODOC in 1992 for hip arthroplasty, proponents and creators of robotic systems for joint arthroplasty claim that implementation of these systems improves accuracy in bone cut selection and improves precision in cut execution [2]. Current robotic and computer-navigated knee arthroplasty systems available on the market today encompass a number of different technologies designed to assist surgeons with implanting components in the optimal alignment for a balanced knee with restored kinematics. With a prevalence of 4.7 million individuals with knee arthroplasties in the US population and increasing annual numbers, the evolution and adoption of technologically assisted surgery have broad potential to impact arthroplasty outcomes for thousands of patients every year [3].

D. L. Kerr (✉) · N. H. Cochrane · A. T. Anastasio · L. T. Charalambous · M. Wu · T. M. Seyler
Department of Orthopaedic Surgery, Duke University Medical Center, Durham, NC, USA
e-mail: david.kerr@duke.edu

F. R. Noyes, S. Barber-Westin (eds.), *Critical Rehabilitation for Partial and Total Knee Arthroplasty*, https://doi.org/10.1007/978-3-030-87003-4_3

3.1.1 Patient Satisfaction and Goals of Robotic Design

Patient satisfaction after total knee arthroplasty may be dependent on a number of patient-specific and technical factors. Despite decades of component design improvements and pre- and postoperative pathway optimization, 10–20% of patients in many studies still endorse dissatisfaction [4–7]. Common causes of dissatisfaction include persistent pain, stiffness, swelling, as well as subjective feelings of poor function [8]. The surgeon's role for maximizing patient satisfaction, in addition to setting appropriate expectations regarding the surgical recovery, rehabilitation process, and functional goals, is to provide a technically precise and well-balanced knee that provides near-native kinematics while minimizing soft-tissue injury and complication risks [9]. Robotic assistance thus aims to facilitate the surgeon's task through evaluation and planning as well as surgical execution.

3.1.2 Surgeon Interest

Unicompartmental knee arthroplasty (UKA) is reported to have higher rates of patient satisfaction and return to sport than TKA but overall is less commonly performed [10, 11]. Surgeons and patients may have concerns regarding the longevity of UKAs compared to TKAs, as analyses of the English/Welsh, Australian, Swedish, and Finnish arthroplasty registries have each revealed lower revision-free survival of UKAs, ranging from 80% to 90% survival rates at 7–10-year follow-up [12–14]. Additional studies of English/Welsh and Nordic registries noted volume-dependent outcomes, with high-volume centers achieving improved UKA survival at 10 years [15, 16]. Whether loosening occurs due to implant design, surgeon technique, or excessive overcorrection or undercorrection of deformity, proponents of robot-assisted arthroplasty claim improved accuracy and precision with component implantation may help surgeons make and execute their intraoperative alignment plan and improve implant survival for patients [17].

3.1.3 Robotic Technologies

Robotic-assisted total knee arthroplasty (RATKA) has been used to describe active (autonomous), semi-active (semi-autonomous, haptic, or tactile systems), and passive systems for assistance with the distal femur and proximal tibia bone cuts in unicompartmental and total knee arthroplasty [18, 19]. Understanding the differences in development, technique, and the unique evidence supporting each technology is important for informed decision-making for both patients and surgeons (Table 3.1).

Passive systems include navigation for surgical planning or active cutting guides and may also provide intraoperative feedback. Adoption of robotic systems overall has progressed slowly as surgeons and patients look for results of early implementation before investing in costly technology with potentially limited returns [20],

Table 3.1 Robotic knee arthroplasty systems with current FDA 510(k) clearance

System	Tsolution-One	Monogram	Mako	CORI	Navio PFS	Velys	ROSA	OMNIbotics
Predecessor	ROBODOC		RIO	Navio				Praxiteles (Praxim)
Company	THINK Surgical	Monogram Orth.	Stryker	Smith & Nephew	Smith & Nephew	Depuy Synthes	Zimmer Biomet	Corin
Headquarters	Fremont, CA	Austin, TX	Mahwah, NJ	Memphis, TN	Memphis, TN	West Chester, PA	Warsaw, IN	Tampa, FL
Previous Developer	Curexo		MAKO Surg. Corp		Blue Belt Tech.	Orthotaxy	Medtech	OMNIlife
	Fremont, CA		Ft. Lauderdale, FL		Plymouth, MN	Paris, FR	Montpellier, FR	East Taunton, MA
FDA 510(k) Clear	2015 Hip, 2019 Knee		2015	2020	2017	2021	2019	2017
Site	Hip, Knee	Hip, Knee	Hip, Knee	Knee	Knee	Knee	Knee, Spine	Knee
Type	Active	Active	Semi-Active	Semi-Active	Semi-Active	Semi-Active	Passive	Passive
Instrument	Burr	Burr	Saw, Burr	Burr	Burr	Saw	Cutting guide	Cutting guide
Pre-Imaging	CT	CT	CT	None	None	None	XR, None	CT
Implant Spec.	Open	Closed	Closed	Closed	Closed	Closed	Closed	Closed

indicating to many the profound impact that robotic arthroplasty has had in orthopedic surgery markets and likely will continue to have for the foreseeable future.

Semi-active systems are currently the most prevalent within the US market and are commonly referred to as haptic or tactile systems, as they utilize robotic guidance while retaining surgeon control within the planned resection [21]. Semi-active systems currently in production include Mako (Stryker, Mahwah, NJ; FDA cleared in 2015), Navio PFS (designed by Blue Belt Technologies, Plymouth, MN, and subsequently bought by Smith & Nephew, Memphis, TN; FDA cleared in 2017), as well as Smith & Nephew's second-generation system, CORI. The Mako system is approved for both hip and knee arthroplasty, has both saw and burr end-instrument capabilities, and is based on a preoperative computed tomography (CT) scan for resection planning. Alternatively, the Navio PFS and subsequently the CORI systems marketed by Smith & Nephew do not require preoperative imaging; rather, surface mapping of the patient's anatomy is performed intraoperatively in conjunction with balance assessment in order to guide resection performed selectively with a burr as the end instrument. Recently, the Velys system (DePuy Synthes, subs. of Johnson & Johnson, Warsaw, IN) received FDA 510(k) clearance in 2021, originally designed by French company Orthotaxy (Paris, France). The Velys system also does not require preoperative imaging. Similar to the Navio PFS and CORI systems, it uses a saw for its end instrument compared to the burr used by the two Smith & Nephew systems. Most semi-active systems use a robotic arm attached to an oscillating saw or burr, together providing a constrained resection path for the surgeon to employ. All the above systems currently in production, Mako, Navio PFS, Cori, and Velys, are closed systems that exclusively use implants from their distributors.

Two other semi-active systems currently in production, ROSA (Zimmer Biomet, Warsaw, IN) and OMNIBotics (Corin, Tampa, FL), use cutting guides as their end instrument, rather than cutting instruments such as saws or burrs used by the other semi-active systems. The ROSA system was originally designed by Medtech (Montpellier, France) for navigational use in orthopedic surgery, including spinal instrumentation, and for knee arthroplasty and is able to guide resection based on preoperative radiographs or be used in an imageless fashion. The OMNIBotics system was also initially developed in France, known as the Praxiteles system by Praxim, before it was purchased by OMNIlife (East Taunton, MA) and subsequently by Corin.

Active, autonomous robotic systems are able to perform bone cuts independently under observation of the surgeon, who first performs the approach and calibration. Active RATKAs are less commonly used, as early results with the CASPAR and ROBODOC systems in Europe and Korea in the 2000s reported prolonged operative times and concerns regarding early postoperative complications [22, 23]. Current autonomous systems include iBlock (formerly Praxiteles; OMNIlife Science, East Taunton, MA) and TSolution-One (formerly ROBODOC; Think Surgical Inc., Fremont, CA; previously Curexo Technology; FDA cleared in 2019). Currently, there is no available clinical data published for the TSolution-One.

3.1.4 Other Technologies

In addition to proper bony resection, soft-tissue and ligamentous balancing is essential for restorative knee function. Instability and stiffness are commonly cited reasons for dissatisfaction by patients after total knee arthroplasty [4–6, 8, 9]. As most prosthetic implants are designed with fixed medial and lateral widths, it is paramount for the surgeon to properly assess and balance the medial and lateral resection gaps. Most commonly this can be performed with variable-thickness blocks that can be subjected to varus and valgus stress to assess for opening or gapping greater on either medial or lateral aspects as an indicator for an inadequately balanced knee. Manual techniques relying on tactile feel may be subject to inter-surgeon variability [24, 25]. New technologies have been developed to assist with this portion of total and unicompartmental knee arthroplasty as well, with products currently commercially available to quantify the force transmitted across the knee. Verasense (Orthosensor Inc., Dania Beach, FL) is a device that provides force data when used in place of the polyethylene liner insert, as well as dynamic measurements of rollback and stability. Verasense may be used with trial components prior to final component implantation to determine if additional bony resection needs to be made or after final component implantation to determine necessity of soft-tissue releases.

In a trial of 84 patients who underwent TKA using Verasense, Cho et al. found that 36% of patients after standard measured resection had a balanced knee with <15 lbs. difference between medial and lateral compartments. After force assessment with Verasense and subsequent modified gap balancing in 66 patients based on Verasense results, 94% of knees were balanced [26]. No comparison was made for gap balancing between Verasense and tactile assessment, and further studies may be helpful in determining the accuracy and reliability of tactile assessment compared to quantitative force measurements with systems such as Verasense. In another study, Geller et al. compared rates of arthrofibrosis requiring manipulation under anesthesia (MUA), a nonsurgical treatment for postoperative stiffness, and found lower rates of MUA in 252 TKAs using Verasense compared to 699 standard TKAs—1.6 vs. 5%, $p = 0.004$ [27]. A clinical trial for Verasense by the authors and Columbia University is ongoing and expected to report patient-reported outcomes from 130 patients enrolled between 2017 and 2020.

3.2 Limitations

While robotic-assisted TKA has made great advances in recent years, there are still some limitations to the technology that are inherent to the cycle of disruptive technology development described by Christensen [28].

The primary barrier to more widespread adoption of this technology is the cost of implementation. The cost of the hardware alone ranges from $400,000 to well over $1,000,000 [20]. Costs are even more prohibitive when considering annual maintenance fees, software upgrades, and per-case disposable costs [20, 29]. Moreover, image-based robotic cases also require advanced preoperative imaging with CT or magnetic resonance imaging (MRI). Finally, Siddiqi et al. offered a thorough cost-benefit analysis including detailed indirect costs that need to be considered in a holistic cost model [20]. As healthcare increasingly trends toward value-based care and bundled payment models, designing comprehensive packages that are inclusive of all ancillary costs will be critical [29].

Working with existing reimbursement schemes, Moschetti et al. performed a Markov decision analysis of robotic unicompartmental knee arthroplasty to explore the current break-even point for robotic knee procedures [30]. The team found that, assuming an image-based system at a cost of $1.362 million, a return on investment can be made once volume surpasses 94 cases per year. For cheaper imageless systems, this break-even point was achieved at 25 cases annually [30]. As such, this technology is presently only a feasible strategy at high-volume centers. Further analyses will need to be performed for TKA and for promising new technology like handheld accelerometer-based navigation systems.

The other important major limitation of robotic-assisted TKA technology is with regard to soft-tissue manipulation. Current versions of orthopedic TKA robots still require the surgeon to perform the dissection and exposure. Once there, systems still require surgeons to retract tissues appropriately to enable cut paths without neurovascular or ligamentous damage [20, 21]. Moreover, current systems cannot actually perform soft-tissue balancing (although they assist in planning gap and ligament balancing) [20, 31]. Future iterations of robotic systems will have better feedback and adaptation mechanisms for mid-cut adjustments and better differentiation of soft-tissue types.

There are other notable limitations when considering this technology. Registration and navigation of the robot require additional or longer incisions for placement of femoral and tibial registration pins [32]. This increases risk for infection, stress risers and periprosthetic fractures, and neurovascular injury due to poor pin placement [20]. Length of surgery is also a concern, as robotic-assisted TKA is still generally longer due to intrinsic workflow delays, OR setup time, implant templating, and intraoperative plan adjustment [20, 21]. Notably, there has been substantial improvement in robotic-assisted TKA efficiency, and there are some studies where surgeons have performed the procedure in comparable time to a conventional TKA [33, 34]. Another concern is that current robotic-assisted TKA systems are implant specific, which limits surgeon options and increases acquisition costs as different surgeons prefer different platforms [21]. Additionally, there are equivocal results on other outcomes such as blood loss, nerve damage, and infection rates, which are all also partially distorted by the learning curves for these techniques [18]. Finally, there are legal concerns, as there is some evidence of an increased rate of litigation with robotic-assisted TKA procedures [35].

While the challenges are not insurmountable, there are still substantial limitations for the widespread adoption of robotic-assisted TKA. Product development with dedicated collaborators will be crucial to expand the use of these systems from a small group of early adopters into standard-of-care practice.

3.3 Outcomes

Whether or not robotic total knee arthroplasty leads to improved radiographic and clinical outcomes remains the subject of significant controversy [36]. Stated broadly, outcomes after robotic-assisted TKA can be grouped into either those related to accuracy and precision of component positioning and alignment or those related to clinical improvement, patient-reported outcomes (PROs), and functionality metrics. These two groups of outcomes are related but occasionally divergent, and where one study may find significant results related to one or both groups, other studies have failed to differentiate. Investigations into accuracy and precision of component positioning and postoperative limb alignment have evaluated both unicompartmental and TKA cohorts.

3.3.1 Radiographic/Alignment Outcomes After Robotic-Assisted TKA

Robotic-assisted TKA has been touted as allowing a surgeon to better replicate the anatomy of the native knee. Banger et al. found improved preservation of native knee anatomy in the coronal, sagittal, and axial planes in robotic-assisted TKA [37]. They did not correlate this finding to PROs. In a randomized controlled trial of 72 patients undergoing either conventional TKA or robotic-assisted implantation, Park et al. evaluated femoral flexion angle (gamma angle) and tibial flexion angle (delta angle) in the lateral x-ray and the femoral flexion angle (alpha angle) in the anteroposterior x-ray postoperatively. Both gamma angle and delta angle were significantly improved both with regard to accuracy to anatomic ideal and precision, with standard deviation being lower in the robotic-assisted cohort across all measured angles. With regard to gamma angle, in particular, the robotic-assisted cohort average was 0.17 degrees, representing the achievement of a near-perfect femoral flexion angle [22]. In congruence with these results, Liow et al. found that there were no mechanical axis outliers in a robot-assisted TKA cohort as compared with a 19.4% rate in a conventional cohort. Furthermore, the robotic-assisted TKA group had 3.23% joint-line malposition outliers as compared to 20.6% in the conventional group [38]. Further bolstering the assertion that robotic-assisted TKA results in fewer radiographic outliers, Yang et al. determined that robotic assistance resulted in significantly fewer postoperative leg alignment outliers with regard to femoral coronal inclination, tibial coronal inclination, femoral sagittal inclination, tibial sagittal inclination, and mechanical axis [39]. This data, taken together, leads to the conclusion that robotic-assisted TKA successfully reduces radiographic outliers with respect to postoperative component alignment.

Several studies have attempted to correlate these radiographic findings to PROs and complication rates. Song et al. prospectively randomized 100 patients who underwent unilateral TKA into a robot-assisted arm and a conventional arm and analyzed mechanical axis alignment, flexion/extension gap balance, and PRO scores across the cohorts. They noted a significant decrease in flexion and extension gap imbalance as well as mechanical axis alignment outliers in the robotic-assisted cohort. We will discuss the outcome metrics from this study in more detail in the following section, but despite the reduction in mechanical axis outliers, there was no improvement in postoperative PRO scores. The robotic-assisted procedure did take 25 minutes longer on average than the conventional but had less postoperative blood drainage [40]. Similarly, Kim et al. compared a single surgeon's robotic-assisted TKA to conventional technique with regard not only to radiographic parameters but also to PROs and complication rates across 1406 patients. These authors failed to find any significant difference between the two cohorts, not only with regard to PROs, survivorship, and complication rates but also with regard to mechanical and radiographic alignment parameters. Thus, they concluded that robotic-assisted TKA was not superior to conventional and, therefore, not cost-effective. These results are poorly generalizable, however, given their single-surgeon sample. It may be reasonable to assume that for an extremely high-volume adult reconstruction surgeon, performing several hundred TKAs yearly, robotic assistance may be unnecessary to achieve adequate alignment. However, for the lower-volume surgeon, robotic assistance may pay dividends in ensuring accuracy and precision of component alignment [41].

3.3.2 Radiographic/Alignment Outcomes After Robotic-Assisted UKA

Studies with methodologies similar to those listed previously have evaluated alignment parameters in unicompartmental knee arthroplasty (UKA) performed using robotic assistance versus the conventional technique. Ollivier et al. found no difference between the two cohorts in regards to lower limb alignment or implant positioning on mediolateral and anteroposterior radiographs. Functionality outcomes differed only marginally between cohorts, and the authors concluded that robotic assistance conferred no real benefit over conventional UKA [42]. In contrast with these results, Bell et al. noticed an improvement in the accuracy of component positioning with robotic-assisted UKA. These authors noted substantial effect sizes, with the percent of cases with femoral component coronal position within 2 degrees of the target position being 70% in the robotic-assisted group versus 28% in the conventional group. These authors did not assess PROs to observe whether or not this discrepancy leads to differential functional outcomes [43].

3.3.3 Radiographic/Alignment Outcomes After Robotic-Assisted TKA Using Adjustable Versus Conventional Cutting Blocks

In a unique study comparing differing techniques within robotic-assisted TKA, Suero et al. compared adjustable cutting blocks to conventional cutting blocks in computer-navigated TKA in 94 patients. These authors found that postoperative mechanical alignment variability and tourniquet time were significantly less in the adjustable cutting block group. Component alignment did not significantly vary between groups [44]. More data is needed to further delineate differences between various protocols for robotic-assisted TKA.

3.4 Clinical/Patient-Reported Outcomes

Patient satisfaction after total knee arthroplasty is dependent on several patient-specific and technical factors. Despite decades of component design improvements and pre- and postoperative pathway optimization, 10–20% of patients in many studies still endorse dissatisfaction [4–7]. Clinical and PROs after robotic-assisted TKA can be related to accuracy and precision of component positioning and alignment; however, there are other contributing factors. Thus, a surgeon's role for maximizing patient satisfaction after TKA is twofold: first, setting appropriate expectations regarding surgical recovery, rehabilitation process, and functional goals and, second, providing a technically precise and well-balanced knee with near-native kinematics while minimizing soft-tissue injury and complication risks [9]. Robotic assistance aims to facilitate the surgeon's task and improve postoperative outcomes through evaluation and planning as well as surgical execution. In this section, we will continue the discussion of outcomes after robotic-assisted TKA by focusing on clinical and PROs.

There are several metrics used to evaluate clinical and patient-reported outcomes. The Oxford Knee Score (OKS) is a knee joint-specific 12-item questionnaire originally developed and validated in 1998 for use in randomized controlled trials in TKA [45]. The OKS has 12 items, five for assessing pain and seven for assessing function. Each item is worth equal weighting [1–5] for a total possible score ranging from 12 to 60. A lower score indicates a better outcome. It is designed specifically for measuring outcomes in knee replacement.

The Knee Injury and Osteoarthritis Outcome Score (KOOS) is a knee joint-specific questionnaire developed in 1998 originally for the purpose of evaluating short-term and long-term symptoms and functioning in subjects with knee injury and osteoarthritis (OA). It was originally validated in patients undergoing anterior cruciate ligament (ACL) reconstruction [46]. The KOOS is a 42-item survey designed to assess people's opinions about the difficulties they experience with activity due to problems with their knees. A higher score indicates a better outcome.

The Western Ontario and McMaster Universities Arthritis Index (WOMAC) was initially developed in 1982 and was first validated for the purpose of evaluating response to treatment in patients with hip and knee OA in 1998 [47, 48]. The WOMAC underwent multiple subsequent revisions and refinements between 1996 and 1999 [49]. The WOMAC is a 24-item questionnaire with three subscales measuring pain (five items), stiffness (two items), and physical function (17 items). A lower score indicates a better outcome.

Finally, the Knee Society Clinical Rating System (KSS) is a knee joint-specific questionnaire originally developed and validated in 1989 for use in assessing the outcome of TKA [47]. The KSS has two components: a knee rating (0–100 points) and function (0–100 points) worth a total of 200 points. The knee rating is divided into pain (0–50 points) and a knee score that assesses range of motion, stability, and alignment (0–50 points). A higher score indicates a better outcome.

Other functional outcomes of interest include the International Knee Documentation Committee [50], the Lower Extremity Functional Scale [51], and the UCLA activity-level rating [52]. Furthermore, many global health scores are available including the Nottingham Health Profile [53], the SF-12 [54], the SF-36 [55], and the Sickness Impact Profile [56].

3.4.1 Clinical and Patient-Reported Outcomes After TKA

The ROBODOC system (Curexo Technology, Fremont, CA) was the first robotic system to be used in orthopedic surgery in 1992. ROBODOC is an active-autonomous, image-based, robotic milling system that can reproduce accurate component placement and an ideal hip-knee-ankle (HKA) mechanical axis (MA) through an image-based preoperative planning system [38, 57]. ROBODOC was subsequently changed to TSolution-One®. As it has been used for several years, there are several studies in the literature that comment on patient satisfaction after RATKA with ROBODOC.

Liow et al. [57] compared patients undergoing RATKA with ROBODOC to those undergoing conventional TKA [57]. Patients in both groups received Zimmer NexGen LPS-Flex posterior stabilized implants. The RATKA group showed significant improvement in outcome scores for several SF-36 parameters (general health, vitality, and role emotional) and a nonsignificant trend toward higher functional scores. However, they did not demonstrate differences in clinical outcome measures of OKS and KSS knee and function scores.

Kim et al. [41] randomized subjects to a robotic-assisted or conventional jig-based TKA [41]. Robotic-assisted TKA was carried out in two steps with CT-based preoperative planning using ORTHODOC (Integrated Surgical Technology Corp., Davis, CA, USA) and robotic-assisted surgery using the ROBODOC surgical assistance. A Duracon® posterior cruciate-substituting total knee prosthesis (Stryker Orthopaedics, Mahwah, NJ, USA) was used in each knee. There was no difference in any clinical outcome measure at the latest follow-up for patients who received robotic-assisted TKAs when compared to those who received conventional TKAs. This included KSS scores, residual pain, WOMAC scores, knee range of motion (ROM), and UCLA activity scores. Furthermore, at a minimum follow-up of 10 years, they found no differences between robotic-assisted TKA and conventional TKA in terms of functional outcome scores, aseptic loosening, overall survivorship, and complications. Their group ultimately did not recommend robotic-assisted surgery, stating that any technique like robotic-assisted surgery which adds cost to the procedure should deliver results that patients can perceive as improvements.

Finally, Song et al. assessed intermediate-term outcomes of patients undergoing RATKA with the ROBODOC in comparison to those undergoing conventional

TKA [40]. They found HSS and WOMAC scores were similar to those previously reported in the literature, with no significant differences between the two.

Within the ROBODOC system, studies have been done to compare outcomes when using the classical (or mechanical) alignment method versus the anatomic (or kinematic) alignment method. Yim et al. [58] compared clinical outcomes between these methods when using ROBODOC with preoperative ORTHODOC planning [58]. They found no significant postoperative differences in knee ROM, HSS, and WOMAC scores. Yeo et al. [59] also evaluated the two alignment methods in patients undergoing ROBODOC-assisted TKA [59]. They also found no significant difference in mean HSS, WOMAC, and KSS scores at final follow-up.

Though there are fewer studies comparing intraoperative alignment methods used during RATKA, there appears to be no difference in clinical outcomes between the two approaches.

MAKO (Stryker, Mahwah, NJ) is a semi-active robotic system and is one of the most prevalent within the US market. It is a haptic or tactile system as it utilizes robotic guidance while retaining surgeon control within the planned resection. Given its recent FDA approval and recent popularity, numerous studies have been published on patient-reported outcomes after RATKA with MAKO. While PROs appear to be relatively similar in the literature focused on RATKA with ROBODOC, the literature demonstrates a trend toward improved PROs when MAKO is used.

Given the brief history of MAKO with its recent FDA approval in 2015, most studies are centered around early postoperative outcomes. Khlopas et al. conducted a prospective randomized controlled trial of early postoperative outcomes in patients undergoing conventional TKA versus those undergoing robotic-arm-assisted TKA with MAKO [60]. Both groups had a cemented Triathlon Cruciate Retaining Total Knee System (Stryker Orthopaedics, Mahwah, NJ) implanted. Functional activity walking and standing scores as well as pain scores were both improved in the RATKA group at 6 weeks and 3 months postoperatively. Importantly, patient satisfaction scores were also improved at 6 weeks and 3 months in the RATKA cohort. Kayani et al. also found improved early postoperative pain scores at four time intervals following surgery [61]. Patients in the RATKA cohort also had decreased opiate analgesia requirements. Finally, Naziri et al. found improved 90-day ROM but comparable complication rates, KSS, and PROs at all early postoperative time points [62]. They found no difference in hospital satisfaction rates.

Marchand et al. in 2017 used the WOMAC patient satisfaction outcome survey to compare 6-month postoperative mean pain, physical function, and total patient satisfaction scores in patients who underwent conventional versus RATKA with MAKO [63]. In their series, patients who underwent robotic-assisted surgery reported significantly better 6-month mean pain and overall satisfaction scores. The same group repeated this study in 2019, assessing 1-year PROs [64]. They found that WOMAC scores were significantly lower in the RATKA group with improved function and decreased pain. Mahoney et al. [65] and Smith et al. [66] both compiled 1-year postoperative clinical outcomes, with both demonstrating clinical improvements of postoperative physical status and function, specifically in KSS score.

Some literature does not specify what robot was used to assist with TKA. Hozack et al. found that patients undergoing RATKA had significantly higher functional activity scores at 6 weeks and 1 year postoperatively [67]. A meta-analysis done by Zhang et al. included seven clinical studies that reported functional outcomes when comparing RATKA using different robotic devices to conventional TKA [68]. Different outcome scores were utilized across the included studies, with the KSS being the most reported followed by Western Ontario and McMaster Universities Osteoarthritis Index (WOMAC) scores. Meta-analysis of outcome data from the studies demonstrated RATKA resulted in a significantly better KSS scores in short to mid-term follow-up.

3.4.2 Clinical and Patient-Reported Outcomes After UKA

There are significantly fewer studies in the literature that assess clinical and PROs after robotic-assisted unicompartmental knee arthroplasty (RAUKA). Gilmour et al. reported on patients undergoing conventional or RAUKA with MAKO [69]. Primary outcomes in the study were OKS and KSS which were not significantly different in the two groups at 2-year follow-up. These findings were supported by Pearle et al. who also reported on patients undergoing RAUKA with MAKO [70]. They found no significant difference in KSS, change in KSS, or Marmor rating between the two cohorts at final follow-up.

Finally, Motesharei et al. compared gait analysis between patients undergoing conventional Oxford UKA and RAUKA with MAKO [71]. At 1-year follow-up, there was a significant difference in the gait of patients in each cohort, with the RAUKA patients demonstrating similar knee excursion compared with native knees, and the conventional Oxford UKA patients demonstrating decreased knee excursion. The authors noted they were unable to specifically attribute this difference to the technique, and other factors may have played a role such as the design of the different implants used for each cohort. Despite these differences, there were no significant differences in OKS and KSS between the two groups.

3.5 Summary

In the coming years, patients and surgeons can expect to see an increase in both the number and variety of robotic technologies commercially available for knee arthroplasty. For both unicompartmental and TKA, the use of robotic assistants to personalize bone resection and knee balancing may be performed in a versatile manner using intraoperative calibration and feedback, with or without the need for preoperative imaging. Since the implementation of early robotic assistants such as ROBODOC, it has been a challenge for many robotic-assistant developers to reduce some of the limitations to broad implementation, particularly with regard to cost, the surgeon's learning curve, and associated prolongation of intraoperative time. As more types of semi-active robotic assistants come to market after their FDA 510(k) clearance in the past 5 years, more patients and surgeons may demonstrate interest in these technologies and refer to the clinical results of early adopters, some of which demonstrate improvements in radiographic, kinematic, and clinical outcomes.

References (EndNote Traveling Library)

1. Gatti CJ, Hallstrom BR, Hughes RE. Surgeon variability in total knee arthroplasty component alignment: a Monte Carlo analysis. Comput Methods Biomech Biomed Engin. 2014;17(15):1738–50.
2. Bargar WL, Bauer A, Börner M. Primary and revision total hip replacement using the Robodoc system. Clin Orthop Relat Res. 1998;354:82–91.
3. Maradit Kremers H, Larson DR, Crowson CS, Kremers WK, Washington RE, Steiner CA, et al. Prevalence of total hip and knee replacement in the United States. J Bone Joint Surg Am. 2015;97(17):1386–97.
4. Bourne RB, Chesworth BM, Davis AM, Mahomed NN, Charron KDJ. Patient satisfaction after total knee arthroplasty: who is satisfied and who is not? Clin Orthop Relat Res. 2010;468(1):57–63.
5. Clement ND, Burnett R. Patient satisfaction after total knee arthroplasty is affected by their general physical well-being. Knee Surg Sports Traumatol Arthrosc. 2013;21(11):2638–46.
6. Nam D, Nunley RM, Barrack RL. Patient dissatisfaction following total knee replacement. The Bone & Joint Journal. 2014;96-B(11_Supple_A):96–100.
7. Von Keudell A, Sodha S, Collins J, Minas T, Fitz W, Gomoll AH. Patient satisfaction after primary total and unicompartmental knee arthroplasty: an age-dependent analysis. Knee. 2014;21(1):180–4.
8. Noble PC, Conditt MA, Cook KF, Mathis KB. The John Insall Award: patient expectations affect satisfaction with total knee arthroplasty. Clin Orthop Relat Res. 2006;452:35–43.
9. Gunaratne R, Pratt DN, Banda J, Fick DP, Khan RJK, Robertson BW. Patient dissatisfaction following total knee arthroplasty: a systematic review of the literature. J Arthroplasty. 2017;32(12):3854–60.
10. Naal FD, Fischer M, Preuss A, Goldhahn J, von Knoch F, Preiss S, et al. Return to sports and recreational activity after unicompartmental knee arthroplasty. Am J Sports Med. 2007;35(10):1688–95.
11. Hopper GP, Leach WJ. Participation in sporting activities following knee replacement: total versus unicompartmental. Knee Surg Sports Traumatol Arthrosc. 2008;16(10):973.
12. Liddle AD, Judge A, Pandit H, Murray DW. Adverse outcomes after total and unicompartmental knee replacement in 101 330 matched patients: a study of data from the National Joint Registry for England and Wales. Lancet. 2014;384(9952):1437–45.
13. W-Dahl A, Robertsson O, Lidgren L, Miller L, Davidson D, Graves S. Unicompartmental knee arthroplasty in patients aged less than 65. Acta Orthop. 2010;81(1):90–4.
14. Koskinen E, Paavolainen P, Eskelinen A, Pulkkinen P, Remes V. Unicondylar knee replacement for primary osteoarthritis: a prospective follow-up study of 1,819 patients from the Finnish Arthroplasty Register. Acta Orthop. 2007;78(1):128–35.
15. Liddle AD, Pandit H, Judge A, Murray DW. Effect of surgical caseload on revision rate following total and unicompartmental knee replacement. JBJS. 2016;98(1):1–8.
16. Badawy M, Fenstad AM, Bartz-Johannessen CA, Indrekvam K, Havelin LI, Robertsson O, et al. Hospital volume and the risk of revision in Oxford unicompartmental knee arthroplasty in the Nordic countries -an observational study of 14,496 cases. BMC Musculoskelet Disord. 2017;18(1):388.

17. Christ AB, Pearle AD, Mayman DJ, Haas SB. Robotic-assisted unicompartmental knee arthroplasty: state-of-the art and review of the literature. J Arthroplasty. 2018;33(7):1994–2001.
18. Lang JE, Mannava S, Floyd AJ, Goddard MS, Smith BP, Mofidi A, et al. Robotic systems in orthopaedic surgery. J Bone Joint Surg Br. 2011;93(10):1296–9.
19. Schneider O, Troccaz J. A six-degree-of-freedom passive arm with dynamic constraints (PADyC) for cardiac surgery application: preliminary experiments. Comput Aided Surg. 2001;6(6):340–51.
20. Siddiqi A, Mont MA, Krebs VE, Piuzzi NS. Not all robotic-assisted total knee arthroplasty are the same. J Am Acad Orthop Surg. 2021;29(2):45–59.
21. Jacofsky DJ, Allen M. Robotics in arthroplasty: a comprehensive review. J Arthroplasty. 2016;31(10):2353–63.
22. Park SE, Lee CT. Comparison of robotic-assisted and conventional manual implantation of a primary total knee arthroplasty. J Arthroplasty. 2007;22(7):1054–9.
23. Siebert W, Mai S, Kober R, Heeckt PF. Technique and first clinical results of robot-assisted total knee replacement. Knee. 2002;9(3):173–80.
24. Elmallah RK, Mistry JB, Cherian JJ, Chughtai M, Bhave A, Roche MW, et al. Can we really "Feel" a balanced total knee arthroplasty? J Arthroplasty. 2016;31(9, Supplement):102–5.
25. D'Lima DD, Patil S, Steklov N, Colwell CW Jr. An ABJS best paper: dynamic intraoperative ligament balancing for total knee arthroplasty. Clin Orthop Relat Res. 2007;463:208–12.
26. Cho KJ, Seon JK, Jang WY, Park CG, Song EK. Objective quantification of ligament balancing using VERASENSE in measured resection and modified gap balance total knee arthroplasty. BMC Musculoskelet Disord. 2018;19(1):266.
27. Geller JA, Lakra A, Murtaugh T. The use of electronic sensor device to augment ligament balancing leads to a lower rate of arthrofibrosis after total knee arthroplasty. J Arthroplasty. 2017;32(5):1502–4.
28. Christensen CM. The innovator's dilemma : when new technologies cause great firms to fail. Boston: Harvard Business Review Press; 2013. xxvii, 252 pages p.
29. Lonner JH, Klement MR. Robotic-assisted medial unicompartmental knee arthroplasty: options and outcomes. J Am Acad Orthop Surg. 2019;27(5):e207–e14.
30. Moschetti WE, Konopka JF, Rubash HE, Genuario JW. Can robot-assisted unicompartmental knee arthroplasty be cost-effective? A Markov decision analysis. J Arthroplasty. 2016;31(4):759–65.
31. Pearle AD, Kendoff D, Musahl V. Perspectives on computer-assisted orthopaedic surgery: movement toward quantitative orthopaedic surgery. J Bone Joint Surg Am. 2009;91 Suppl 1:7–12.
32. Kayani B, Konan S, Ayuob A, Onochie E, Al-Jabri T, Haddad FS. Robotic technology in total knee arthroplasty: a systematic review. EFORT Open Rev. 2019;4(10):611–7.
33. Kayani B, Konan S, Huq SS, Tahmassebi J, Haddad FS. Robotic-arm assisted total knee arthroplasty has a learning curve of seven cases for integration into the surgical workflow but no learning curve effect for accuracy of implant positioning. Knee Surg Sports Traumatol Arthrosc. 2019;27(4):1132–41.
34. Grau L, Lingamfelter M, Ponzio D, Post Z, Ong A, Le D, et al. Robotic arm assisted total knee arthroplasty workflow optimization, operative times and learning curve. Arthroplast Today. 2019;5(4):465–70.
35. Davies BL, Rodriguez y Baena FM, Barrett AR, Gomes MP, Harris SJ, Jakopec M, et al. Robotic control in knee joint replacement surgery. Proc Inst Mech Eng H. 2007;221(1):71–80.
36. Shatrov J, Parker D. Computer and robotic – assisted total knee arthroplasty: a review of outcomes. J Exp Orthop. 2020;7(1):70.
37. Banger MS, Johnston WD, Razii N, Doonan J, Rowe PJ, Jones BG, et al. Robotic arm-assisted bi-unicompartmental knee arthroplasty maintains natural knee joint anatomy compared with total knee arthroplasty: a prospective randomized controlled trial. Bone Joint J. 2020;102-B(11):1511–8.

38. Liow MH, Xia Z, Wong MK, Tay KJ, Yeo SJ, Chin PL. Robot-assisted total knee arthroplasty accurately restores the joint line and mechanical axis. A prospective randomised study. J Arthroplasty. 2014;29(12):2373–7.
39. Yang HY, Seon JK, Shin YJ, Lim HA, Song EK. Robotic total knee arthroplasty with a cruciate-retaining implant: a 10-year follow-up study. Clin Orthop Surg. 2017;9(2):169–76.
40. Song EK, Seon JK, Yim JH, Netravali NA, Bargar WL. Robotic-assisted TKA reduces postoperative alignment outliers and improves gap balance compared to conventional TKA. Clin Orthop Relat Res. 2013;471(1):118–26.
41. Kim YH, Yoon SH, Park JW. Does robotic-assisted TKA result in better outcome scores or long-term survivorship than conventional TKA? A randomized. Controlled Trial Clin Orthop Relat Res. 2020;478(2):266–75.
42. Ollivier M, Parratte S, Lunebourg A, Viehweger E, Argenson JN. The John Insall Award: no functional benefit after unicompartmental knee arthroplasty performed with patient-specific instrumentation: a randomized trial. Clin Orthop Relat Res. 2016;474(1):60–8.
43. Bell SW, Anthony I, Jones B, MacLean A, Rowe P, Blyth M. Improved accuracy of component positioning with robotic-assisted unicompartmental knee arthroplasty: data from a prospective, randomized controlled study. J Bone Joint Surg Am. 2016;98(8):627–35.
44. Suero EM, Plaskos C, Dixon PL, Pearle AD. Adjustable cutting blocks improve alignment and surgical time in computer-assisted total knee replacement. Knee Surg Sports Traumatol Arthrosc. 2012;20(9):1736–41.
45. Dawson J, Fitzpatrick R, Murray D, Carr A. Questionnaire on the perceptions of patients about total knee replacement. J Bone Joint Surg Br. 1998;80(1):63–9.
46. Roos EM, Toksvig-Larsen S. Knee injury and Osteoarthritis Outcome Score (KOOS) - validation and comparison to the WOMAC in total knee replacement. Health Qual Life Outcomes. 2003;1:17.
47. Insall JN, Dorr LD, Scott RD, Scott WN. Rationale of the knee society clinical rating system. Clin Orthop Relat Res. 1989;248:13–4.
48. Bellamy N, Buchanan WW, Goldsmith CH, Campbell J, Stitt LW. Validation study of WOMAC: a health status instrument for measuring clinically important patient relevant outcomes to antirheumatic drug therapy in patients with osteoarthritis of the hip or knee. J Rheumatol. 1988;15(12):1833–40.
49. Bellamy N. WOMAC: a 20-year experiential review of a patient-centered self-reported health status questionnaire. J Rheumatol. 2002;29(12):2473–6.
50. Collins NJ, Misra D, Felson DT, Crossley KM, Roos EM. Measures of knee function: International Knee Documentation Committee (IKDC) Subjective Knee Evaluation Form, Knee Injury and Osteoarthritis Outcome Score (KOOS), Knee Injury and Osteoarthritis Outcome Score Physical Function Short Form (KOOS-PS), Knee Outcome Survey Activities of Daily Living Scale (KOS-ADL), Lysholm Knee Scoring Scale, Oxford Knee Score (OKS), Western Ontario and McMaster Universities Osteoarthritis Index (WOMAC), Activity Rating Scale (ARS), and Tegner Activity Score (TAS). Arthritis Care Res (Hoboken). 2011;63 Suppl 11:S208–28.
51. Binkley JM, Stratford PW, Lott SA, Riddle DL. The Lower Extremity Functional Scale (LEFS): scale development, measurement properties, and clinical application. North American Orthopaedic Rehabilitation Research Network. Phys Ther. 1999;79(4):371–83.
52. Naal FD, Impellizzeri FM, Leunig M. Which is the best activity rating scale for patients undergoing total joint arthroplasty? Clin Orthop Relat Res. 2009;467(4):958–65.
53. Dunbar MJ, Robertsson O, Ryd L, Lidgren L. Appropriate questionnaires for knee arthroplasty. Results of a survey of 3600 patients from the Swedish Knee Arthroplasty Registry. J Bone Joint Surg Br. 2001;83(3):339–44.
54. Ware J Jr, Kosinski M, Keller SD. A 12-item short-form health survey: construction of scales and preliminary tests of reliability and validity. Med Care. 1996;34(3):220–33.
55. Ware JE Jr, Sherbourne CD. The MOS 36-item short-form health survey (SF-36). I. Conceptual framework and item selection. Med Care. 1992;30(6):473–83.

56. Bergner M, Bobbitt RA, Carter WB, Gilson BS. The sickness impact profile: development and final revision of a health status measure. Med Care. 1981;19(8):787–805.
57. Liow MHL, Chin PL, Pang HN, Tay DK, Yeo SJ. THINK surgical TSolution-one((R)) (Robodoc) total knee arthroplasty. SICOT J. 2017;3:63.
58. Yim JH, Song EK, Khan MS, Sun ZH, Seon JK. A comparison of classical and anatomical total knee alignment methods in robotic total knee arthroplasty: classical and anatomical knee alignment methods in TKA. J Arthroplasty. 2013;28(6):932–7.
59. Yeo JH, Seon JK, Lee DH, Song EK. No difference in outcomes and gait analysis between mechanical and kinematic knee alignment methods using robotic total knee arthroplasty. Knee Surg Sports Traumatol Arthrosc. 2019;27(4):1142–7.
60. Khlopas A, Sodhi N, Hozack WJ, Chen AF, Mahoney OM, Kinsey T, et al. Patient-reported functional and satisfaction outcomes after robotic-arm-assisted total knee arthroplasty: early results of a prospective multicenter investigation. J Knee Surg. 2020;33(7):685–90.
61. Kayani B, Konan S, Tahmassebi J, Pietrzak JRT, Haddad FS. Robotic-arm assisted total knee arthroplasty is associated with improved early functional recovery and reduced time to hospital discharge compared with conventional jig-based total knee arthroplasty: a prospective cohort study. Bone Joint J. 2018;100-B(7):930–7.
62. Naziri Q, Cusson BC, Chaudhri M, Shah NV, Sastry A. Making the transition from traditional to robotic-arm assisted TKA: what to expect? A single-surgeon comparative-analysis of the first-40 consecutive cases. J Orthop. 2019;16(4):364–8.
63. Marchand RC, Sodhi N, Khlopas A, Sultan AA, Harwin SF, Malkani AL, et al. Patient satisfaction outcomes after robotic arm-assisted Total knee arthroplasty: a short-term evaluation. J Knee Surg. 2017;30(9):849–53.
64. Marchand RC, Sodhi N, Anis HK, Ehiorobo J, Newman JM, Taylor K, et al. One-year patient outcomes for robotic-arm-assisted versus manual total knee arthroplasty. J Knee Surg. 2019;32(11):1063–8.
65. Mahoney O, Kinsey T, Sodhi N, Mont MA, Chen AF, Orozco F, et al. Improved component placement accuracy with robotic-arm assisted total knee arthroplasty. J Knee Surg. 2020.
66. Smith AF, Eccles CJ, Bhimani SJ, Denehy KM, Bhimani RB, Smith LS, et al. Improved patient satisfaction following robotic-assisted total knee arthroplasty. J Knee Surg. 2021;34(7):730–8.
67. Hozack WJ. Multicentre analysis of outcomes after robotic-arm assisted total knee arthroplasty. Orthop Proc. 2018;100-B(SUPP_12):38.
68. Zhang J, Ndou WS, Ng N, Gaston P, Simpson PM, Macpherson GJ, et al. Robotic-arm assisted total knee arthroplasty is associated with improved accuracy and patient reported outcomes: a systematic review and meta-analysis. Knee Surg Sports Traumatol Arthrosc. 2021.
69. Gilmour A, MacLean AD, Rowe PJ, Banger MS, Donnelly I, Jones BG, et al. Robotic-arm-assisted vs conventional unicompartmental knee arthroplasty. The 2-year clinical outcomes of a randomized controlled trial. J Arthroplasty. 2018;33(7S):S109–S15.
70. Pearle AD, van der List JP, Lee L, Coon TM, Borus TA, Roche MW. Survivorship and patient satisfaction of robotic-assisted medial unicompartmental knee arthroplasty at a minimum two-year follow-up. Knee. 2017;24(2):419–28.
71. Motesharei A, Rowe P, Blyth M, Jones B, Maclean A. A comparison of gait one year post operation in an RCT of robotic UKA versus traditional Oxford UKA. Gait Posture. 2018;62:41–5.

Advanced Surgical Techniques for Tibiofemoral Unicompartmental Knee Replacement

4

Frank R. Noyes

4.1 Indications

Unicompartmental knee arthroplasty (UKA) is a valid treatment option for patients in whom severe joint damage and complete loss of joint space are present in one compartment. This chapter focuses on tibiofemoral compartment UKA and represents a summary of a previous comprehensive work on this topic [1]. The author has previously published a similar chapter on patellofemoral UKA [2]. In appropriate patient candidates, the advantages of UKA compared with total knee arthroplasty (TKA) include less blood loss, smaller incisions, decreased soft tissue injury, preservation of bone stock, return to higher levels of function, fewer complications, shortened hospital stays, and an overall faster recovery [3–7].

The primary indication for UKA is symptomatic isolated painful arthritis marked by moderate to severe joint line pain and/or stiffness that limits daily activities. Pain and swelling may occur while resting, either during the day or at night. Failure of a lengthy course of nonoperative treatment has occurred that included non-steroidal anti-inflammatory medications (NSAID), steroid injections, physical therapy, and weight control.

Our experience with this operation has usually involved patients less than 60 years of age. It is important to note that several investigations have reported that neither age [8–15] nor gender [12, 15–18] appears to influence outcomes in modern studies.

The majority of UKA candidates will have undergone prior procedures such as chondroplasty, meniscectomy, microfracture, autologous chondrocyte implantation (ACI), and osteochondral autograft transfer. Several investigations have shown that patients with anterior cruciate ligament (ACL) deficiency may undergo a

F. R. Noyes (✉)
Cincinnati SportsMedicine and Orthopaedic Center, The Noyes Knee Institute, Cincinnati, OH, USA

F. R. Noyes, S. Barber-Westin (eds.), *Critical Rehabilitation for Partial and Total Knee Arthroplasty*, https://doi.org/10.1007/978-3-030-87003-4_4

successful concomitant ACL reconstruction with UKA [14, 19–24]. It is important that the patient has realistic expectations regarding what this operation may and may not accomplish. At our center, most patients are able to walk without support within approximately 2–3 weeks postoperatively, and the majority return to daily activities within 4–6 weeks. Light, low-impact activities such as walking, swimming, golfing, light hiking, and bicycling can often be performed by 3 months. However, running and high-impact athletic or occupational activities are not advised, and it is essential that the patient understands and accepts these limitations [25].

4.2 Contraindications

Preexisting joint arthritis in another compartment of the knee is the principal contraindication to UKA because of the noteworthy evidence that this is the leading cause of failure [15, 17, 26–30]. Patients with moderate to advanced articular cartilage deterioration and/or moderate to severe joint space narrowing on standing posteroanterior (PA) radiographs in two or three compartments are not candidates. Anterior or patellofemoral knee pain, with or without moderate patellofemoral joint narrowing or arthritic damage, is not an absolute contraindication [13, 31–34]. However, persistent patellar pain on stairs, kneeling, and light activity will persist after UKA, and most patients with these concurrent symptoms will choose TKA.

Other contraindications include uncorrected excessive varus or valgus malalignment (greater than 3°), knee ligament instability, knee hyperextension of 10° or more, inflammatory arthritis, and prior infection. Patients with complex regional pain syndrome, diabetes, knee arthrofibrosis (excessive extension or flexion contracture), chondrocalcinosis, rheumatoid arthritis, or neuromuscular disorders affecting limb control are not considered candidates. Patients who are obese (body mass index [BMI] greater than 32) are not considered candidates for UKA, although recent reports noted no significant differences in survival rates according to BMI subcategories [35–39].

Osteopenia (bone mineral density T score between −1.0 and −2.5 standard deviations below normal) and osteoporosis (T score less than −2.5) are contraindications for this operation owing to the potential risk of subsidence of the implants. Other contraindications include failure to treat the patient with all possible conservative measures, noncompliance with rehabilitation, and unrealistic expectations for future activity levels.

A few reports have shown poorer results when medial UKA was done in patients with only partial loss of tibiofemoral joint space and articular cartilage [40–43]. Ultimately, the final decision to perform UKA or TKA is made during surgery after all of the joint surfaces have been visualized. The patient should be informed and consent obtained to perform either procedure.

4.3 Implant Design

UKAs may be generally categorized according to the bone-cut preparation (resurfacing or inset) and bearing surface (mobile or fixed). Resurfacing implants require minimal bone resection, while inset implants require angular cutting similar to TKA. Bearing surfaces are usually all polyethylene or modular and include fixed bearing and mobile bearing. The initial UKA implants, such as the Marmor (Smith & Nephew, Memphis, TN) and St Georg Sled (Waldemar Link, Hamburg, Germany), were fixed bearing with all-polyethylene tibial inserts. Problems with these prostheses included subsidence in both the femoral condyle and tibial plateau, aseptic loosening, and wear due to suboptimal design [44]. Subsequently, implants were redesigned to distribute loads onto the cortical rim and had a minimum thickness of the tibial insert of more than 6 millimeters. Metal-backed components were introduced, requiring greater bone resection. The Miller-Galante (Zimmer, Warsaw, IN) is a well-known metal-backed, fixed-bearing implant with a modular polyethylene insert.

Mobile-bearing implant designs were introduced in attempts to reduce the stress exerted on the tibial surface. These implants, such as the Oxford (Biomet, Bridgend, UK), have a metal femoral component that articulates with a polyethylene meniscal component and a flat metal tibial surface. A porous-coated prosthesis was developed in order to induce bone growth and provide better fixation. For instance, the cementless Oxford Phase 3 has a layer of porous titanium with calcium hydroxyapatite under its components. Mobile-bearing implants are subject to dislocation of the mobile insert from the tibial base.

4.4 Robotic Technology

It is well known and documented that early UKA failures are frequently caused by inaccurate positioning of the components that leads to undercorrection or overcorrection of the final limb alignment. Excessive malalignment of the tibial component (>3°) or posterior tibial slope (>7°) may cause component loosening, fractures, and increased bone stresses [45–49]. Robotic-assisted surgical navigation was introduced in the early 2000s in order to improve accuracy in UKA (postoperative limb alignment, component positioning, and soft tissue balancing) using less invasive techniques. There are two types of robotic surgery systems: haptic (or tactile) and autonomous. Haptic systems require active participation of the surgeon to complete the entire operation, while autonomous robotic systems complete the operation after the surgeon has performed the approach and set up the machine. Haptic systems constrain the motion of the cutting tool to only the preplanned volume or area of resection. Preoperative three-dimensional models of the patient's knee (created with computed tomography [CT] scans) are merged with referenced bony surfaces during surgery to form a final model of the actual anatomy of the patient. The component placement and exact cutting zones are determined. As the surgeon resects these areas, the robotic arm provides auditory and tactile feedback, limiting the tip of the rotating burr to just the predefined cutting area. The MAKOplasty Partial Knee Resurfacing System that uses the Robotic Arm Interactive Orthopedic System (RIO) (Stryker, Kalamazoo, MI) and the Acrobot system (The Acrobot Company, London, UK) are examples of commercially available haptic systems.

Many studies have compared short-term outcomes between various navigation and conventional UKA techniques [50–62]. Negrin et al. [61] conducted a systematic review of 15 articles published between 2005 and 2019 and concluded that the majority reported improved accuracy position in robotic-assisted cases. Nair and associates [63] identified 15 studies published from 2003 to 2011 and also found that navigation methods improved component alignment and position and reduced radiographic outliers compared with conventional systems. Both of these reviews reported few significant differences in clinical outcomes, which is not surprising considering that the majority of studies had a follow-up of 2 years or less. A meta-analysis was conducted by Weber et al. [64] of ten studies (levels II and III) involving 258 medial UKAs implanted with navigation and 295 medial UKAs implanted with conventional techniques. The study reported that there were more outliers in the conventional group compared with the navigation group for all variables assessed, including mechanical axis (30% and 11%, respectively), femoral antero-posterior (AP) alignment (17% and 5%, respectively), femoral lateral alignment (41% and 18%, respectively), tibial AP alignment (14% and 8%, respectively), and tibial slope (22% and 9%, respectively). Chin et al. [51] performed meta-analyses on 13 studies published from 2005 to 2019 and concluded that robotic-assisted UKA produced superior radiological and short-term clinical outcomes compared with conventional UKA.

Mofidi et al. [55] calculated accuracy rates by comparing intraoperative planned and postoperative radiographic measurements in 232 knees that underwent medial UKA using the MAKOplasty system. Accuracy rates of the femoral prosthesis were 2.8° ± 2.5° in the coronal plane and 3.6° ± 3.3° in the sagittal plane. Accuracy rates of the tibial component were 2.2° ± 1.75° in the coronal plane and 2.4° ± 2° in the sagittal plane. The authors concluded there was a high degree of agreement between intraoperatively planned prosthesis alignment and postoperatively measured alignment. Proper cementation technique was considered crucial in achieving accurate alignment.

Matsui et al. [65] found that a portable navigation system improved the accuracy of the implantation of the tibial component of Oxford Phase 3 medial UKA in 70 patients. The incidence of outliers in the coronal plane was 9.3% in the study group compared with 41% in the conventional implantation group ($P < 0.0001$). There was no difference in the incidence of outliers in the sagittal plane. Suda et al. [66] also reported superior accuracy of a portable navigation system compared with conventional implantation in 51 patients. This study reported that all of the navigation group implants were aligned within 3.0° of the target coronal and sagittal implant alignment. In the conventional group, 76.5% and 88.2% of the implants were aligned within 3.0° of the target coronal and sagittal implants, respectively ($P < 0.05$).

4.5 Clinical Examination

A thorough history is required that includes documentation of prior surgical procedures, conservative treatment measures, and all knee joint injuries. Symptoms are typically experienced most often during stair climbing, walking on uneven ground, and kneeling or squatting.

The comprehensive physical examination includes a complete patellofemoral examination to assess patellar tilt, subluxation, mobility, Q angle, and lower limb rotational alignment (femoral internal torsion, tibial external torsion). The patella and all surrounding tissues are palpated to localize pain. The medial and lateral joint lines are also inspected for any tenderness, indicative of tibiofemoral joint involvement that may contraindicate UKA. The patient's gait, range of knee motion, lower extremity and hip muscle strength, and neurovascular status are evaluated. All knee ligaments are tested.

Radiographs include standing AP at 0° of knee flexion, lateral at 30° of knee flexion, weight-bearing PA at 45° of knee flexion, and patellofemoral axial views. Double-stance full-standing radiographs of both lower extremities, from the femoral heads to the ankle joints, are obtained in knees in which varus or valgus lower extremity alignment is detected on clinical examination. Magnetic resonance imaging (MRI) is required in certain cases to determine the cartilage status of the entire knee joint, along with all other soft tissue structures.

4.6 Surgical Technique

The UKA operative technique described in this chapter uses an implant that is positioned using three-dimensional modeling and computer-assisted robotic surgical navigation [45]. Before surgery, customized CT scans are obtained with the patient lying supine with a motion rod attached to the operative leg. Although the author has used various UKA prostheses, the precision obtained from the RIO UKA system for preoperative planning and surgical implantation appears to offer distinct benefits and has been incorporated in his practice since 2008 and provides the surgical experience discussed in this chapter.[1]

A detailed description of the surgical technique for the RIO UKA is available at http://www.makosurgical.com/physicians/products/rio and will not be repeated in this chapter. However, there are technical and operative details that should be stressed. It is important that the surgeon and technician are thoroughly familiar with the detailed procedures and follow the exact steps that include preoperative planning of the alignment and size of the tibial and femoral implants. The surgeon must perform an adequate surgical exposure, remove bone osteophytes and retained meniscus tissues, place retractors that curve around the posterior tibia to protect the neurovascular structures, perform precise registration of anatomic landmarks for the RIO software, achieve soft tissue balancing of extension and flexion gaps with

[1] The author has no conflict of interest directly or indirectly with this implant or robotic system.

appropriate adjustment of tibial and femoral implants, and perform meticulous cement fixation of implants.

The usual preoperative planning steps are taken before surgery. These include a 5-day scrub with chlorhexidine. A detailed history for prior deep venous thrombosis (DVT) episodes, including personal and family history or other DVT risk factors, is undertaken. In the absence of DVT risk factors, aspirin (81 mg twice a day) is used for 21 days postoperatively. Other chemical forms of anticoagulant therapy are not required unless specific risk factors, such as prior DVT or pulmonary embolism, are present. The patient should be mobilized and active the first day after surgery and thereafter.

The operative limb is signed by the surgeon before the patient receives appropriate antibiotic intravenous medication. A time-out is performed in the operating room with the signed limb signature visible and verbal agreement of patient name, birth date, preoperative antibiotics, allergies, and operative procedure planned by surgeons and operative staff. During the operative procedure, a sequential calf pressure device is used along with antiembolism stockings on the opposite limb.

The patient positioning shown in Fig. 4.1 involves the De Mayo Knee Positioner (Innovative Medical Products, Inc., Plainville, CT) to control the knee flexion position. The opposite extremity has a posterior thigh pad that, along with reflex of the hip portion of the surgical bed, maintains 10° of hip flexion and decreases tension on the femoral nerve.

After appropriate draping with the knee at 45° flexion, a limited medial (or lateral) parapatellar incision is made that extends in the quadriceps tendon 3–5 cm above the patella to allow sufficient lateral or medial patella glide for exposure. An examination of the knee joint confirms the expected pathology and ensures no unexpected joint arthritis is present in the other knee compartments. There are often reactive and scarred fat pad tissues that require removal along with retained meniscus tissues of the involved compartment. Osteophytes are not removed at this point because they are helpful in identifying tibial and femoral geometry in the

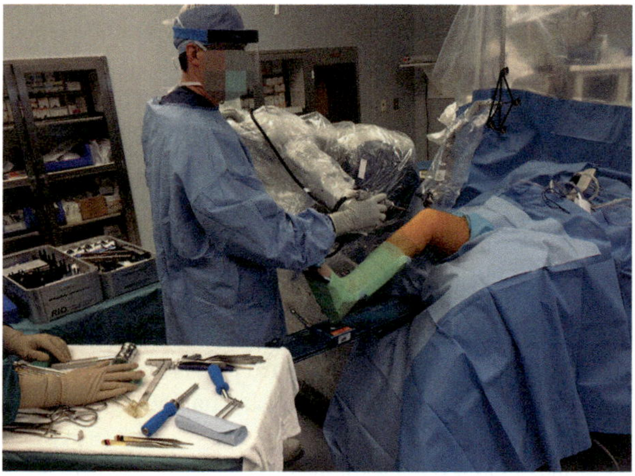

Fig. 4.1 The operative positioning of the lower limb, along with the Robotic Arm Interactive Orthopedic System. (Reprinted with permission from Noyes and Barber-Westin [1])

registration process. The tibial and femoral arrays are placed at a sufficient distance from the knee joint (Fig. 4.2) in order not to obstruct the surgeon's view. The author routinely uses a headlight to completely view the interior of the knee joint. The registration process is meticulous and follows the detailed MAKOplasty Partial Knee Application User Guide 206388 Rev 01 and Surgical Technique and Planning Guide #201844 (Stryker).

After the removal of osteophytes, the joint balancing step is completed that captures data, providing the tibiofemoral compartment spacing or opening at multiple knee flexion angles under a mild varus or valgus loading (Figs. 4.3 and 4.4). This allows for proper medial or lateral ligament soft tissue tension, with attention directed to prevent overstuffing of the tibiofemoral compartment, particularly at higher angles of joint flexion. The preoperative virtual positioning of the tibiofemoral components in all three planes includes fine-tuning of the tibial slope that is performed at this point to provide a normal soft tissue balance of extension and numerous knee flexion gaps. The planned operative bone resection is mapped and validated prior to commencing with the operative procedure. This includes fine-tuning of the medial-lateral and internal-external positions of the implant using the software to compute and verify that the femoral component tracks in a central position over the tibial component throughout the entire flexion-extension range of knee motion (Fig. 4.5). This step also confirms there is proper sizing of the tibial and femoral implants. The RIO is positioned in the operative field and registered (Fig. 4.6).

The operative plan starts first with the femoral bone resection, followed by tibial bone resection (Fig. 4.7). The trial components are placed with the selected tibial polyethylene trial, and determination is made that there is correct anatomic prosthesis alignment during full knee flexion and extension. The surgeon ensures that the anterior femoral tip is flush with the cartilage surface and not proud. Verification of restoration of normal medial or lateral ligament stability and joint opening is performed. Retained posterior meniscus fragments are removed with arthroscopic instruments using headlight illumination. The cementing technique follows

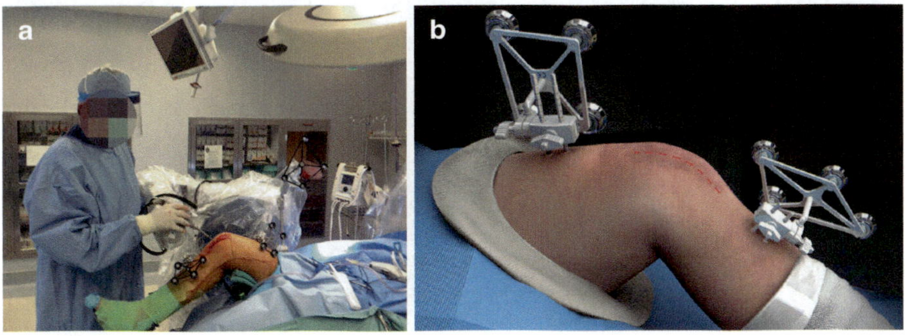

Fig. 4.2 (**a**) Operative view and (**b**) illustration of the femoral and tibial arrays and checkpoints (**b**, courtesy of Stryker Orthopaedics, Fort Lauderdale, FL). (Reprinted with permission from Noyes and Barber-Westin [1])

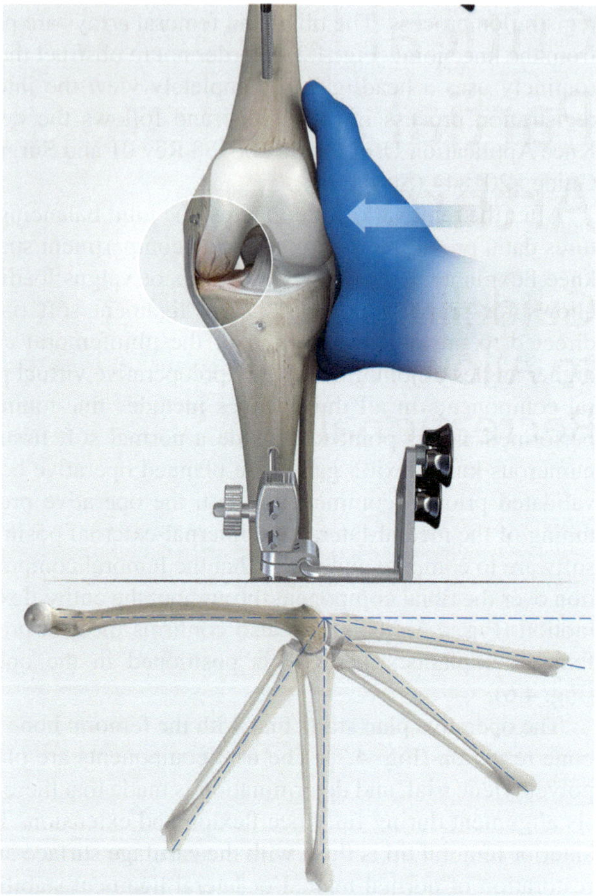

Fig. 4.3 Remove overhanging medial osteophytes and then capture a minimum of four poses while applying a valgus stress to passively correct the coronal deformity. The magnitude of the valgus stress must be such that it opens up the collapsed medial compartment and tensions the medial collateral ligament to achieve the desired degree of correction and joint stability. Caution must be exercised to not overcorrect the deformity. In the case of a lateral UKA, capture poses while applying a varus stress. The poses captured multiple times starting at extension, mid-flexion, flexion, and full flexion (or at 0°, 10°, and every 20° up to 120°) (courtesy of Stryker Orthopaedics, Fort Lauderdale, FL). (Reprinted with permission from Noyes and Barber-Westin [1])

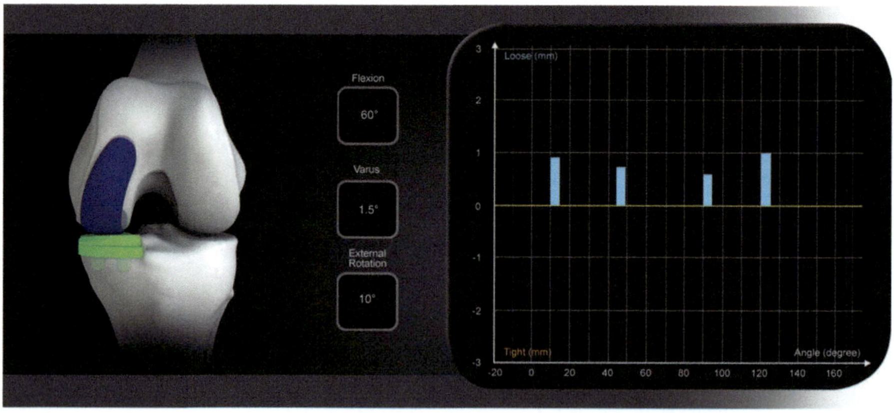

Fig. 4.4 Fine-tune the femoral and tibial implant placement to ensure joint gaps are 0–1.5 mm of looseness through range of motion and good central loading exists between the femoral and tibial components (courtesy of Stryker Orthopaedics, Fort Lauderdale, FL). (Reprinted with permission from Noyes and Barber-Westin [1])

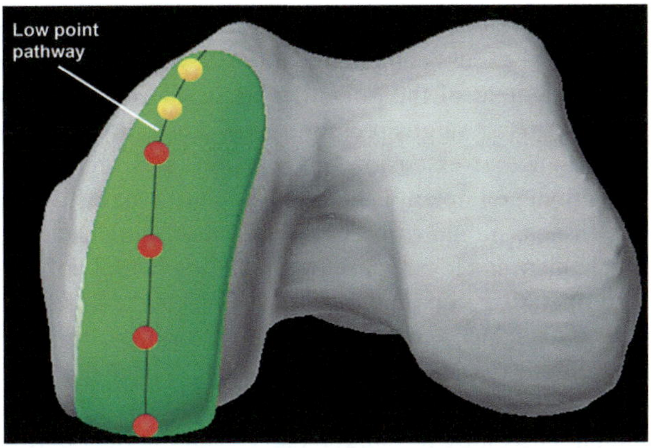

Fig. 4.5 Once the joint is balanced, fine-tune the medial-lateral position and internal-external rotation of the femoral component to ensure that the femoral component tracks centrally over the tibial component through the patient's range of motion (courtesy of Stryker Orthopaedics, Fort Lauderdale, FL). (Reprinted with permission from Noyes and Barber-Westin [1])

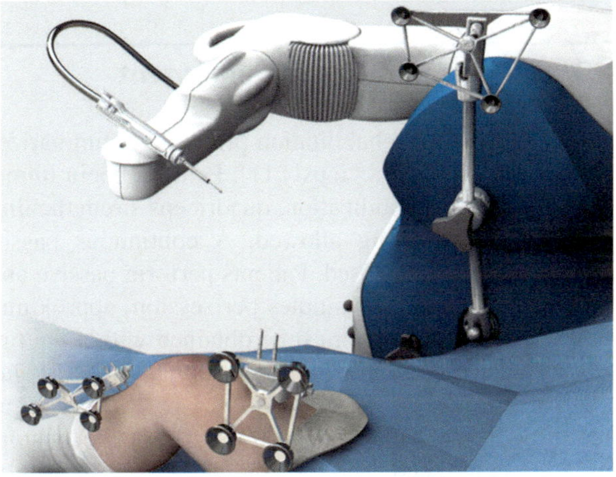

Fig. 4.6 Position the RIO in the operative field and perform registration and verification of the robotic arm (courtesy of Stryker Orthopaedics, Fort Lauderdale, FL). (Reprinted with permission from Noyes and Barber-Westin [1])

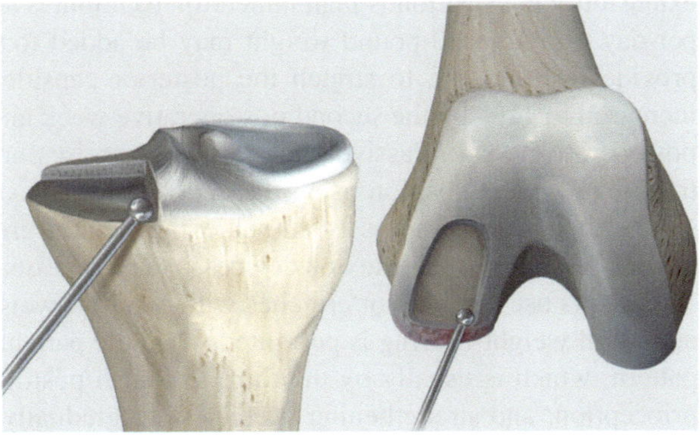

Fig. 4.7 Resect the femoral and tibial surfaces and then create peg holes and keels (courtesy of Stryker Orthopaedics, Fort Lauderdale, FL). (Reprinted with permission from Noyes and Barber-Westin [1])

meticulous steps of irrigation, drying of surfaces, tibial prosthesis placement, and removal of excess cement under direct visualization. Femoral prosthesis cementing and placement of the polyethylene tibial component are done with the joint held under varus or valgus pressure at 60° knee flexion. After verification of the soft tissue balance at extension, mid-flexion, and high-flexion knee positions, the final polyethylene implant is placed. The tourniquet is deflated and meticulous hemostasis ensues, along with intravenous transamic acid administration. The extensor mechanism is closed, and the medial or lateral soft tissue structures are balanced. The operative steps in closure are designed to prevent excessive medial or lateral soft tissue tension, with the goal of restoring a normal medial or lateral patella glide at 0° and 20° knee flexion. An adductor nerve block is commonly performed postoperatively, and in the majority of cases, the patient remains as an outpatient. The patient is seen by the surgeon and rehabilitation staff the next day in the outpatient clinic to initiate the postoperative rehabilitation protocol.

4.7 Postoperative Management

The postoperative rehabilitation protocol is summarized in Table 4.1 and has been described in detail previously [1]. Patients begin immediate range of knee motion (ROM), patellar mobilization, quadriceps strengthening, and balance training with partial weight-bearing allowed. A continuous passive motion machine is not required or routinely used. Patients perform passive and active ROM exercises in a seated position for 10 minutes per session, approximately six times per day. Full passive knee extension must be obtained within the first 7 days to avoid excessive scarring. Patellar mobilization is important to restore a normal medial-lateral glide and prevent contracture of soft tissue patellar retinacular structures. If the patient has difficulty regaining at least 0° by the seventh postoperative day, an overpressure program is initiated. The foot and ankle are propped on a towel or other device to elevate the hamstrings and gastrocnemius that allows the knee to drop into full extension. This position is maintained for 10 minutes and repeated four to six times per day. A 10- to 20-pound weight may be added to the distal thigh and knee to provide overpressure to stretch the posterior capsule. Knee flexion is gradually increased to 110° by the second postoperative week and 135° by the third to fourth postoperative week. Passive knee flexion exercises are performed initially in the traditional seated position using the opposite lower extremity to provide overpressure. Other methods to assist in achieving flexion greater than 90° include chair rolling, wall slides, knee flexion devices, and passive quadriceps stretching exercises.

Patients use a walker or crutches with 50–75% weight-bearing allowed as tolerated. Full weight-bearing is permitted when the patient demonstrates a normal gait pattern, which is usually by the third to fourth postoperative week. Balance, proprioception, and strengthening exercises are gradually increased as supervised by the therapist through approximately the 12th postoperative week. At this time, objective isokinetic tests for quadriceps and hamstring isometric muscle strength and power are used to determine if continued muscle strengthening is required to

Table 4.1 Noyes Knee Institute rehabilitation protocol for unicompartmental arthroplasty

	Postoperative weeks					
	1–2	3–4	5–6	7–8	9–12	13–26
Range of motion minimum goals:						
0°–110°	X					
0°–135°		X				
Weight-bearing:						
50–75% body weight, with assistive devices	X					
100% body weight, wean from assistive devices		X				
Patella mobilization	X	X	X	X		
Modalities:						
Electrical muscle stimulation	X	X	X			
Pain/edema management (cryotherapy)	X	X	X	X	X	X
Stretching:						
Hamstring, gastrocnemius-soleus	X	X	X	X	X	X
Iliotibial band, quadriceps					X	X
Strengthening:						
Ankle pumps (plantar flexion with resistance band)	X	X				
Quadriceps isometrics, straight leg raises	X	X	X	X	X	X
Knee extension quadriceps, active/active-assisted	X					
Closed-chain: toe-raises, wall-sits, mini-squats		X	X	X	X	X
Knee flexion hamstring curls (0°–90°)		X	X	X	X	X
Knee extension quadriceps (90°–30°)		X	X	X	X	X
Hip abduction-adduction, multi-hip	X	X	X	X	X	X
Leg press (70°–10°)		X	X	X	X	X
Upper body weight training			X	X	X	X
Core training			X	X	X	X
Balance/gait/proprioceptive training:						
Weight shifting, balance board (two-legged), cup walking, tandem stance	X	X	X			
Mini-trampoline, balance board (single-legged; stable vs. unstable surface), single-leg stance				X	X	
Conditioning:						
Upper body conditioner	X	X	X	X	X	
Stationary bicycling (high seat, low resistance)		X	X	X	X	X
Aquatic program (water walking, depth at thigh or waist)			X	X	X	X
Swimming (straight leg kicking)				X	X	X
Stair-climbing machine (low resistance, low stroke)				X	X	X
Ski machine (short stride and level, low resistance)				X	X	X
Elliptical machine				X	X	X
Walking					X	X
Fitness center training:						
25 minutes strengthening, 25 minutes cardiovascular training, 10 minutes flexibility. Achieve AHA guidelines.[a] Watch for swelling, pain						X

[a]American Heart Association guidelines: physical activity per week: 150–300 minutes moderate intensity or 75–150 minutes vigorous intensity. Strengthening all major muscle groups ≥2 days/week

return the patient to normal parameters. It is noted that some patients have significant atrophy of all muscle groups of the lower extremity (hip, knee, and ankle) during the disuse period prior to UKA surgery. This problem may delay full recovery, and it may take up to 12 months to fully return to normal parameters. Objective tests to perform to determine strength and neuromuscular indices are detailed in Chap. 11, and our return-to-sport criteria are shown in Chap. 9. As with total knee arthroplasty patients, many UKA patients desire a highly functional knee [67], which is only possible with return of normal neuromuscular parameters. An individualized strengthening and aerobic conditioning program is developed as required. It is viewed as a high priority to return patients to a heart-healthy aerobic conditioning program that involves the ability to perform 30 minutes of vigorous activity five times a week, because such exercise has proven effects on cardiovascular health, diabetics, stroke avoidance, and overall mental well-being.

4.8 Complications and Leading Causes of Failure

The progression of tibiofemoral or patellofemoral arthritis and implant loosening are the most common causes of failure or unsatisfactory results [15, 17, 26–30, 68, 69]. A study of 418 failed UKAs from the French Hip and Knee Society reported that loosening was the main reason for failure (occurring in 45%), followed by progression of osteoarthritis (OA) (15%) and wear (12%) [30]. These findings were similar to those reported in the Swedish, Finnish [70], and Australian registries. The operations were performed between 1978 and 2009 and included medial UKA in 88%. The majority of bearing designs were fixed (80%), and cement was used for 85% of the femoral components and 70% of the tibial components. These rates of failure far exceed what is reported in more modern UKA studies and, in particular, with robotic instrumentation.

In a study of 1746 UKAs performed in the Kaiser Permanente National Total Joint Registry from 2002 to 2009, Bini et al. [71] reported that implant type, patient age, and yearly surgeon volume were significantly associated with revision rates. A patient less than 55 years of age had a significantly higher revision rate of 11.7% (39 of 332) compared with those aged 55 to 65 (4.4%; 28 of 642) and those over 65 (2.6%; 20 of 772; $P < 0.001$). The Preservation All-Poly tibial UKA had a greater risk of revision compared with the Zimmer UKA (9.5% and 1.1%, respectively; $P < 0.001$). The revision rates for surgeons who performed 12 or fewer UKAs per year were significantly higher than the revision rates for surgeons who performed more than 12 UKAs per year (6.4% and 3.2%, respectively; $P < 0.01$).

Component loosening [15, 17, 26–28, 72–76] and bearing dislocation [72, 76–80] are two other leading causes of failure. The effect of BMI [17] and patient age have produced mixed results in terms of risks of failure.

Prosthesis-related bone loss (postoperative decrease in bone mineral density [BMD]) reported after TKA [81, 82] has been believed to be related to strain shielding. Strain shielding may promote reduction of bone density and bone resorption, while overload promotes excessive formation of bone that causes an increase in bone density and may induce fatigue damage [83]. Loss of bone may lead to periprosthetic fracture or weakening of the implant fixation, resulting in loosening and implant failure [82, 84]. To date, only one clinical study assessed BMD after UKA. Richmond et al. [85] followed 50 medial UKAs (Oxford or Genesis) with CT osteodensitometry 1 and 2 years postoperatively. These authors reported mean cancellous BMD decreased only 1.9% on the medial side and 1.1% on the lateral side. Mean cortical BMD decreased 0.4% on the medial side and 0.5% on the lateral side. There were no differences between the implant designs in early BMD changes.

4.9 Survivorship Rates

The survivorship rates reported after medial UKA are shown in Table 4.2 [8, 12, 15, 17, 29, 36, 39, 74, 76, 77, 86–97]. An overview of clinical outcomes after medial UKA has been previously published [1]. The Oxford UKA has been the most widely studied of all medial UKA prostheses. Labek et al. [98] conducted a systematic review of literature published from 1988 to 2008 that described outcomes of the Oxford UKA. The investigators found that the average results published by the inventor team were significantly better with regard to revision rates than those published by independent studies or worldwide registries. The revision rate from the developing team was 2.7 times lower than the rates published in independent studies and 4.4 times lower than registry data from Sweden and Denmark. These authors cautioned that "the average surgeon should be aware of the fact that the outcome published by the inventing center appears to be hardly reproducible in average patient care and other institutions" [98]. Ten-year survival rates from independent studies ranged from 75% to 95%, while rates from the inventor team ranged from 93% to 95%.

The question of whether individuals with bilateral severe medial OA should undergo simultaneous or staged UKA has been addressed in three studies [99–101]. Chen and coworkers [99] followed a group of 171 patients for 2 years postoperatively. The patients were invited to choose between the two options, and the majority (72.5%) elected a simultaneous procedure. There were no differences in complications or short-term outcomes with regard to AKS or Oxford scores. The cumulative operating time and length of hospital stay were shorter for simultaneous procedures, and the overall cost for this option was lower. There were no serious complications in either group; all patients received enoxaparin 40 mg once daily and pneumatic calf pumps for prophylaxis of venous thromboembolic events. Chan et al. [100] reported significant differences in major complications between 318 simultaneous and 160 staged medial UKA knees. There were 13 such complications in the simultaneous group and none in the staged group; however, no chemoprophylaxis was used for thromboembolic events that accounted for ten of the 13 complications. Berend et al. [101] reported no major complications in 70 knees that underwent simultaneous UKA and 282 knees that had staged bilateral UKAs. These investigators used chemoprophylaxis (discretion of the medical management providers) and mechanical compression boots to prevent thromboembolic events. The

Table 4.2 Survival rates of medial unicompartmental arthroplasty

Citation	Prosthesis	Knees (n); mean f.u.	Survival end points	Survival rates			
				5–7 years	8–10 years	15 years	20 years
Boissonneault et al. [86]	Oxford	92; 5 years	Revision	94%	--	--	--
Kim et al. [87]	Oxford	246; 7.4 years	Revision or exchange of implant	--	92%	--	--
Matharu et al. [12]	Oxford	459; 4.4 years	Conversion TKA	94% - 93%	--	--	--
Greco et al. [8]	Oxford	425; 6.1 years	Revision	96%	86%	--	--
Yoshida et al. [76]	Oxford	1251; 5.2 years	Revision	98% - 98%	95%	--	--
Murray et al. [39]	Oxford	2438; 4.6 years	Removal or exchange of implant	95–100%, depending on BMI	93–95%, depending on BMI	--	--
Alnachoukati et al. [36]	Oxford	825; 9.7 years	Revision	--	85%	--	--
Emerson et al. [88]	Oxford	213; 10.0 years	Revision	--	88%	--	--
Kristensen et al. [15]	Oxford	659; 4.6 years	Removal or exchange of implant	--	85%	--	--
Argenson et al. [29]	Miller-Galante	160; 20 years	Revision	--	94%	83%	74%
Rachha et al. [89]	Miller-Galante	56; 10.7 years	Revision	--	95%	--	--
Pennington et al. [90]	Miller-Galante	46; 11 years	Revision	--	92%	--	--
Foran et al. [91]	Miller-Galante	62; 19 years	Revision	--	--	93%	90%
Parratte et al. [92]	Miller-Galante	35; 9.7 years	Revision	--	81%	70%	--
Berger et al. [93]	Miller-Galante	59; 13 years	Revision	--	98%	96%	--
Hamilton et al. [17]	Preservation	517; 4.9 years	Revision	92%	--	--	--
Bruni et al. [74]	Preservation	33; 8 years	Revision	--	83%	--	--
Liebs et al. [94]	Preservation	430; 6 years	Revision	93% - 90%	90%	--	--
Bhattacharya et al. [95]	Preservation	97; 3.7 years	Revision or waiting for revision	91%	--	--	--
Biswas et al. [96]	Zimmer Uni Knee	88; 4 years	Revision or loosening on x-ray	--	96%	--	--
Burger et al. [68]	Restoris MCK System, Mako	802; 4.9 years	Revision	97.8%	--	--	--
Bruce et al. [97]	Uniglide	184; 10–12 years	Revision	94%	89%	--	--

BMI body mass index, *TKA* total knee arthroplasty

Table 4.3 Survival rates of lateral unicompartmental arthroplasty

Citation	Prosthesis	Knees (n); mean f.u.	Survival end points	Survival rates		
				5–7 years	8–10 years	15–20 years
Baker et al. [102]	Multiple 66% mobile bearing	2052; NA	Revision	93% - 93%	--	--
Kennedy et al. [103]	Oxford Domed	325; 7 years	Revision	--	85%	--
Walker et al. [104]	Oxford Domed	363; 3 years	Revision	85%	--	--
Fornell et al. [105]	Oxford Domed	41; 4 years	Revision	97.5%	--	--
Weston-Simmons et al. [106]	Oxford Domed	265; 4.1 years	Revision	94% - 92%	92%	--
Edmiston et al. [107]	Zimmer or Miller-Galante	65; 6.8 years	Revision	94%	--	--
Liebs and Herzberg [94]	Preservation Mobile bearing	128; 6 years	Revision	92% - 83%	83%	--
Smith et al. [108]	AMC Uniglide fixed bearing	101; 4.5 years	Revision	95% - 91%	--	--
Heyse et al. [18]	Genesis (Accuris)	50; 10.8 years	Revision	--	92%	92%
Deroche et al. [109]	HLS Evolution	39; 17.9 years	Removal or revision	--	--	82% - 79%
Lustig et al. [110]	HLS Evolution fixed bearing	54; 14.2 years	Revision, implant removal, loosening, implant ipsilateral medial UKA	---	89%	86%
Tu et al. [111]	Sled	121; 5 years	Revision	99.2%	--	--
Burger et al. [68]	Restoris MCK System, Mako	171; 4.3 years	Revision	97.6%	--	--

simultaneous group had shorter cumulative operating room time and hospital stay and a higher AKS function score, a mean of 19.4 months postoperatively. There was a selection bias in that patients who received simultaneous procedures were younger and less obese.

The survivorship rates reported after lateral UKA are shown in Table 4.3 [18, 68, 94, 102–111]. An overview of clinical outcomes has been previously published [1]. The largest series reported at the time of writing from Baker et al. [102] compared survivorship rates between 2052 lateral UKAs and 30,795 medial UKAs from the National Joint Registry of England and Wales. The 7-year rates were comparable

(93% for lateral and 91% for medial), and only age (younger than 55 years) significantly affected the results. Several studies [18, 94, 106, 112–115] reported 10-year survival rates from 83% to 100%, and three investigations [18, 114, 115] produced 15-year rates that ranged from 80% to 92%.

In an analysis of athletic activity levels before and after surgery, Walker et al. [116] reported that 98% of 45 patients were able to return to sports activities a mean of 3 years after undergoing an Oxford Domed (Biomet, Bridgend UK) UKA. The majority were participating in low-impact activities. There were no significant differences in SF-36 scores between the patients and a matched healthy control population. Canetti et al. [117] reported that patients who received a robotic-assisted lateral UKA returned to recreational activities faster than those who underwent the conventional technique (4.2 ± 1.9 months and 10.5 ± 6.7 months, respectively, $P < 0.01$).

Clinical outcomes have been mixed regarding lateral UKA performed for posttraumatic OA secondary to tibial plateau fracture [114, 118]. Lustig et al. [114] reported survivorship rates of 100% at 10 years and 80% at 15 years in a small series of 13 patients followed a mean of 10.2 years postoperatively. The mean AKS knee score improved from 51 points before surgery to 88 points at follow-up, with similar improvements noted in the mean AKS function score. However, Sah and Scott [118] found inferior outcomes in AKS scores in ten patients treated for posttraumatic OA compared with 38 patients who underwent lateral UKA for primary OA. Although none of the knees had been revised a mean of 5.2 years postoperatively (range, 2–15 years), five of the ten patients in the posttraumatic OA group reported only fair satisfaction with their outcome. All 38 patients in the primary OA group reported excellent satisfaction.

4.10 Illustrative Cases

Case 1 A 52-year-old man presented with chronic left knee pain in the medial tibiofemoral compartment that occurred with all daily activities and prevented any light recreational sports. He previously underwent a medial meniscectomy and then failed a course of conservative treatment of physical therapy and NSAID medications. The physical examination showed an absence of clinical findings related to the patellofemoral and lateral tibiofemoral compartments. Standing 45° PA radiographs showed loss of the medial tibiofemoral compartment space (Fig. 4.8a). The patient underwent a MAKO medial UKA, with correction of the varus angulation to neutral. The preoperative planning of the procedure is shown in Fig. 4.8b–d. An important part of the procedure was the determination of the amount of medial joint opening that allowed the appropriate adjustment of the tibiofemoral gap, avoiding undue compartment loads and balancing the medial soft tissue restraints (Fig. 4.8e). The postoperative radiographs are shown in Fig. 4.8f–g.

Case 2 A 46-year-old woman presented with right lateral knee pain and lateral tibiofemoral arthritis. She had a 20-minute walking tolerance. She previously

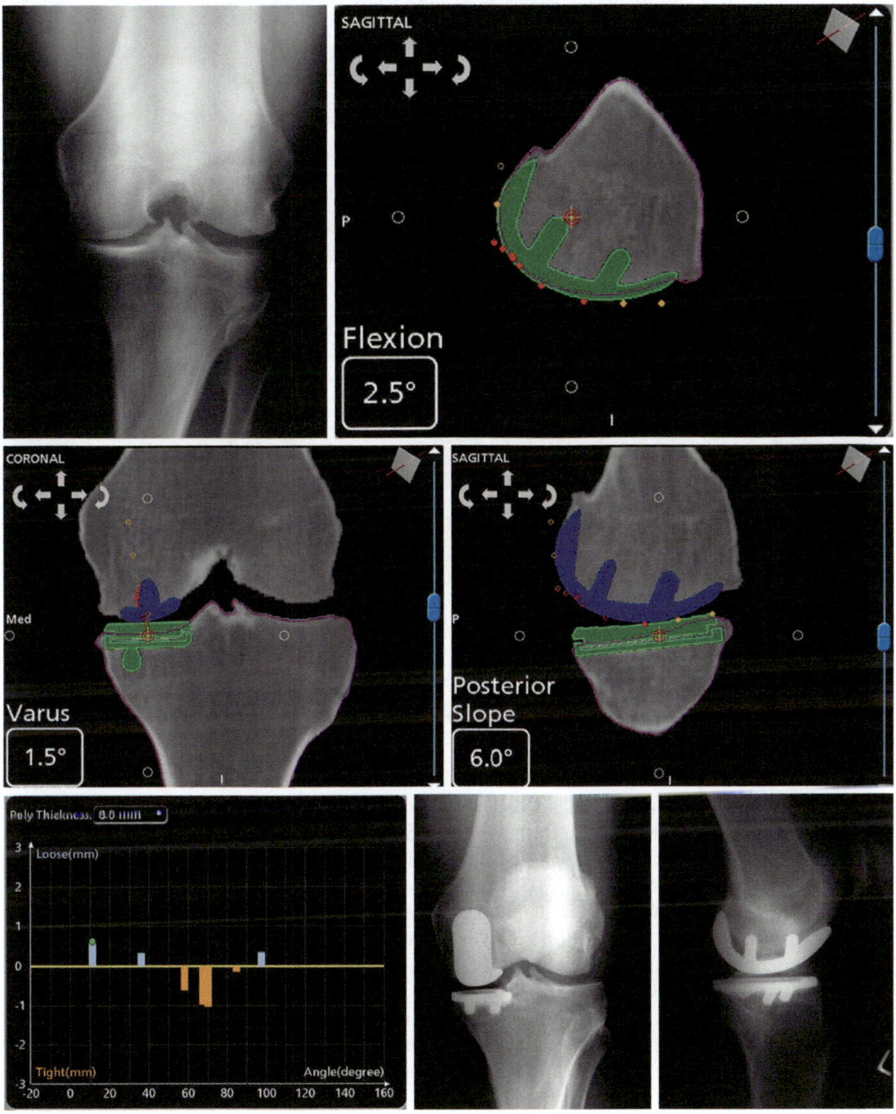

Fig. 4.8 Case 1. (Reprinted with permission from Noyes and Barber-Westin [1])

underwent a lateral meniscus transplant that was successful in alleviating her knee pain for 6 years. The patient elected to undergo lateral UKA after the transplant failed and a 45° radiograph showed loss of the lateral tibiofemoral compartment space (Fig. 4.9a). A lateral UKA using the MAKOplasty technique was performed. The preoperative planning and placement of the prosthesis are shown in Fig. 4.9b–d. The postoperative radiographs are shown in Fig. 4.9e, f.

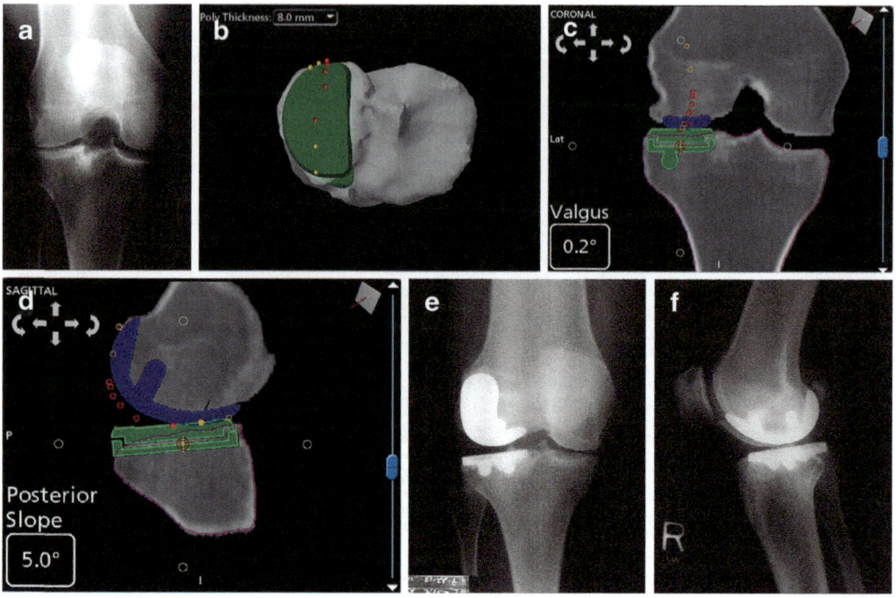

Fig. 4.9 Case 2. (Reprinted with permission from Noyes and Barber-Westin [1])

References

1. Noyes FR, Barber-Westin SD. Unicompartmental knee replacement for varus or valgus malalignment. In: Noyes FR, Barber-Westin SD, editors. Noyes' knee disorders: surgery, rehabilitation, clinical outcomes. 2nd ed. Philadelphia: Elsevier; 2017. p. 882–910. https://doi.org/10.1016/b978-0-323-32903-3.00030-5.
2. Noyes FR, Barber-Westin SD. Unicompartmental patellofemoral replacement. In: Noyes FR, Barber-Westin SD, editors. Noyes' knee disorders: surgery, rehabilitation, clinical outcomes. 2nd ed. Philadelphia: Elsevier; 2017. p. 1036–57. https://doi.org/10.1016/b978-0-323-32903-3.00037-8.
3. Clement ND, Bell A, Simpson P, Macpherson G, Patton JT, Hamilton DF. Robotic-assisted unicompartmental knee arthroplasty has a greater early functional outcome when compared to manual total knee arthroplasty for isolated medial compartment arthritis. Bone Joint Res. 2020;9(1):15–22. https://doi.org/10.1302/2046-3758.91.Bjr-2019-0147.R1.
4. Kleeblad LJ, van der List JP, Zuiderbaan HA, Pearle AD. Larger range of motion and increased return to activity, but higher revision rates following unicompartmental versus total knee arthroplasty in patients under 65: a systematic review. Knee Surg Sports Traumatol Arthrosc. 2018;26(6):1811–22. https://doi.org/10.1007/s00167-017-4817-y.
5. Lum ZC, Crawford DA, Lombardi AV Jr, Hurst JM, Morris MJ, Adams JB, Berend KR. Early comparative outcomes of unicompartmental and total knee arthroplasty in severely obese patients. Knee. 2018;25(1):161–6. https://doi.org/10.1016/j.knee.2017.10.006.
6. Migliorini F, Tingart M, Niewiera M, Rath B, Eschweiler J. Unicompartmental versus total knee arthroplasty for knee osteoarthritis. Eur J Orthop Surg Traumatol. 2019;29(4):947–55. https://doi.org/10.1007/s00590-018-2358-9.
7. Wilson HA, Middleton R, Abram SGF, Smith S, Alvand A, Jackson WF, Bottomley N, Hopewell S, Price AJ. Patient relevant outcomes of unicompartmental versus total

knee replacement: systematic review and meta-analysis. BMJ (Clinical research ed). 2019;364:l352. https://doi.org/10.1136/bmj.l352.

8. Greco NJ, Lombardi AV Jr, Price AJ, Berend ME, Berend KR. Medial Mobile-bearing unicompartmental knee arthroplasty in young patients aged less than or equal to 50 years. J Arthroplasty. 2018;33(8):2435–9. https://doi.org/10.1016/j.arth.2018.03.069.
9. Lee M, Chen J, Shi Lu C, Lo NN, Yeo SJ. No differences in outcomes scores or survivorship of unicompartmental knee arthroplasty between patients younger or older than 55 years of age at minimum 10-year followup. Clin Orthop Relat Res. 2019;477(6):1434–46. https://doi.org/10.1097/corr.0000000000000737.
10. Kennedy JA, Matharu GS, Hamilton TW, Mellon SJ, Murray DW. Age and outcomes of medial meniscal-bearing unicompartmental knee arthroplasty. J Arthroplasty. 2018;33(10):3153–9. https://doi.org/10.1016/j.arth.2018.06.014.
11. Hamilton TW, Pandit HG, Jenkins C, Mellon SJ, Dodd CAF, Murray DW. Evidence-based indications for Mobile-bearing unicompartmental knee arthroplasty in a consecutive cohort of thousand knees. J Arthroplasty. 2017;32(6):1779–85. https://doi.org/10.1016/j.arth.2016.12.036.
12. Matharu G, Robb C, Baloch K, Pynsent P. The Oxford medial unicompartmental knee replacement: survival and the affect of age and gender. Knee. 2012;19(6):913–7. https://doi.org/10.1016/j.knee.2012.03.004.
13. Pandit H, Jenkins C, Gill HS, Smith G, Price AJ, Dodd CA, Murray DW. Unnecessary contraindications for mobile-bearing unicompartmental knee replacement. J Bone Joint Surg. 2011;93(5):622–8. https://doi.org/10.1302/0301-620X.93B5.26214.
14. Weston-Simons JS, Pandit H, Jenkins C, Jackson WF, Price AJ, Gill HS, Dodd CA, Murray DW. Outcome of combined unicompartmental knee replacement and combined or sequential anterior cruciate ligament reconstruction: a study of 52 cases with mean follow-up of five years. J Bone Joint Surg. 2012;94(9):1216–20. https://doi.org/10.1302/0301-620X.94B9.28881.
15. Kristensen PW, Holm HA, Varnum C. Up to 10-year follow-up of the Oxford medial partial knee arthroplasty--695 cases from a single institution. J Arthroplasty. 2013;28(9 Suppl):195–8. https://doi.org/10.1016/j.arth.2013.05.010.
16. Dyrhovden GS, Lygre SHL, Badawy M, Gøthesen Ø, Furnes O. Have the causes of revision for total and unicompartmental knee arthroplasties changed during the past two decades? Clin Orthop Relat Res. 2017;475(7):1874–86. https://doi.org/10.1007/s11999-017-5316-7.
17. Hamilton WG, Ammeen DJ, Hopper RH Jr. Mid-term survivorship of minimally invasive unicompartmental arthroplasty with a fixed-bearing implant: revision rate and mechanisms of failure. J Arthroplasty. 2014;29(5):989–92. https://doi.org/10.1016/j.arth.2013.10.010.
18. Heyse TJ, Khefacha A, Peersman G, Cartier P. Survivorship of UKA in the middle-aged. Knee. 2012;19(5):585–91. https://doi.org/10.1016/j.knee.2011.09.002.
19. Iriberri I, Suau S, Payán L, Aragón JF. Long-term deterioration after one-stage unicompartmental knee arthroplasty and anterior cruciate ligament reconstruction. Musculoskelet Surg. 2019;103(3):251–6. https://doi.org/10.1007/s12306-018-0582-4.
20. Volpin A, Kini SG, Meuffels DE. Satisfactory outcomes following combined unicompartmental knee replacement and anterior cruciate ligament reconstruction. Knee Surg Sports Traumatol Arthrosc. 2018;26(9):2594–601. https://doi.org/10.1007/s00167-017-4536-4.
21. Ventura A, Legnani C, Terzaghi C, Iori S, Borgo E. Medial unicondylar knee arthroplasty combined to anterior cruciate ligament reconstruction. Knee Surg Sports Traumatol Arthrosc. 2017;25(3):675–80. https://doi.org/10.1007/s00167-015-3808-0.
22. Tian S, Wang B, Wang Y, Ha C, Liu L, Sun K. Combined unicompartmental knee arthroplasty and anterior cruciate ligament reconstruction in knees with osteoarthritis and deficient anterior cruciate ligament. BMC Musculoskelet Disord. 2016;17:327. https://doi.org/10.1186/s12891-016-1186-5.
23. Tinius M, Hepp P, Becker R. Combined unicompartmental knee arthroplasty and anterior cruciate ligament reconstruction. Knee Surg Sports Traumatol Arthrosc. 2012;20(1):81–7. https://doi.org/10.1007/s00167-011-1528-7.

24. Krishnan SR, Randle R. ACL reconstruction with unicondylar replacement in knee with functional instability and osteoarthritis. J Orthop Surg Res. 2009;4:43. https://doi.org/10.1186/1749-799X-4-43.
25. Kleeblad LJ, Strickland SM, Nwachukwu BU, Kerkhoffs G, Pearle AD. Satisfaction with return to sports after unicompartmental knee arthroplasty and what type of sports are patients doing. Knee. 2020;27(2):509–17. https://doi.org/10.1016/j.knee.2019.11.011.
26. Ernstbrunner L, Imam MA, Andronic O, Perz T, Wieser K, Fucentese SF. Lateral unicompartmental knee replacement: a systematic review of reasons for failure. Int Orthop. 2018;42(8):1827–33. https://doi.org/10.1007/s00264-017-3662-4.
27. Mohammad HR, Strickland L, Hamilton TW, Murray DW. Long-term outcomes of over 8,000 medial Oxford phase 3 unicompartmental knees-a systematic review. Acta Orthop. 2018;89(1):101–7. https://doi.org/10.1080/17453674.2017.1367577.
28. Citak M, Cross MB, Gehrke T, Dersch K, Kendoff D. Modes of failure and revision of failed lateral unicompartmental knee arthroplasties. Knee. 2015;22(4):338–40. https://doi.org/10.1016/j.knee.2015.03.008.
29. Argenson JN, Blanc G, Aubaniac JM, Parratte S. Modern unicompartmental knee arthroplasty with cement: a concise follow-up, at a mean of twenty years, of a previous report. J Bone Joint Surg Am. 2013;95(10):905–9. https://doi.org/10.2106/JBJS.L.00963.
30. Epinette JA, Brunschweiler B, Mertl P, Mole D, Cazenave A, French Society for H, Knee. Unicompartmental knee arthroplasty modes of failure: wear is not the main reason for failure: a multicentre study of 418 failed knees. Orthop Traumatol Surg Res. 2012;98(6 Suppl):S124–30. https://doi.org/10.1016/j.otsr.2012.07.002.
31. Burger JA, Dooley MS, Kleeblad LJ, Zuiderbaan HA, Pearle AD. What is the impact of patellofemoral joint degeneration and malalignment on patient-reported outcomes after lateral unicompartmental knee arthroplasty? Bone Joint J. 2020;102-b(6):727–35. https://doi.org/10.1302/0301-620x.102b6.Bjj-2019-1429.R1.
32. Burger JA, Kleeblad LJ, Laas N, Pearle AD. The influence of preoperative radiographic patellofemoral degenerative changes and malalignment on patellofemoral-specific outcome scores following fixed-bearing medial unicompartmental knee arthroplasty. J Bone Joint Surg Am. 2019;101(18):1662–9. https://doi.org/10.2106/jbjs.18.01385.
33. Hamilton TW, Pandit HG, Maurer DG, Ostlere SJ, Jenkins C, Mellon SJ, Dodd CAF, Murray DW. Anterior knee pain and evidence of osteoarthritis of the patellofemoral joint should not be considered contraindications to mobile-bearing unicompartmental knee arthroplasty: a 15-year follow-up. Bone Joint J. 2017;99-B(5):632–9. https://doi.org/10.1302/0301-620X.99B5.BJJ-2016-0695.R2.
34. Song MH, Kim BH, Ahn SJ, Yoo SH, Kang SW, Oh KT. Does the appearance of the patellofemoral joint at surgery influence the clinical result in medial unicompartmental knee arthroplasty? Knee. 2013;20(6):457–60. https://doi.org/10.1016/j.knee.2013.05.005.
35. Affatato S, Caputo D, Bordini B. Does the body mass index influence the long-term survival of unicompartmental knee prostheses? A retrospective multi-centre study. Int Orthop. 2019;43(6):1365–70. https://doi.org/10.1007/s00264-018-4217-z.
36. Alnachoukati OK, Barrington JW, Berend KR, Kolczun MC, Emerson RH, Lombardi AV Jr, Mauerhan DR. Eight hundred twenty-five medial mobile-bearing unicompartmental knee arthroplasties: the first 10-year US multi-center survival analysis. J Arthroplasty. 2018;33(3):677–83. https://doi.org/10.1016/j.arth.2017.10.015.
37. Cavaignac E, Lafontan V, Reina N, Pailhe R, Wargny M, Laffosse JM, Chiron P. Obesity has no adverse effect on the outcome of unicompartmental knee replacement at a minimum follow-up of seven years. Bone Joint J. 2013;95-B(8):1064–8. https://doi.org/10.1302/0301-620X.95B8.31370.
38. Kuipers BM, Kollen BJ, Bots PC, Burger BJ, van Raay JJ, Tulp NJ, Verheyen CC. Factors associated with reduced early survival in the Oxford phase III medial unicompartment knee replacement. Knee. 2010;17(1):48–52. https://doi.org/10.1016/j.knee.2009.07.005.
39. Murray DW, Pandit H, Weston-Simons JS, Jenkins C, Gill HS, Lombardi AV, Dodd CA, Berend KR. Does body mass index affect the outcome of unicompartmental knee replacement? Knee. 2013;20(6):461–5. https://doi.org/10.1016/j.knee.2012.09.017.

40. Hamilton TW, Pandit HG, Inabathula A, Ostlere SJ, Jenkins C, Mellon SJ, Dodd CA, Murray DW. Unsatisfactory outcomes following unicompartmental knee arthroplasty in patients with partial thickness cartilage loss: a medium-term follow-up. Bone Joint J. 2017;99-b(4):475–82. https://doi.org/10.1302/0301-620x.99b4.Bjj-2016-1061.R1.
41. Maier MW, Kuhs F, Streit MR, Schuhmacher P, Walker T, Ewerbeck V, Gotterbarm T. Unicompartmental knee arthroplasty in patients with full versus partial thickness cartilage loss (PTCL): equal in clinical outcome but with higher reoperation rate for patients with PTCL. Arch Orthop Trauma Surg. 2015;135(8):1169–75. https://doi.org/10.1007/s00402-015-2236-4.
42. Pandit H, Gulati A, Jenkins C, Barker K, Price AJ, Dodd CA, Murray DW. Unicompartmental knee replacement for patients with partial thickness cartilage loss in the affected compartment. Knee. 2011;18(3):168–71. https://doi.org/10.1016/j.knee.2010.05.003.
43. Niinimaki TT, Murray DW, Partanen J, Pajala A, Leppilahti JI. Unicompartmental knee arthroplasties implanted for osteoarthritis with partial loss of joint space have high reoperation rates. Knee. 2011;18(6):432–5. https://doi.org/10.1016/j.knee.2010.08.004.
44. Maduekwe UI, Zywiel MG, Bonutti PM, Johnson AJ, Delanois RE, Mont MA. Scientific evidence for the use of modern unicompartmental knee arthroplasty. Expert Rev Med Devices. 2010;7(2):219–39. https://doi.org/10.1586/erd.09.65.
45. Conditt MA, Roche MW. Minimally invasive robotic-arm-guided unicompartmental knee arthroplasty. J Bone Joint Surg Am. 2009;91 Suppl 1:63–8. https://doi.org/10.2106/JBJS.H.01372.
46. Hernigou P, Deschamps G. Posterior slope of the tibial implant and the outcome of unicompartmental knee arthroplasty. J Bone Joint Surg Am. 2004;86-A(3):506–11.
47. Sawatari T, Tsumura H, Iesaka K, Furushiro Y, Torisu T. Three-dimensional finite element analysis of unicompartmental knee arthroplasty--the influence of tibial component inclination. J Orthop Res. 2005;23(3):549–54. https://doi.org/10.1016/j.orthres.2004.06.007.
48. Lonner JH, John TK, Conditt MA. Robotic arm-assisted UKA improves tibial component alignment: a pilot study. Clin Orthop Relat Res. 2010;468(1):141–6. https://doi.org/10.1007/s11999-009-0977-5.
49. Kasodekar VB, Yeo SJ, Othman S. Clinical outcome of unicompartmental knee arthroplasty and influence of alignment on prosthesis survival rate. Singapore Med J. 2006;47(9):796–802.
50. Alvand A, Khan T, Jenkins C, Rees JL, Jackson WF, Dodd CAF, Murray DW, Price AJ. The impact of patient-specific instrumentation on unicompartmental knee arthroplasty: a prospective randomised controlled study. Knee Surg Sports Traumatol Arthrosc. 2018;26(6):1662–70. https://doi.org/10.1007/s00167-017-4677-5.
51. Chin BZ, Tan SSH, Chua KCX, Budiono GR, Syn NL, O'Neill GK. Robot-assisted versus conventional total and unicompartmental knee arthroplasty: a meta-analysis of radiological and functional outcomes. J Knee Surg. 2020. https://doi.org/10.1055/s-0040-1701440.
52. Fu J, Wang Y, Li X, Yu B, Ni M, Chai W, Hao L, Chen J. Robot-assisted vs. conventional unicompartmental knee arthroplasty : systematic review and meta-analysis (Roboterassistierte vs. konventionelle unikompartimentäre Knieendoprothese : Systematisches Review und Metaanalyse). Orthopade. 2018;47(12):1009–17. https://doi.org/10.1007/s00132-018-3604-x.
53. Gaudiani MA, Samuel LT, Kamath AF, Courtney PM, Lee GC. Robotic-assisted versus manual unicompartmental knee arthroplasty: contemporary systematic review and meta-analysis of early functional outcomes. 2020. J Knee Surg https://doi.org/10.1055/s-0040-1701455.
54. Motesharei A, Rowe P, Blyth M, Jones B, Maclean A. A comparison of gait one year post operation in an RCT of robotic UKA versus traditional Oxford UKA. Gait Posture. 2018;62:41–5. https://doi.org/10.1016/j.gaitpost.2018.02.029.
55. Mofidi A, Plate JF, Lu B, Conditt MA, Lang JE, Poehling GG, Jinnah RH. Assessment of accuracy of robotically assisted unicompartmental arthroplasty. Knee Surg Sports Traumatol Arthrosc. 2014;22(8):1918–25. https://doi.org/10.1007/s00167-014-2969-6.
56. Lim MH, Tallay A, Bartlett J. Comparative study of the use of computer assisted navigation system for axial correction in medial unicompartmental knee arthroplasty. Knee Surg Sports Traumatol Arthrosc. 2009;17(4):341–6. https://doi.org/10.1007/s00167-008-0655-2.

57. Rosenberger RE, Fink C, Quirbach S, Attal R, Tecklenburg K, Hoser C. The immediate effect of navigation on implant accuracy in primary mini-invasive unicompartmental knee arthroplasty. Knee Surg Sports Traumatol Arthrosc. 2008;16(12):1133–40. https://doi.org/10.1007/s00167-008-0618-7.
58. Seon JK, Song EK, Park SJ, Yoon TR, Lee KB, Jung ST. Comparison of minimally invasive unicompartmental knee arthroplasty with or without a navigation system. J Arthroplasty. 2009;24(3):351–7. https://doi.org/10.1016/j.arth.2007.10.025.
59. Weber P, Utzschneider S, Sadoghi P, Pietschmann MF, Ficklscherer A, Jansson V, Muller PE. Navigation in minimally invasive unicompartmental knee arthroplasty has no advantage in comparison to a conventional minimally invasive implantation. Arch Orthop Trauma Surg. 2012;132(2):281–8. https://doi.org/10.1007/s00402-011-1404-4.
60. Konyves A, Willis-Owen CA, Spriggins AJ. The long-term benefit of computer-assisted surgical navigation in unicompartmental knee arthroplasty. J Orthop Surg Res. 2010;5:94. https://doi.org/10.1186/1749-799X-5-94.
61. Negrín R, Ferrer G, Iñiguez M, Duboy J, Saavedra M, Larraín NR, Jabes N, Barahona M. Robotic-assisted surgery in medial unicompartmental knee arthroplasty: does it improve the precision of the surgery and its clinical outcomes? Systematic review J Robot Surg. 2020. https://doi.org/10.1007/s11701-020-01162-8.
62. Thilak J, Thadi M, Mane PP, Sharma A, Mohan V, Babu BC. Accuracy of tibial component positioning in the robotic arm assisted versus conventional unicompartmental knee arthroplasty. J Orthop. 2020;22:367–71. https://doi.org/10.1016/j.jor.2020.08.022.
63. Nair R, Tripathy G, Deysine GR. Computer navigation systems in unicompartmental knee arthroplasty: a systematic review. Am J Orthop (Belle Mead NJ). 2014;43(6):256–61.
64. Weber P, Crispin A, Schmidutz F, Utzschneider S, Pietschmann MF, Jansson V, Muller PE. Improved accuracy in computer-assisted unicondylar knee arthroplasty: a meta-analysis. Knee Surg Sports Traumatol Arthrosc. 2013;21(11):2453–61. https://doi.org/10.1007/s00167-013-2370-x.
65. Matsui Y, Fukuoka S, Masuda S, Matsuura M, Masada T, Fukunaga K. Accuracy of tibial component placement in unicompartmental knee arthroplasty performed using an accelerometer-based portable navigation system. Knee Surg Sports Traumatol Arthrosc. 2020;28(12):3733–9. https://doi.org/10.1007/s00167-019-05752-4.
66. Suda Y, Takayama K, Ishida K, Hayashi S, Hashimoto S, Niikura T, Matsushita T, Kuroda R, Matsumoto T. Improved implant alignment accuracy with an accelerometer-based portable navigation system in medial unicompartmental knee arthroplasty. Knee Surg Sports Traumatol Arthrosc. 2020;28(9):2917–23. https://doi.org/10.1007/s00167-019-05669-y.
67. Waldstein W, Kolbitsch P, Koller U, Boettner F, Windhager R. Sport and physical activity following unicompartmental knee arthroplasty: a systematic review. Knee Surg Sports Traumatol Arthrosc. 2017;25(3):717–28. https://doi.org/10.1007/s00167-016-4167-1.
68. Burger JA, Kleeblad LJ, Laas N, Pearle AD. Mid-term survivorship and patient-reported outcomes of robotic-arm assisted partial knee arthroplasty. Bone Joint J. 2020;102-b(1):108–16. https://doi.org/10.1302/0301-620x.102b1.Bjj-2019-0510.R1.
69. van der List JP, Zuiderbaan HA, Pearle AD. Why do medial unicompartmental knee arthroplasties fail today? J Arthroplasty. 2016;31(5):1016–21. https://doi.org/10.1016/j.arth.2015.11.030.
70. Niinimaki T, Eskelinen A, Makela K, Ohtonen P, Puhto AP, Remes V. Unicompartmental knee arthroplasty survivorship is lower than TKA survivorship: a 27-year Finnish registry study. Clin Orthop Relat Res. 2014;472(5):1496–501. https://doi.org/10.1007/s11999-013-3347-2.
71. Bini S, Khatod M, Cafri G, Chen Y, Paxton EW. Surgeon, implant, and patient variables may explain variability in early revision rates reported for unicompartmental arthroplasty. J Bone Joint Surg Am. 2013;95(24):2195–202. https://doi.org/10.2106/JBJS.L.01006.
72. Vasso M, Corona K, D'Apolito R, Mazzitelli G, Panni AS. Unicompartmental knee arthroplasty: modes of failure and conversion to Total knee arthroplasty. Joints. 2017;5(1):44–50. https://doi.org/10.1055/s-0037-1601414.

73. Schroer WC, Barnes CL, Diesfeld P, LeMarr A, Ingrassia R, Morton DJ, Reedy M. The Oxford unicompartmental knee fails at a high rate in a high-volume knee practice. Clin Orthop Relat Res. 2013;471(11):3533–9. https://doi.org/10.1007/s11999-013-3174-5.
74. Bruni D, Akkawi I, Iacono F, Raspugli GF, Gagliardi M, Nitri M, Grassi A, Zaffagnini S, Bignozzi S, Marcacci M. Minimum thickness of all-poly tibial component unicompartmental knee arthroplasty in patients younger than 60 years does not increase revision rate for aseptic loosening. Knee Surg Sports Traumatol Arthrosc. 2013;21(11):2462–7. https://doi.org/10.1007/s00167-013-2578-9.
75. Bergeson AG, Berend KR, Lombardi AV Jr, Hurst JM, Morris MJ, Sneller MA. Medial mobile bearing unicompartmental knee arthroplasty: early survivorship and analysis of failures in 1000 consecutive cases. J Arthroplasty. 2013;28(9 Suppl):172–5. https://doi.org/10.1016/j.arth.2013.01.005.
76. Yoshida K, Tada M, Yoshida H, Takei S, Fukuoka S, Nakamura H. Oxford phase 3 unicompartmental knee arthroplasty in Japan--clinical results in greater than one thousand cases over ten years. J Arthroplasty. 2013;28(9 Suppl):168–71. https://doi.org/10.1016/j.arth.2013.08.019.
77. Burger JA, Kleeblad LJ, Sierevelt IN, Horstmann WG, Nolte PA. Bearing design influences short- to mid-term survivorship, but not functional outcomes following lateral unicompartmental knee arthroplasty: a systematic review. Knee Surg Sports Traumatol Arthrosc. 2019;27(7):2276–88. https://doi.org/10.1007/s00167-019-05357-x.
78. Kim SJ, Postigo R, Koo S, Kim JH. Causes of revision following Oxford phase 3 unicompartmental knee arthroplasty. Knee Surg Sports Traumatol Arthrosc. 2014;22(8):1895–901. https://doi.org/10.1007/s00167-013-2644-3.
79. Lim HC, Bae JH, Song SH, Kim SJ. Oxford phase 3 unicompartmental knee replacement in Korean patients. J Bone Joint Surg. 2012;94(8):1071–6. https://doi.org/10.1302/0301-620X.94B8.29372.
80. Choy WS, Kim KJ, Lee SK, Yang DS, Lee NK. Mid-term results of oxford medial unicompartmental knee arthroplasty. Clin Orthop Surg. 2011;3(3):178–83. https://doi.org/10.4055/cios.2011.3.3.178.
81. Li MG, Nilsson KG. Changes in bone mineral density at the proximal tibia after total knee arthroplasty: a 2-year follow-up of 28 knees using dual energy X-ray absorptiometry. J Orthop Res. 2000;18(1):40–7. https://doi.org/10.1002/jor.1100180107.
82. Soininvaara TA, Miettinen HJ, Jurvelin JS, Suomalainen OT, Alhava EM, Kroger HP. Periprosthetic tibial bone mineral density changes after total knee arthroplasty: one-year follow-up study of 69 patients. Acta Orthop Scand. 2004;75(5):600–5. https://doi.org/10.1080/00016470410001493.
83. Frost HM. A 2003 update of bone physiology and Wolff's Law for clinicians. Angle Orthod. 2004;74(1):3–15. https://doi.org/10.1043/0003-3219(2004)074<0003:AUOBPA>2.0.CO;2.
84. Meireles S, Completo A, Antonio Simoes J, Flores P. Strain shielding in distal femur after patellofemoral arthroplasty under different activity conditions. J Biomech. 2010;43(3):477–84. https://doi.org/10.1016/j.jbiomech.2009.09.048.
85. Richmond BI, Hadlow SV, Lynskey TG, Walker CG, Munro JT. Proximal tibial bone density is preserved after unicompartmental knee arthroplasty. Clin Orthop Relat Res. 2013;471(5):1661–9. https://doi.org/10.1007/s11999-013-2784-2.
86. Boissonneault A, Pandit H, Pegg E, Jenkins C, Gill HS, Dodd CA, Gibbons CL, Murray DW. No difference in survivorship after unicompartmental knee arthroplasty with or without an intact anterior cruciate ligament. Knee Surg Sports Traumatol Arthrosc. 2013;21(11):2480–6. https://doi.org/10.1007/s00167-012-2101-8.
87. Kim KT, Lee S, Kim TW, Lee JS, Boo KH. The influence of postoperative tibiofemoral alignment on the clinical results of unicompartmental knee arthroplasty. Knee Surg Relat Res. 2012;24(2):85–90. https://doi.org/10.5792/ksrr.2012.24.2.85.
88. Emerson RH, Alnachoukati O, Barrington J, Ennin K. The results of Oxford unicompartmental knee arthroplasty in the United States: a mean ten-year survival analysis.

Bone Joint J. 2016;98-b(10 Supple B):34–40. https://doi.org/10.1302/0301-620x.98b10.Bjj-2016-0480.R1.
89. Rachha R, Veravalli K, Sood M. Medium term results of the Miller-Galante knee arthroplasty with 10 year survivorship. Acta Orthop Belg. 2013;79(2):197–204.
90. Pennington DW, Swienckowski JJ, Lutes WB, Drake GN. Unicompartmental knee arthroplasty in patients sixty years of age or younger. J Bone Joint Surg Am. 2003;85-A(10):1968–73.
91. Foran JR, Brown NM, Della Valle CJ, Berger RA, Galante JO. Long-term survivorship and failure modes of unicompartmental knee arthroplasty. Clin Orthop Relat Res. 2013;471(1):102–8. https://doi.org/10.1007/s11999-012-2517-y.
92. Parratte S, Argenson JN, Pearce O, Pauly V, Auquier P, Aubaniac JM. Medial unicompartmental knee replacement in the under-50s. J Bone Joint Surg. 2009;91(3):351–6. https://doi.org/10.1302/0301-620X.91B3.21588.
93. Berger RA, Meneghini RM, Sheinkop MB, Della Valle CJ, Jacobs JJ, Rosenberg AG, Galante JO. The progression of patellofemoral arthrosis after medial unicompartmental replacement: results at 11 to 15 years. Clin Orthop Relat Res. 2004;428:92–9. 00003086-200411000-00015 [pii]. https://doi.org/10.1097/01.blo.0000147700.89433.a5.
94. Liebs TR, Herzberg W. Better quality of life after medial versus lateral unicondylar knee arthroplasty. Clin Orthop Relat Res. 2013;471(8):2629–40. https://doi.org/10.1007/s11999-013-2966-y.
95. Bhattacharya R, Scott CE, Morris HE, Wade F, Nutton RW. Survivorship and patient satisfaction of a fixed bearing unicompartmental knee arthroplasty incorporating an all-polyethylene tibial component. Knee. 2012;19(4):348–51. https://doi.org/10.1016/j.knee.2011.04.009.
96. Biswas D, Van Thiel GS, Wetters NG, Pack BJ, Berger RA, Della Valle CJ. Medial unicompartmental knee arthroplasty in patients less than 55 years old: minimum of two years of follow-up. J Arthroplasty. 2014;29(1):101–5. https://doi.org/10.1016/j.arth.2013.04.046.
97. Bruce DJ, Hassaballa M, Robinson JR, Porteous AJ, Murray JR, Newman JH. Minimum 10-year outcomes of a fixed bearing all-polyethylene unicompartmental knee arthroplasty used to treat medial osteoarthritis. Knee. 2020;27(3):1018–27. https://doi.org/10.1016/j.knee.2020.02.018.
98. Labek G, Sekyra K, Pawelka W, Janda W, Stockl B. Outcome and reproducibility of data concerning the Oxford unicompartmental knee arthroplasty: a structured literature review including arthroplasty registry data. Acta Orthop. 2011;82(2):131–5. https://doi.org/10.3109/17453674.2011.566134.
99. Chen JY, Lo NN, Jiang L, Chong HC, Tay DK, Chin PL, Chia SL, Yeo SJ. Simultaneous versus staged bilateral unicompartmental knee replacement. Bone Joint J. 2013;95-B(6):788–92. https://doi.org/10.1302/0301-620X.95B6.30440.
100. Chan WC, Musonda P, Cooper AS, Glasgow MM, Donell ST, Walton NP. One-stage versus two-stage bilateral unicompartmental knee replacement: a comparison of immediate post-operative complications. J Bone Joint Surg. 2009;91(10):1305–9. https://doi.org/10.1302/0301-620X.91B10.22612.
101. Berend KR, Morris MJ, Skeels MD, Lombardi AV Jr, Adams JB. Perioperative complications of simultaneous versus staged unicompartmental knee arthroplasty. Clin Orthop Relat Res. 2011;469(1):168–73. https://doi.org/10.1007/s11999-010-1492-4.
102. Baker PN, Jameson SS, Deehan DJ, Gregg PJ, Porter M, Tucker K. Mid-term equivalent survival of medial and lateral unicondylar knee replacement: an analysis of data from a National Joint Registry. J Bone Joint Surg. 2012;94(12):1641–8. https://doi.org/10.1302/0301-620X.94B12.29416.
103. Kennedy JA, Mohammad HR, Yang I, Mellon SJ, Dodd CAF, Pandit HG, Murray DW. Oxford domed lateral unicompartmental knee arthroplasty. Bone Joint J. 2020;102-b(8):1033–40. https://doi.org/10.1302/0301-620x.102b8.Bjj-2019-1330.R2.
104. Walker T, Zahn N, Bruckner T, Streit MR, Mohr G, Aldinger PR, Clarius M, Gotterbarm T. Mid-term results of lateral unicondylar mobile bearing knee arthroplasty: a multicentre study of 363 cases. Bone Joint J. 2018;100-b(1):42–9. https://doi.org/10.1302/0301-620x.100b1.Bjj-2017-0600.R1.

105. Fornell S, Prada E, Barrena P, García-Mendoza A, Borrego E, Domecq G. Mid-term outcomes of mobile-bearing lateral unicompartmental knee arthroplasty. Knee. 2018;25(6):1206–13. https://doi.org/10.1016/j.knee.2018.05.016.
106. Weston-Simons JS, Pandit H, Kendrick BJ, Jenkins C, Barker K, Dodd CA, Murray DW. The mid-term outcomes of the Oxford Domed Lateral unicompartmental knee replacement. Bone Joint J. 2014;96-B(1):59–64. https://doi.org/10.1302/0301-620X.96B1.31630.
107. Edmiston TA, Manista GC, Courtney PM, Sporer SM, Della Valle CJ, Levine BR. Clinical outcomes and survivorship of lateral unicompartmental knee arthroplasty: does surgical approach matter? J Arthroplasty. 2018;33(2):362–5. https://doi.org/10.1016/j.arth.2017.09.009.
108. Smith JR, Robinson JR, Porteous AJ, Murray JR, Hassaballa MA, Artz N, Newman JH. Fixed bearing lateral unicompartmental knee arthroplasty--short to midterm survivorship and knee scores for 101 prostheses. Knee. 2014;21(4):843–7. https://doi.org/10.1016/j.knee.2014.04.003.
109. Deroche E, Batailler C, Lording T, Neyret P, Servien E, Lustig S. High survival rate and very low Wear of lateral unicompartmental arthroplasty at long term: a case series of 54 cases at a mean follow-up of 17 years. J Arthroplasty. 2019;34(6):1097–104. https://doi.org/10.1016/j.arth.2019.01.053.
110. Lustig S, Lording T, Frank F, Debette C, Servien E, Neyret P. Progression of medial osteoarthritis and long term results of lateral unicompartmental arthroplasty: 10 to 18 year follow-up of 54 consecutive implants. Knee. 2014;21 Suppl 1:S26–32. https://doi.org/10.1016/S0968-0160(14)50006-3.
111. Tu Y, Ma T, Wen T, Yang T, Xue L, Xue H. Does Unicompartmental knee replacement offer improved clinical advantages over total knee replacement in the treatment of isolated lateral osteoarthritis? A matched cohort analysis from an independent center. J Arthroplasty. 2020;35(8):2016–21. https://doi.org/10.1016/j.arth.2020.03.021.
112. Lustig S, Elguindy A, Servien E, Fary C, Munini E, Demey G, Neyret P. 5- to 16-year follow-up of 54 consecutive lateral unicondylar knee arthroplasties with a fixed-all polyethylene bearing. J Arthroplasty. 2011;26(8):1318–25. https://doi.org/10.1016/j.arth.2011.01.015.
113. Pennington DW, Swienckowski JJ, Lutes WB, Drake GN. Lateral unicompartmental knee arthroplasty: survivorship and technical considerations at an average follow-up of 12.4 years. J Arthroplasty. 2006;21(1):13–7. https://doi.org/10.1016/j.arth.2004.11.021.
114. Lustig S, Parratte S, Magnussen RA, Argenson JN, Neyret P. Lateral unicompartmental knee arthroplasty relieves pain and improves function in posttraumatic osteoarthritis. Clin Orthop Relat Res. 2012;470(1):69–76. https://doi.org/10.1007/s11999-011-1963-2.
115. Argenson JN, Parratte S, Bertani A, Flecher X, Aubaniac JM. Long-term results with a lateral unicondylar replacement. Clin Orthop Relat Res. 2008;466(11):2686–93. https://doi.org/10.1007/s11999-008-0351-z.
116. Walker T, Gotterbarm T, Bruckner T, Merle C, Streit MR. Return to sports, recreational activity and patient-reported outcomes after lateral unicompartmental knee arthroplasty. Knee Surg Sports Traumatol Arthrosc. 2015;23(11):3281–7. https://doi.org/10.1007/s00167-014-3111-5.
117. Canetti R, Batailler C, Bankhead C, Neyret P, Servien E, Lustig S. Faster return to sport after robotic-assisted lateral unicompartmental knee arthroplasty: a comparative study. Arch Orthop Trauma Surg. 2018;138(12):1765–71. https://doi.org/10.1007/s00402-018-3042-6.
118. Sah AP, Scott RD. Lateral unicompartmental knee arthroplasty through a medial approach. Study with an average five-year follow-up. J Bone Joint Surg Am. 2007;89(9):1948–54. https://doi.org/10.2106/JBJS.F.01457.

Effect of Preoperative Rehabilitation on Clinical Outcomes and Function After Knee Arthroplasty

5

Sue Barber-Westin and Frank R. Noyes

5.1 Introduction

Experienced clinicians are well aware that many patient candidates for total knee arthroplasty (TKA) have noteworthy issues related to muscle atrophy and weakness and loss of normal range of motion (ROM). Osteoarthritis (OA) involves the deterioration of the entire knee joint and includes a decline in muscle strength as pain becomes prominent with recreational, work, and daily activities. Shorter et al. [1] reviewed current published information regarding skeletal muscle wasting and OA. These authors discussed the beneficial effects of exercise to maintain muscle mass and function to delay TKA and suggested mechanisms such as promoting microRNA expression in joint tissues. Callahan et al. [2] studied sex-specific cellular and molecular functional changes and adaptations to chronic disuse atrophy in older adults with symptomatic knee OA compared with matched normal volunteers. This study reported major changes in cross-sectional muscle areas, fiber morphology, and other molecular changes associated with OA and also noted important sex-dependent effects in skeletal muscle fiber size and fiber type distribution.

Since 1993, multiple investigations have been conducted to determine if exercise intervention done before TKA could improve lower extremity muscle strength, function, and patient-reported outcome measures (PROMs) before surgery and positively impact postoperative outcomes. This chapter reviews 13 randomized controlled trials (RCTs) [3–15] and summarizes findings from six review studies [16–21]. The effects of exercise programs on muscle strength (quadriceps, hamstrings, hip) and function measured either objectively or with PROMs are described,

S. Barber-Westin (✉)
Noyes Knee Institute, Cincinnati, OH, USA
e-mail: sbwestin@csmref.org

F. R. Noyes
Cincinnati SportsMedicine and Orthopaedic Center, The Noyes Knee Institute,
Cincinnati, OH, USA

F. R. Noyes, S. Barber-Westin (eds.), *Critical Rehabilitation for Partial and Total Knee Arthroplasty*, https://doi.org/10.1007/978-3-030-87003-4_5

both before and after TKA. Other investigations that either combined all data from knee and hip arthroplasty [22–24], did not perform comparisons between the study and control groups [25], only determined length of hospital stay and discharge disposition [26], or were underpowered to detect statistically significant differences between study and control groups [27–29] were not included.

5.2 Randomized Controlled Trials

A summary of the preoperative programs and outcome measures from the 13 RCTs is shown in Table 5.1. All studies except two [3, 12] conducted sample size power calculations to determine the minimum number of subjects required. The intervention programs varied with regard to all factors, including frequency and duration of the program, as well as specific exercise protocols. Only three programs consisted of daily exercise, and the majority required patients to attend supervised therapy or exercise sessions. Ten studies conducted testing after training was completed and before TKA was performed. Eleven investigations conducted testing after surgery that ranged from 1 to 12 months postoperatively.

Muscle strength was determined in eight studies using either isometric or isokinetic dynamometers or the one repetition-maximum test. A variety of other objective measures were conducted, including timed up-and-go (TUG), walk, stair-climb, and sit-to-stand tests (see Chap. 9 for test descriptions). PROMs were collected in all studies except one and included American Knee Society (AKS), Hospital Anxiety and Depression Scale (HAD), Knee Injury and Osteoarthritis Outcome Score (KOOS), Oxford Knee Score (OKS), Western Ontario and McMaster Universities Osteoarthritis Index (WOMAC), and pain visual analogue scales (VAS).

5.3 Effect of Trials on Strength and Function Before Surgery

Three of ten studies that measured results before TKA was performed reported significant effects of preoperative rehabilitation on multiple factors (Table 5.2). Calatayud et al. [4] found significant improvements in ten variables; data for the objective tests are shown in Table 5.3. This study employed a rigorous program that included high-intensity, supervised training 3 days a week for 8 weeks. The program began with a 15-minute warm-up, followed by an exercise protocol of five sets of ten repetitions of seated leg press, knee extension, leg curl, and hip abduction. Intensity was based on the patient's ability to execute ten repetition maximum. Then, subjects performed four sets of 30 seconds of double-leg stance and four sets of 15 seconds of single-leg stance on an unstable device. The program resulted in significant improvements in quadriceps, hamstrings, and hip abduction strength, as well as function in the TUG and stair-climb tests. Knee flexion and extension improved by a mean of approximately 10° and 8°, respectively.

Skoffer et al. [6] reported significant differences between study and control groups in quadriceps and hamstrings isometric muscle strength ($P < 0.01$), TUG

Table 5.1 Randomized controlled trials with preoperative exercise programs

Study	N		Preoperative program		Outcome measures		
	Study	Control	Duration	Exercises	Time	Objective	PROMs
Jahic et al. [3]	10	10	3 ×/day for 6 weeks at home	Quadriceps strengthening, flexibility, resistance training (details NA)	Baseline, after training and before surgery, 3–6–12 months po	None	AKS Knee score and Function score
Tungtrongjit et al. [10]	30	30	3 ×/day for 3 weeks at home	Knee extension, in chair, no weight, 10 reps	Baseline, after training and before surgery, 1–3–6 months po	Isometric quadriceps strength	WOMAC, pain VAS
Gstoettner et al. [11]	15	20	1 ×/week for 6 weeks in clinic 1 ×/day for 6 weeks at home	Warm-up, flexibility, proprioception program: slide step forward/backward, step forward/backward, single-leg stance, squats; floor to unstable platform	Baseline, after training and before surgery, 6 weeks po	Biodex stability system, 60-m walk, stair climb	WOMAC, KSS Knee and Function
Calatayud et al. [4]	22	22	3 ×/week for 8 weeks in clinic	High intensity program: 5 sets × 10 reps of leg press, knee extension, ham curls, hip abduction; double and single-leg stance on Bosu, step-ups, calf raises, flexibility	Baseline, after training and before surgery, 1 and 3 months po	Isometric strength, ROM, TUG, stair climb	WOMAC, pain VAS, SF-36
Eil et al. [5]	24	26	2 ×/week for 6 weeks in clinic	Stationary bike, ankle pumps, isometric quadriceps, straight leg raise, heel slides, hamstring stretch	Baseline, 6 week and 3 months po	ROM	KOOS
Skoffer et al. [6]	29	21	3 ×/week for 4 weeks in clinic	Stationary bike, PREs: leg press, knee extension, knee flexion, hip extension/abduction/adduction, and stretching	Baseline, after training and before surgery, 1–6–12 weeks po	30-second chair-stand, TUG, 10 MWT, 6 MWT, isokinetic (60°/s) and isometric quadriceps and hamstrings strength, ROM	KOOS, pain VAS
Matassi et al. [7]	61	61	5 ×/week for 6 weeks at home	Flexibility, isometric quadriceps, isotonic quadriceps and hamstring, step-ups	Baseline, 6 weeks-6–12 months po	ROM	AKS

(continued)

Table 5.1 (continued)

Study	N		Preoperative program		Outcome measures		
	Study	Control	Duration	Exercises	Time	Objective	PROMs
van Leeuwen et al. [8]	7	9	2–3 ×/week for 6 weeks in clinic 2–3 ×/week at home	PREs leg press, leg extension in clinic; step-ups, squats at home	Baseline, after training and before surgery, 6 and 12 weeks po	Isometric quadriceps and hamstrings strength, sit-to-stand test, 6 MWT, stair climb	WOMAC
Villadsen et al. [9]	41	40	2 ×/week for ~8 weeks (12 sessions minimum) in clinic	Stationary bike, 2–3 sets x 10 reps of 4 neuromuscular exercises (core stability, postural orientation, muscle strength, function)	Baseline and after training. No postoperative assessment	20-m walk, sit-to-stand, muscle power of quadriceps, hip extensors, hip abductors	KOOS
Swank et al. [12]	37	36	3 ×/week for 4–8 weeks; clinic and home	Exercises with resistance band: squats, leg extension, leg curl, multi-hip; foot plantar flexion, dorsiflexion; step ups forward/lateral	Baseline and after training. No postoperative assessment	6 MWT, sit-to-stand, stair climb, quadriceps and hamstrings isokinetic strength 60°/s	None
Williamson et al. [13]	60	61	1 ×/week for 6 weeks in clinic	Quadriceps isometrics, straight leg raises, sit to stand, stair climbing, knee extension with theraband, balance board training	Baseline, 7–12–16 weeks po	50-m walk	OKS, WOMAC, HAD
Rooks et al. [14]	14	15	3 ×/week for 6 weeks in community fitness facility	Pool-based exercises 1st 3 weeks; then land-based cardio, strength, flexibility	Baseline, after training and before surgery, 8 and 26 weeks po	1-rep max quadriceps strength, functional reach, TUG	WOMAC, SF-36
Beaupre et al. [15]	65	66	3 ×/week for 4 weeks in clinic	Quadriceps isometrics, straight leg raises, knee extension (ankle weight), knee flexion with tubing for resistance	Baseline, after training and before surgery, 3–6–12 months po	Quadriceps and hamstrings isometric strength, ROM	WOMAC, SF-36

AKS American Knee Society, *HAD* Hospital Anxiety and Depression Scale, *KOOS* Knee Injury and Osteoarthritis Outcome Score, *MWT* minute walk test, *NA* not available, *OKS* Oxford Knee Score, *PRE* progressive resistive exercises, *PROMs* patient-reported outcome measures, *RCT* randomized controlled trial, *ROM* range of motion, *T* time, *TUG* timed up and go, *VAS* visual analogue scale, *WOMAC* Western Ontario and McMaster Universities Osteoarthritis Index

Table 5.2 Significant effects of programs on objective testing and PROMs compared with control group before surgery

Study	Strength			TUG	Stair climb	Sit-to-stand	Walk tests	ROM	Other objective	Patient-reported outcome measures
	Quad	Ham	Hip							
Jahic et al. [3]	--	--	--	--	--	--	--	--	--	AKS Knee and Function scores: **yes**
Tungtrongjit et al. [10]	No effect	--	--	--	--	--	--	--	--	WOMAC, pain VAS: no effect
Gstoettner et al. [11]	--	--	--	--	No effect	--	No effect	--	Biodex stability stance: no effect	WOMAC, AKS Knee and Function scores: no effect
Calatayud et al. [4]	**Yes**	**Yes**	**Yes**	**Yes**	**Yes**	--	--	**Yes**	--	WOMAC, SF-36, pain VAS: **yes**
Skoffer et al. [6]	**Yes isometric**	**Yes isometric**	--	**Yes**	--	**Yes**	No effect	No effect	--	KOOS: no, pain VAS: **yes**
van Leeuwen et al. [8]	No effect	No effect	--	--	No effect	No effect	No effect	--	--	WOMAC: no effect
Villadsen et al. [9]	No effect	No effect	No effect	--	--	**Yes**	--	--	--	KOOS: no effect
Swank et al. [12]	**Yes**	No effect	--	--	**Yes**	**Yes**	No effect	--	--	--
Rooks et al. [14]	No effect	--	--	No effect	--	--	--	--	Functional reach: no effect	WOMAC, SF-36: no effect
Beaupre et al. [15]	No effect	No effect	--	--	--	--	--	No effect		WOMAC, SF-36: no effect

AKS American Knee Society, *HAD* Hospital Anxiety and Depression Scale, *KOOS* Knee Injury and Osteoarthritis Outcome Score, *OKS* Oxford Knee Score, *TUG* timed up and go, *VAS* visual analogue scale, *WOMAC* Western Ontario and McMaster Universities Osteoarthritis Index
-- indicates test not done, bold indicates significant difference between intervention and control groups

Table 5.3 Significant mean improvements reported after an 8-week high-intensity preoperative training program before TKA[a]

Variable	Testing time	Control group	Intervention group	Between-group difference	*P* value
Range of motion: flexion (°)	Baseline	104.2	104.0	0.2	NS
	Before TKA	102.8	114.4	−11.6	0.005
Range of motion: extension (°)	Baseline	14.0	14.4	−0.4	NS
	Before TKA	14.9	6.6	8.3	<0.0001
Timed up and go (s)	Baseline	8.5	8.6	−0.1	NS
	Before TKA	9.0	6.7	2.3	<0.0001
Stair climb (s)	Baseline	11.2	11.0	0.1	NS
	Before TKA	11.4	7.2	4.2	<0.0001
Isometric knee flexion (kg)	Baseline	9.1	9.2	−0.1	NS
	Before TKA	8.2	17.6	−9.4	<0.0001
Isometric knee extension (kg)	Baseline	23.5	23.5	0	NS
	Before TKA	22.0	37.8	−15.8	<0.0001
Isometric hip abduction (kg)	Baseline	7.2	7.3	−0.1	NS
	Before TKA	7.1	13.4	−6.3	<0.0001

[a]From Calatayud et al. [4]
NS not significant

($P = 0.03$), and the sit-to-stand (chair-stand) test ($P = 0.001$), as well as pain VAS ($P < 0.0001$). In this investigation, subjects trained 3 days a week for 4 weeks under supervised conditions. The program was 60 minutes in length and included stationary bicycling, followed by three sets of eight to 12 repetitions of maximum resistance on leg press, knee extension, knee flexion, hip extension, hip abduction, and hip adduction machines. Even so, the authors acknowledged the need for further exploration of a longer training program to produce even greater gains in these indices.

Swank et al. [12] reported improvements in quadriceps isokinetic strength ($P = 0.01$), stair-climb test ($P < 0.05$), and sit-to-stand test ($P < 0.05$) after a home-based program that involved training three times a week for 4–8 weeks. The time period was determined according to the time available before TKA was scheduled; there was a mean of 13.4 sessions (range, 10–16) completed by the 37 patients. This program involved nine lower body exercises with resistance bands of squats, hip flexion-extension, hip abduction-adduction, ankle plantar flexion-dorsiflexion, and knee extension-flexion. The initial training was set at a low level to ensure completion for the first 4 weeks, and then patients were encouraged to increase the intensity of the band resistance. The patients also performed forward and lateral step training and flexibility exercises. Knee extension isokinetic peak torque (60°/s) improved in the study group from 54.4 ± 5.6 Nm to 60.0 ± 5.4 Nm, while the control group had a decrease in these values from 56.8 ± 5.8 Nm to 50.7 ± 5.5 Nm ($P = 0.01$, group/time interaction). The authors recommended increased supervision for future studies because patient training logs indicated a lack of adherence to the intended progression of the program.

Jahic et al. [3] only measured AKS scores in a small pilot study consisting of 20 patients who completed a home-based program of quadriceps strengthening, flexibility, and resistance training three times a day for 6 weeks. The details of this program were not provided. These investigators reported significant differences between the intervention and control groups for the mean AKS Knee (46.4 ± 8.0 and 35.7 ± 5.58, respectively; $P < 0.05$) and Function (40.5 ± 7.25 and 29.5 ± 7.25, respectively; $P < 0.05$) scores.

5.4 Effect of Trials on Strength and Function After Surgery

Only three of 11 studies reported significant effects of the preoperative programs on both objective and PROM measures after TKA was performed (Table 5.4). Calatayud et al. [4] reported significant differences between the intervention and control groups for all variables studied at 1 and 3 months postoperatively, shown in Table 5.5. Skoffer et al. [6] found significant differences in changes from baseline to 6- and 12-week postoperative time periods between study and control in 30-second chair-stand, TUG, and quadriceps and hamstrings isokinetic and isometric tests (Table 5.6). There were no significant differences between groups in the 6- and 10-minute walking tests, KOOS, or pain VAS scores.

Tungtrongjit et al. [10] reported significant differences in quadriceps isometric strength between intervention and control groups at 1 month (5.5 ± 2.9 kg and 4.0 ± 2.7 kg, respectively; $P = 0.01$) and 3 months postoperatively (7.5 + 2.9 and 5.3 + 3.4, respectively; $P = 0.006$). Pain VAS scores were significantly superior in the intervention group compared with the control group at 1 month (2.9 ± 1.5 and 3.8 ± 1.4, respectively; $P = 0.03$) and 3 months postoperatively (1.6 + 1.3 and 2.6 + 1.4, respectively; $P = 0.003$). There were also significantly superior WOMAC total, pain, stiffness, and function scores in the intervention group at 1 and 3 months postoperatively ($P < 0.001$ to <0.02). There were no significant differences between groups for any variable at 6 months postoperatively. This program only included knee extensions (three sets of ten repetitions) performed without weight three times a day for 3 weeks.

Jahic et al. [3] found significant differences between the intervention and control groups in the AKS Knee score at 3 months (76.7 ± 6.83 and 57.9 ± 7.05, $P = 0.0001$) and 6 months (79.1 ± 6.97 and 69.1 ± 7.34, $P = 0.006$). There were no differences in the AKS Function score at any postoperative time period.

No study determined the number of patients that returned to recreational, sports, or work activities postoperatively. The effect of prerehabilitation on longer postoperative outcomes was only assessed in three studies (12 postoperative months in two studies [3, 7] and six postoperative months in one study [10]), and none of these reported group differences at the final follow-up evaluation.

Table 5.4 Significant effect of programs on objective testing and PROMs compared with control group after surgery[a]

Study	Strength			TUG	Stair climb	Sit-to-stand	Walk tests	ROM	Other objective	Patient-reported outcome measures
	Quad	Ham	Hip							
Jahic et al. [3]	--	--	--	--	--	--	--	--	--	AKS Knee and Function scores: **3 and 6 months po**
Tungtrongjit et al. [10]	**1 and 3 months po**	--	--	--	--	--	--	--		WOMAC and pain VAS: **1 and 3 months po**
Gstoettner et al. [11]	--	--	--	--	No effect	--	No effect	--	Biodex stability stance: 6 weeks po: no effect	WOMAC, AKS Knee and Function scores: no effect
Calatayud et al. [4]	**3 months po**	**1 and 3 months po**	**1 and 3 months po**	**1 and 3 months po**	**1 and 3 months po**	--	--	**1 and 3 months po**	--	WOMAC, SF-36, pain VAS: **1 and 3 months po**
Eil et al. [5]	--	--	--	--	--	--	--	No effect	--	KOOS: no effect
Skoffer et al. [6]	**6 and 12 weeks po**	**6 and 12 weeks po**	--	**6 and 12 weeks po**	--	**6 and 12 weeks po**	No effect	No effect	--	KOOS, pain VAS: no effect
Matassi et al. [7]	--	--	--	--	--	--	--	No effect	--	AKS: no effect
van Leeuwen et al. [8]	No effect	No effect	--	--	No effect	No effect	No effect	--	--	WOMAC: no effect
Williamson et al. [13]	--	--	--	--	--	--	No effect	--	--	WOMAC, OKS, HAD: no effect
Rooks et al. [14]	No effect	--	--	No effect	--	--	--	--	Functional reach: no effect	WOMAC, SF-36: no effect
Beaupre et al. [15]	No effect	No effect	--	--	--	--	--	No effect	--	WOMAC, SF-36: no effect

AKS American Knee Society, *HAD* Hospital Anxiety and Depression Scale, *KOOS* Knee Injury and Osteoarthritis Outcome Score, *OKS* Oxford Knee Score, *TUG* timed up and go, *VAS* visual analogue scale, *WOMAC* Western Ontario and McMaster Universities Osteoarthritis Index

[a]For variables with significant differences, the time postoperatively is shown

-- indicates test not done, bold indicates significant difference between intervention and control group

Table 5.5 Significant mean differences between control and intervention groups after TKA[a]

Variable	Testing time	Control group	Intervention group	Between-group difference	*P* value
Range of motion: flexion (°)	1 month po	82.3	88.8	−6.5	0.005
	3 months po	96.4	101.2	−4.8	0.005
Range of motion: extension (°)	1 month po	16.9	11.1	5.8	<0.0001
	3 months po	13.9	8.2	5.6	<0.0001
Timed up and go (s)	1 month po	9.4	7.3	2.1	<0.0001
	3 months po	8.7	7.0	1.7	<0.0001
Stair climb (s)	1 month po	11.4	7.2	3.6	<0.0001
	3 months po	12.7	9.1	4.2	<0.0001
Isometric knee flexion (kg)	1 month po	3.9	8.7	−4.8	<0.0001
	3 months po	4.4	9.4	−5.0	<0.0001
Isometric knee extension (kg)	1 month po	7.7	8.9	−1.2	NS
	3 months po	14.3	22.8	−8.5	<0.0001
Isometric hip abduction (kg)	1 month po	4.8	7.7	−2.9	<0.0001
	3 months po	5.0	7.8	−2.8	<0.0001
Pain VAS	1 month po	4.2	2.5	1.7	<0.0001
	3 months po	2.9	1.4	1.5	<0.0001
WOMAC	1 month po	42.4	28.4	14.0	<0.0001
	3 months po	30.7	25.0	5.8	<0.0001
WOMAC pain	1 month po	5.1	4.0	1.1	<0.0001
	3 months po	3.8	2.9	0.9	<0.0001
WOMAC stiffness	1 month po	4.2	2.8	1.4	<0.0001
	3 months po	3.2	2.2	0.9	<0.0001
WOMAC function	1 month po	31.6	20.5	11.0	<0.0001
	3 months po	22.7	18.8	3.9	<0.0001
SF-36 physical functioning	1 month po	46.9	51.4	−4.4	<0.0001
	3 months po	53.0	55.7	−2.7	<0.0001

[a]From Calatayud et al. [4]
NS not significant

5.5 Systematic Reviews and Meta-analyses

A summary of the major findings of three meta-analyses [16–18] and three systematic reviews [19–21] on the topic of preoperative rehabilitation before TKA is shown in Table 5.7. All three systematic reviews and one of the meta-analyses [18] failed to find consistent significant improvements in all postoperative outcome measures from the preoperative programs. However, pooled data from two or the recent meta-analyses that included many more recent studies reported some benefits from preoperative programs. Moyer et al. [17] reported significant improvements in the intervention groups compared with the control groups in postoperative PROMs of function (standardized mean difference [SMD] = 0.32, 95% confidence interval [CI] = 0.06–0.57, $P = 0.01$) and quadriceps strength (SMD = 0.42, 95% CI = 0.16–0.68, $P = 0.002$). There were no significant differences in VAS pain, anxiety, or hamstrings strength. Chen et al. [16] reported significant improvements in the intervention groups compared with the control groups in the sit-to-stand test (mean difference [MD] = 1.68, 95% CI = 1.25–2.10, $P < 0.05$) and in total knee ROM

Table 5.6 Significant mean differences between control and intervention groups after TKA[a]

Variable	Testing time	Control group Mean ± SD (change from baseline)	Intervention group Mean ± SD (change from baseline)	*P* value[b]
30-s chair stand test (rep)	Baseline	10.4 ± 3.3	10.8 ± 5.1	--
	6 weeks po	9.6 ± 4.4 (−1.1)	13.3 ± 5.0 (2.5)	0.004
	12 weeks po	11.0 ± 4.4 (0.2)	14.7 ± 4.7 (3.9)	0.001
Timed-up-and-go test (s)	Baseline	9.3 ± 3.0	9.1 ± 2.6	--
	6 weeks po	10.0 ± 2.4 (0.8)	8.3 ± 2.3 (−0.7)	0.02
	12 weeks po	8.9 ± 2.1 (−0.1)	7.9 ± 2.3 (−1.2)	0.05
Isokinetic knee extension 60°/s (Nm/kg)	Baseline	0.9 ± 0.3	0.8 ± 0.4	--
	6 weeks po	0.6 ± 0.2 (−0.3)	0.7 ± 0.2 (−0.1)	0.003
	12 weeks po	0.7 ± 0.2 (−0.2)	0.9 ± 0.3 (0)	0.002
Isokinetic knee flexion 60°/s (Nm/kg)	Baseline	0.5 ± 0.2	0.5 ± 0.3	--
	6 weeks po	0.4 ± 0.2 (−0.1)	0.5 ± 0.2 (0)	0.004
	12 weeks po	0.4 ± 0.2 (−0.1)	0.5 ± 0.2 (0.01)	0.002
Isometric knee flexion (Nm/kg)	Baseline	1.0 ± 0.4	1.0 ± 0.3	--
	6 weeks po	0.6 ± 0.3 (−0.4)	0.9 ± 0.3 (−0.2)	0.002
	12 weeks po	0.8 ± 0.3 (−0.3)	1.0 ± 0.3 (0)	<0.001
Isometric knee extension (Nm/kg)	Baseline	0.6 ± 0.3	0.6 ± 0.3	--
	6 weeks po	0.5 ± 0.2 (0)	0.7 ± 0.3 (0.1)	0.02
	12 weeks po	0.6 ± 0.2 (−0.1)	0.7 ± 0.3 (0.1)	0.04

[a]From Skoffer et al. [36]
[b]*P* values based on the difference between groups in the change from baseline values

(MD = 3.62, 95% CI = 0.05–7.19, $P < 0.05$). There were no differences found for quadriceps strength, knee extension, knee flexion, 6-minute walk test, or WOMAC scores.

The problems inherent with analyzing pooled data from studies with low quality of evidence and vastly different programs were noted by all of these investigations. Many of the early studies were underpowered to detect significant differences between intervention and control groups, and few used objective tests to measure knee function. As previously mentioned, the intervention programs varied with regard to all factors, including frequency and duration of the program, as well as specific exercise protocols.

5.6 Conclusions

We believe data from recent studies suggests that a preoperative TKA rehabilitation program has the potential to improve both objective and subjective knee functions. The investigations from Calatayud et al. [4] and Skoffer et al. [6] reported

Table 5.7 Results of systematic reviews and meta-analyses

Study, type	N studies	Years studies published	Overall findings of preoperative programs on postoperative outcomes
Chen et al. [16] Meta-analysis	16	2004–2016	Exercise groups had significantly reduced length of hospital stay and superior sit-to-stand test. No significant differences between groups for quadriceps strength, 6-minute walk test, knee flexion, knee extension, or WOMAC scores
Moyer et al. [17] Meta-analysis	19	2000–2016	Intervention groups had significantly reduced length of hospital stay and better quadriceps strength and function-related PROMs at 3 months postoperatively compared with control groups
Hoogeboom et al. [18] Meta-analysis	9	1993–2008	No benefit of preoperative exercise on functional recovery or PROMs. None of the studies met authors' predetermined criteria for high therapeutic validity
Chesham et al. [19] Systematic review	10	2004–2014	Multiple methodological problems, all programs differed, 50% of studies showed no effect preoperative program, 50% showed a few superior outcomes in intervention groups
Kwok et al. [20] Systematic review	11	1995–2014	Few differences existed in outcomes between the intervention and control groups. Most studies were underpowered and the quality of evidence was moderate or poor
Jordan et al. [21] Systematic review	11	1993–2012	No evidence for improvement in PROMs and little evidence of improvement in objective measures. Poor study quality

PROMs patient-reported outcome measures, *WOMAC* Western Ontario and McMaster Universities Osteoarthritis Index

significant differences between intervention and control groups for multiple variables both before and after TKA. These investigations employed rigorous, supervised programs that trained patients 3 days a week for 4–8 weeks. Multiple sets of progressive resistive exercises for knee and hip strengthening appear to be mandatory for these types of improvements. Current recommendations to achieve muscle hypertrophy include using resistance training loads of 60–70% of one repetition maximum (1-RM) [30]. The problem is that these higher loads are frequently not tolerable in TKA candidates. Blood flow restriction training (BFRT) with low-resistance loads (such as 30% of 1-RM) has been advocated as an adjunct to rehabilitation in patients with severe lower extremity muscular atrophy [31, 32]. BFRT investigations have evaluated safety and complications and concluded that this treatment modality is safe and no more likely to result in an adverse event when compared with standard exercises [31–34]. Still, clinicians need to be aware of pre-existing or risk factors before recommending BFRT, especially in the TKA population. The most frequent patient complaints are delayed muscle soreness and fatigue, and close supervision is necessary to monitor cuff pressures, exercises, and patient safety. There must be no evidence of history of varicose veins, deep venous thrombosis or pulmonary embolism, myocardial infarction, stroke, or unstable cardiac disease. The patient must not be on heart medications or demonstrate hypertension (>140/90) or cardiac disorders of any type, including tachycardia (>100 bpm) [35]. Future studies are required to determine the efficacy of modern and unique training methods such as BFRT to further improve the efficacy of preoperative TKA rehabilitation.

References

1. Shorter E, Sannicandro AJ, Poulet B, Goljanek-Whysall K. Skeletal muscle wasting and its relationship with osteoarthritis: a mini-review of mechanisms and current interventions. Curr Rheumatol Rep. 2019;21(8):40.
2. Callahan DM, Tourville TW, Miller MS, Hackett SB, Sharma H, Cruickshank NC, Slauterbeck JR, Savage PD, Ades PA, Maughan DW, Beynnon BD, Toth MJ. Chronic disuse and skeletal muscle structure in older adults: sex-specific differences and relationships to contractile function. Am J Physiol Cell Physiol. 2015;308(11):C932–43. https://doi.org/10.1152/ajpcell.00014.2015.
3. Jahic D, Omerovic D, Tanovic AT, Dzankovic F, Campara MT. The effect of prehabilitation on postoperative outcome in patients following primary total knee arthroplasty. Med Arch. 2018;72(6):439–43. https://doi.org/10.5455/medarh.2018.72.439-443.
4. Calatayud J, Casaña J, Ezzatvar Y, Jakobsen MD, Sundstrup E, Andersen LL. High-intensity preoperative training improves physical and functional recovery in the early post-operative periods after total knee arthroplasty: a randomized controlled trial. Knee Surg Sports Traumatol Arthrosc. 2017;25(9):2864–72. https://doi.org/10.1007/s00167-016-3985-5.
5. Eil MSM, Ismail MAS, Shokri AA, Ab Rahman S. Preoperative physiotherapy and short-term functional outcomes of primary total knee arthroplasty. Singapore Med J. 2016;57(3):138.
6. Skoffer B, Dalgas U, Mechlenburg I. Progressive resistance training before and after total hip and knee arthroplasty: a systematic review. Clin Rehabil. 2015;29(1):14–29. https://doi.org/10.1177/0269215514537093.
7. Matassi F, Duerinckx J, Vandenneucker H, Bellemans J. Range of motion after total knee arthroplasty: the effect of a preoperative home exercise program. Knee Surg Sports Traumatol Arthrosc. 2014;22(3):703–9.
8. van Leeuwen DM, de Ruiter CJ, Nolte PA, de Haan A. Preoperative strength training for elderly patients awaiting total knee arthroplasty. Rehabil Res Pract. 2014;2014:462750. https://doi.org/10.1155/2014/462750.
9. Villadsen A, Overgaard S, Holsgaard-Larsen A, Christensen R, Roos EM. Immediate efficacy of neuromuscular exercise in patients with severe osteoarthritis of the hip or knee: a secondary analysis from a randomized controlled trial. J Rheumatol. 2014;41(7):1385–94. https://doi.org/10.3899/jrheum.130642.
10. Tungtrongjit Y, Weingkum P, Saunkool P. The effect of preoperative quadriceps exercise on functional outcome after total knee arthroplasty. J Med Assoc Thai. 2012;95 Suppl 10:S58–66.
11. Gstoettner M, Raschner C, Dirnberger E, Leimser H, Krismer M. Preoperative proprioceptive training in patients with total knee arthroplasty. Knee. 2011;18(4):265–70. https://doi.org/10.1016/j.knee.2010.05.012.
12. Swank AM, Kachelman JB, Bibeau W, Quesada PM, Nyland J, Malkani A, Topp RV. Prehabilitation before total knee arthroplasty increases strength and function in older adults with severe osteoarthritis. J Strength Cond Res. 2011;25(2):318–25. https://doi.org/10.1519/JSC.0b013e318202e431.

13. Williamson L, Wyatt MR, Yein K, Melton JT. Severe knee osteoarthritis: a randomized controlled trial of acupuncture, physiotherapy (supervised exercise) and standard management for patients awaiting knee replacement. Rheumatology (Oxford). 2007;46(9):1445–9. https://doi.org/10.1093/rheumatology/kem119.
14. Rooks DS, Huang J, Bierbaum BE, Bolus SA, Rubano J, Connolly CE, Alpert S, Iversen MD, Katz JN. Effect of preoperative exercise on measures of functional status in men and women undergoing total hip and knee arthroplasty. Arthritis Rheum. 2006;55(5):700–8. https://doi.org/10.1002/art.22223.
15. Beaupre LA, Lier D, Davies DM, Johnston DB. The effect of a preoperative exercise and education program on functional recovery, health related quality of life, and health service utilization following primary total knee arthroplasty. J Rheumatol. 2004;31(6):1166–73.
16. Chen H, Li S, Ruan T, Liu L, Fang L. Is it necessary to perform prehabilitation exercise for patients undergoing total knee arthroplasty: meta-analysis of randomized controlled trials. Phys Sportsmed. 2018;46(1):36–43. https://doi.org/10.1080/00913847.2018.1403274.
17. Moyer R, Ikert K, Long K, Marsh J. The value of preoperative exercise and education for patients undergoing total hip and knee arthroplasty: a systematic review and meta-analysis. JBJS reviews. 2017;5(12):e2. https://doi.org/10.2106/JBJS.RVW.17.00015.
18. Hoogeboom TJ, Oosting E, Vriezekolk JE, Veenhof C, Siemonsma PC, de Bie RA, van den Ende CH, van Meeteren NL. Therapeutic validity and effectiveness of preoperative exercise on functional recovery after joint replacement: a systematic review and meta-analysis. PLoS One. 2012;7(5):e38031. https://doi.org/10.1371/journal.pone.0038031.
19. Chesham RA, Shanmugam S. Does preoperative physiotherapy improve postoperative, patient-based outcomes in older adults who have undergone total knee arthroplasty? A systematic review. Physiother Theory Pract. 2017;33(1):9–30. https://doi.org/10.1080/09593985.2016.1230660.
20. Kwok IH, Paton B, Haddad FS. Does pre-operative physiotherapy improve outcomes in primary total knee arthroplasty? - a systematic review. J Arthroplasty. 2015;30(9):1657–63. https://doi.org/10.1016/j.arth.2015.04.013.
21. Jordan JM, Helmick CG, Renner JB, Luta G, Dragomir AD, Woodard J, Fang F, Schwartz TA, Abbate LM, Callahan LF, Kalsbeek WD, Hochberg MC. Prevalence of knee symptoms and radiographic and symptomatic knee osteoarthritis in African Americans and Caucasians: the Johnston County Osteoarthritis Project. J Rheumatol. 2007;34(1):172–80.
22. Cavill S, McKenzie K, Munro A, McKeever J, Whelan L, Biggs L, Skinner EH, Haines TP. The effect of prehabilitation on the range of motion and functional outcomes in patients following the total knee or hip arthroplasty: a pilot randomized trial. Physiother Theory Pract. 2016;32(4):262–70. https://doi.org/10.3109/09593985.2016.1138174.
23. Wang L, Lee M, Zhang Z, Moodie J, Cheng D, Martin J. Does preoperative rehabilitation for patients planning to undergo joint replacement surgery improve outcomes? A systematic review and meta-analysis of randomised controlled trials. BMJ Open. 2016;6(2):e009857. https://doi.org/10.1136/bmjopen-2015-009857.
24. Cabilan CJ, Hines S, Munday J. The effectiveness of prehabilitation or preoperative exercise for surgical patients: a systematic review. JBI Database System Rev Implement Rep. 2015;13(1):146–87. https://doi.org/10.11124/jbisrir-2015-1885.
25. Topp R, Swank AM, Quesada PM, Nyland J, Malkani A. The effect of prehabilitation exercise on strength and functioning after total knee arthroplasty. PM R. 2009;1(8):729–35. https://doi.org/10.1016/j.pmrj.2009.06.003.
26. Chughtai M, Shah NV, Sultan AA, Solow M, Tiberi JV, Mehran N, North T, Moskal JT, Newman JM, Samuel LT, Bhave A, Mont MA. The role of prehabilitation with a telerehabilitation system prior to total knee arthroplasty. Ann Transl Med. 2019;7(4):68. https://doi.org/10.21037/atm.2018.11.27.
27. Brown K, Topp R, Brosky JA, Lajoie AS. Prehabilitation and quality of life three months after total knee arthroplasty: a pilot study. Percept Mot Skills. 2012;115(3):765–74. https://doi.org/10.2466/15.06.10.PMS.115.6.765-774.

28. McKay H, Tsang G, Heinonen A, MacKelvie K, Sanderson D, Khan KM. Ground reaction forces associated with an effective elementary school based jumping intervention. Br J Sports Med. 2005;39(1):10–4. https://doi.org/10.1136/bjsm.2003.008615.
29. Walls RJ, McHugh G, O'Gorman DJ, Moyna NM, O'Byrne JM. Effects of preoperative neuromuscular electrical stimulation on quadriceps strength and functional recovery in total knee arthroplasty. A pilot study. BMC Musculoskelet Disord. 2010;11:119. https://doi.org/10.1186/1471-2474-11-119.
30. American College of Sports M. American College of Sports Medicine position stand. Progression models in resistance training for healthy adults. Med Sci Sports Exerc. 2009;41(3):687–708. https://doi.org/10.1249/MSS.0b013e3181915670.
31. Barber-Westin S, Noyes FR. Blood flow-restricted training for lower extremity muscle weakness due to knee pathology: a systematic review. Sports Health. 2019;11(1):69–83. https://doi.org/10.1177/1941738118811337.
32. Hughes L, Paton B, Rosenblatt B, Gissane C, Patterson SD. Blood flow restriction training in clinical musculoskeletal rehabilitation: a systematic review and meta-analysis. Br J Sports Med. 2017;51(13):1003–11. https://doi.org/10.1136/bjsports-2016-097071.
33. Minniti MC, Statkevich AP, Kelly RL, Rigsby VP, Exline MM, Rhon DI, Clewley D. The safety of blood flow restriction training as a therapeutic intervention for patients with musculoskeletal disorders: a systematic review. Am J Sports Med. 2019. 363546519882652. https://doi.org/10.1177/0363546519882652.
34. DePhillipo NN, Kennedy MI, Aman ZS, Bernhardson AS, O'Brien LT, LaPrade RF. The role of blood flow restriction therapy following knee surgery: expert opinion. Arthroscopy. 2018;34(8):2506–10. https://doi.org/10.1016/j.arthro.2018.05.038.
35. Mattocks KT, Jessee MB, Mouser JG, Dankel SJ, Buckner SL, Bell ZW, Owens JG, Abe T, Loenneke JP. The application of blood flow restriction: lessons from the laboratory. Curr Sports Med Rep. 2018;17(4):129–34. https://doi.org/10.1249/jsr.0000000000000473.
36. Skoffer B, Maribo T, Mechlenburg I, Hansen PM, Soballe K, Dalgas U. Efficacy of preoperative progressive resistance training on postoperative outcomes in patients undergoing total knee arthroplasty. Arthritis Care Res. 2016;68(9):1239–51. https://doi.org/10.1002/acr.22825.

Postoperative Rehabilitation Part I: Strategies and Protocol to Avoid Complications and Return to Daily Activities in Postoperative Weeks 1–12

6

Timothy Heckmann, Frank R. Noyes, and Sue Barber-Westin

6.1 Introduction

This is the first of two chapters that detail our total knee arthroplasty (TKA) postoperative rehabilitation program, whose overall goal is to return patients to an active lifestyle to enhance their overall quality of life. The goals in the first 12 postoperative weeks are to resolve pain and swelling and restore adequate range of knee motion (ROM), gait, and balance. Sufficient muscle strength should be present to allow pain-free activities of daily living as well as return to light work and low-impact aerobic activities such as walking, bicycling, and swimming. Complications may be avoided by following the recommended protocol and closely monitoring the patient's progress. Chapter 7 provides additional rehabilitation recommendations for strengthening and aerobic conditioning for patients desiring to return to sports and other more strenuous physical activities, as well as our return to activity testing guidelines.

The topic of postoperative rehabilitation after TKA has received tremendous attention, especially in the last decade. General findings from recent systematic reviews and meta-analyses are shown in Table 6.1 [1–11]. In 2020, the American Physical Therapy Association (APTA) published position statements regarding preoperative and postoperative therapy concepts, and these are summarized in Table 6.2 [12]. The APTA also described prognostic factors that could have an effect on postoperative outcomes, including body mass index, depression, preoperative physical findings, age, gender, use of tobacco products, patient support systems, and comorbidities, and these are shown in Table 6.3 [12]. Nearly all clinical rehabilitation

T. Heckmann · S. Barber-Westin (✉)
Noyes Knee Institute, Cincinnati, OH, USA
e-mail: tpheckmann@mercy.com; sbwestin@csmref.org

F. R. Noyes
Cincinnati SportsMedicine and Orthopaedic Center, The Noyes Knee Institute, Cincinnati, OH, USA

F. R. Noyes, S. Barber-Westin (eds.), *Critical Rehabilitation for Partial and Total Knee Arthroplasty*, https://doi.org/10.1007/978-3-030-87003-4_6

Table 6.1 TKA outpatient postoperative rehabilitation: conclusions from systematic reviews

Citation	Study purpose	No. and type of studies	Dates databases searched	Conclusions
Yue et al. [11]	Compare effectiveness of NMES, TENS, EA quadriceps strength and function	17 RCT	Inception to 10/17	NMES associated with higher quadriceps strength and objective function. Benefits maximal when performed 1–2 ×/day for 3–6 weeks. TENS analgesia benefit over control interventions. Only two studies on EA
Bragonzoni et al. [2]	Determine changes in proprioception and balance	13 any type	1/08–2/18	No consensus exists regarding improvement or worsening in proprioception before or after TKA. Improvements in balance noted by seven studies. High variability in methods, rehabilitation programs, and timeline of follow-up
Domínguez-Navarro et al. [5]	Determine changes in proprioception and balance	7 RCT	Inception to 12/17	Moderate to significant effect of balance and proprioception training on balance and self-reported function (KOOS, KSS, WOMAC)
Doma et al. [4]	Study effects of balance training in patients ≥65 years	12 RCT	Inception to 1/18	Greater improvements in walking capacity, balance-specific performance measures, subjective measures of physical function, and ROM for programs that emphasize balance training compared with conventional programs
Dávila Castrodad et al. [3]	Analyze study design, rehabilitation methods, and outcomes	20 any type	1/13–12/18	Early rehabilitation, telerehabilitation, outpatient therapy, high intensity, and high velocity exercise may be successful. Weight-bearing biofeedback, NMES, and balance control important. Future studies should provide more detail of the rehabilitation methodology
Wang et al. [9]	Determine effectiveness of technology-assisted rehabilitation	17 RCT	Inception to 11/18	Effects too small for clinical significance regarding effects of technology-assisted rehabilitation (especially telerehabilitation) on improvement of function and pain compared with conventional rehabilitation
Pfeufer et al. [7]	Determine effectiveness of biofeedback on outcomes	11 any type	Inception to 5/18	Biofeedback effective improving gait symmetry, reducing pain, increasing activity levels
Buhagiar et al. [1]	Compare outcomes of clinic-based versus home-based programs	5 RCT	Inception to 6/18	Low- to moderate-quality evidence showed no difference between programs in 6-min walk test (10 and 52 wks po), OKS pain, function (10 and 52 wks po), QOL (10–52 wks po), knee ROM

(continued)

Table 6.1 (continued)

Citation	Study purpose	No. and type of studies	Dates databases searched	Conclusions
Kuijer et al. [6]	Determine effect rehabilitation on return to work and sports	None found any type	Inception to 3/17	No studies were found that evaluated the effect of postoperative rehabilitation on return to work or sports
Yang et al. [10]	Evaluate effect CPM	16 RCT	1/2000 to 5/18	No effect on CPM on improving ROM or functional outcomes

CPM continuous passive motion, *EA* electroacupuncture, *KOOS* Knee Injury and Osteoarthritis Score, *KSS* Knee Society Score, *NMES* neuromuscular electrical stimulation, *OKS* Oxford Knee Score, *po* postoperative, *QOL* quality of life, *RCT* randomized controlled trials, *ROM* range of motion, *TENS* transcutaneous electrical nerve stimulation, *wks* weeks, *WOMAC* Western Ontario and McMaster Universities Osteoarthritis Index

studies have focused on the first 12–14 postoperative weeks, and a summary of the major findings of several of these is shown in Table 6.4 [13–28].

Currently, the majority of TKA are outpatient procedures unless the patient has complications related to pain management or anesthesia, which necessitates an overnight hospital stay. We see all patients in our clinic well before surgery, at which time they are provided with extensive verbal, written, and video instructions to prepare them for the procedure [12]. These include postoperative diet, wound care, medications, activity, exercises, cryotherapy, and measures to prevent deep venous thrombosis. Note is made of patients who present with limitations in ROM, and they are advised that additional therapeutic measures may be required to achieve full knee extension and flexion (at least 0–130°) postoperatively. It is also important that the social aspects of the surgical procedure be understood and family responsibilities assigned in terms of the initial postoperative care at home and transportation of the patient to the outpatient rehabilitation facility.

Our patients are instructed to begin knee ROM, ankle pumps, gastroc-soleus stretching, quadriceps isometrics, cryotherapy, compression, and elevation immediately or as soon as possible after surgery. Patients are seen in our clinic on the second or third postoperative day by the surgeon and therapist [12]. Our protocol consists of clinic-based patient visits twice per week for the first four postoperative weeks, once per week during postoperative weeks 5–8, and every other week during postoperative weeks 9–12. The patient sees the surgeon at the third postoperative week for x-rays and an evaluation. If a complication is detected at that time in ROM or muscle dysfunction, additional clinic visits and therapeutic measures will be prescribed. In addition, a home exercise program is provided that is to be conducted every day for the first 12 postoperative weeks. We typically use simple printed exercise sheets to assist in reminding the patient of the exercises to be accomplished. There are also programs such as Medbridge (https://www.medbridgeeducation.com) that allow the therapist to construct a template of exercises that are available to the patient via a mobile app. The home exercise program allows customization of

Table 6.2 Recommendations for rehabilitation after TKA from the APTA 2020 Clinical Practice Guideline[a]

Intervention	No. of studies reviewed	Practice recommendations
Preoperative education	4	Provide and include, at a minimum: patient expectations during hospitalization and factors influencing discharge planning and disposition, postoperative rehabilitation program, safe transferring techniques, use of assistive devices, and fall prevention
Preoperative exercise program	9	Design programs and teach patients to implement strengthening and flexibility exercises
Physical therapy postoperative timing	2	Should start within 24 hours of surgery and prior to discharge
Continuous passive motion device	12	Should NOT be used after primary, uncomplicated TKA
Postoperative ROM exercises	5	Teach and encourage patients to implement passive, active-assistive, and active ROM exercises
Immediate postoperative knee flexion during rest for blood loss and swelling	5	To reduce in the first 7 days after surgery, teach patients to position the knee in some degree of flexion (30°–90°) while resting
Cryotherapy	10	Teach patients and other caregivers the use of cryotherapy; encourage for early postoperative pain management
Neuromuscular electrical stimulation	5	Use to improve quadriceps muscle strength, gait performance, performance-based outcomes, and patient-reported outcomes
Physical activity	11	Develop an early mobility plan and teach patients the importance of early mobility and appropriate progression of PA based on safety, functional tolerance, and physiological response
Motor function training (balance, walking, movement, symmetry)	6	Should be included after TKA
Resistance and intensity of strengthening exercise	4	Design, implement, teach, and progress in high-intensity strength training and exercise programs within 7 days after surgery to improve function, strength, and ROM
Postoperative physical therapy supervision	2	Should be provided, with the optimal setting determined by patient safety, mobility, and environmental and personal factors
Group-based versus individual-based therapy	3	May use group-based or individual-based physical therapy sessions

APTA American Physical Therapy Association, *PA* physical activity, *ROM* range of motion, *TKA* total knee arthroplasty
[a]From Jette et al. [12]

exercises, based on individual patient requirements, and videos are provided of all exercises to enhance correct form. Our entire protocol for the first 12 postoperative weeks is summarized in Table 6.5.

Table 6.3 Prognostic factors to take into consideration for outcomes after TKA from the APTA 2020 Clinical Practice Guideline[a]

Prognostic factor	No. of studies reviewed	Postoperative outcomes
Body mass index (high)	12	Associated more complications, worse outcomes
Depression	3	Associated worse outcomes
Preoperative ROM	4	Positively associated po ROM; minimal effect physical function, quality of life
Preoperative physical function	16	Positively associated physical function
Preoperative strength	2	Positively associated physical function
Age	17	Data mixed PROMS, performance-based, and impairment-based outcomes
Diabetes	6	Not associated worse functional outcomes
Number of comorbidities	8	Greater degree of comorbidity associated worse PROMS
Gender	16	Associated positive and negative effects on outcomes
Tobacco, active use	0	Associated less than optimal functional outcomes
Patient support, lack of	0	Associated less than optimal functional outcomes

APTA American Physical Therapy Association, *BMI* body mass index, *PO* postoperative, *PROMS* patient-reported outcome measures, *ROM* range of motion
[a]From Jette et al. [12]

6.2 Modalities

In the immediate postoperative period, knee joint effusion and swelling of the operative limb must be carefully monitored and controlled. Our patients receive intravenous Decadron at the time of surgery (unless contraindications exist such as diabetes), which significantly decreases postoperative limb swelling. Meticulous surgical techniques, joint hemostasis, and compression dressings without joint drainage are used. Frequently, an anti-inflammatory oral medication is indicated for residual swelling or joint effusion. In the initial outpatient setting, we use electrogalvanic stimulation (EGS) or high-voltage galvanic stimulation (HVGS) with ice, compression, and elevation. EGS/HVGS uses the concept of like charges repelling. The knee joint effusion has a negative electrical charge, and therefore, placement of the negative electrodes at the knee and the positive (dispersive) electrode on either the low back or opposite thigh will assist the body in removing the fluid from the joint. Newer electrical modalities have programs which have active treatment electrodes that do not require the use of a separate dispersive electrode. The treatment duration is approximately 30 minutes, and patients are encouraged to use this portable modality three to six times per day. The intensity is set each time to patient tolerance.

When knee joint effusion is controlled, neuromuscular electrical stimulation (NMES) is used to facilitate and enhance quadriceps contraction [11, 12, 27, 28]. One electrode is placed over the vastus medialis oblique (VMO), and the second electrode is placed on the central to lateral aspect of the upper third of the

Table 6.4 Summary of recent comparative clinical studies of postoperative TKA rehabilitation

Citation	N	Trial and assessment tests PO time periods		Major findings, exercise group compared with control group	
		Trial	Tests	Intervention	Findings
Bade et al. [13]	162, RCT	11 weeks	3, 6, 12 months	High-intensity versus low-intensity rehabilitation protocols	No differences in outcomes for several objective tests, WOMAC, SF-12, and quadriceps and hamstring strength
Bruun-Olsen et al. [14]	57, RCT	12–14 weeks	12–15 weeks, 9 months	Walking skill program	Superior 6 MWT results only; no difference in timed stair climbing, timed stands, ROM, and KOOS scores
Christiansen et al. [15]	26, RCT	6 weeks	6, 26 weeks	Weight-bearing biofeedback training in addition to standard rehabilitation	Program increased knee extension moments during walking and reduced time to perform SST. No effect on gait analysis functional weight-bearing symmetry on walking or knee extension moments during SST
Hsu et al. [16]	34, comparative study	24 weeks	24 weeks	Circuit training program in women	Significantly superior improvements in stride length, step velocity, excursion active ROM, KOOS scores, and SF-36 scores
Hsu et al. [17]	29, comparative study	24 weeks	24, 36 weeks	Resistance training program in women	Improved knee extensor and flexor isokinetic strength at 60°/s, distance in 6 MWT, KOOS scores. However, improvements not significantly superior to control group
Husby et al. [18]	41, RCT	9 weeks	10 weeks, 12 months	Maximal strength training (80–90% 1-RM)	Significant and superior improvements in leg press and knee extension 1-RM values both test periods. No difference pain, 6 MWT, or KOOS scores

(continued)

Table 6.4 (continued)

Citation	N	Trial and assessment tests PO time periods		Major findings, exercise group compared with control group	
		Trial	Tests	Intervention	Findings
Jakobsen et al. [19]	82, RCT	7 weeks	8, 26 weeks	Progressive strength training in addition to standard rehabilitation	No difference in outcomes for 6 MWT, isometric knee extension strength, KOOS scores, Oxford scores, pain, and ROM
Karaman et al. [20]	46, RCT	6 weeks	6 weeks	Pilates-based exercises in addition to standard rehabilitation	Superior improvements in Berg balance test and SF-36 scores
Li et al. [21]	107, RCT	14 weeks	14 weeks	Tai chi chuan exercises	Superior outcomes for WOMAC physical function score, 6 MWT, and SF-36 scores. No difference in WOMAC pain score or ROM
Liao et al. [22]	130, RCT	8 weeks	8, 32 weeks	Balance exercises in addition to standard rehabilitation	Superior improvements in balance (functional reach and single-leg stance), gait speed, timed up-and-go test, 30-s timed chair-stand test, stair-climb test, and WOMAC physical function score
Molla et al. [23]	40, RCT	7 weeks	7, 9 weeks	Early resistive exercises in addition to standard rehabilitation	Superior balance scores (Romberg, Star Excursion, Berg)
Paravlic et al. [44]	26, RCT	4 weeks	4 weeks	Motor imagery in addition to standard rehabilitation	Lower deterioration in quadriceps isometric strength, SST, gait speed under single and dual task conditions
Piva et al. [45]	44, RCT	6 months	6 months	Comprehensive behavioral intervention (intense exercises and education program)	Resulted in less pain, higher SF-36 physical function scores, superior single-leg stance test scores

(continued)

Table 6.4 (continued)

Citation	N	Trial and assessment tests PO time periods		Major findings, exercise group compared with control group	
		Trial	Tests	Intervention	Findings
Piva et al. [24]	240, RCT	12 weeks	3 and 6 months	Exercise programs (clinical based or community based)	Resulted in superior scores on performance tests and patient-reported outcome measures
Sattler et al. [25]	60, RCT	2 weeks	2 days, 2 weeks, 4 months	Pedaling-based protocol	Superior to a standard rehabilitation protocol in 6 MWT, OKS, EQ-5D
Schache et al. [26]	105, RCT	8 weeks	6, 26 weeks	Hip abductor strengthening in addition to standard rehabilitation	No difference in improvements in hip strength or KOOS, LEFS, or SF-12 scores
Stevens-Lapsley et al. [27]	66, RCT	6 weeks	3.5, 6.5, 13, 26, 52 weeks	Quadriceps muscle NMES in addition to standard rehabilitation	Superior muscle strength, ROM, 6 MWT, stair-climb test, TUG test at 3.5 weeks postoperatively, but no differences at 52 weeks postoperatively
Yoshida et al. [28]	66, RCT	2 weeks	2, 4 weeks	Motor-level NMES and sensory-level NMES in additional to standard rehabilitation	Superior maximum voluntary isometric contraction and 2 MWT early postoperatively

SF-36 Short Form 36, *KOOS* Knee Injury and Osteoarthritis Outcome Score, *LEFS* Lower Extremity Functional Scale, *MWT* min walk test, *OKS* Oxford Knee Score, *NMES* neuromuscular electrical stimulation, *RCT* randomized controlled trial, *ROM* range of motion, *SST* sit-to-stand test, *WOMAC* Western Ontario and McMaster Universities Osteoarthritis Index

quadriceps muscle belly. The treatment duration is 15–20 minutes. The patient actively contracts the quadriceps muscle simultaneously with the machine's stimulation. NMES is continued until the muscle grade is rated as good.

Biofeedback is also useful in enhancing the active quadriceps contraction if the patient is having difficulty initiating an active quadriceps contraction. It may also be used to facilitate hamstring relaxation if the patient has difficulty achieving full knee extension due to knee pain or muscle spasm. The surface electrode may be placed over the selected muscle component to provide positive feedback to the patient and clinician regarding the quality of active or voluntary muscle contraction or, conversely, muscle relaxation. The electrode may also be positioned over the hamstring muscle belly while the patient performs ROM exercises. When used for

9 weeks postoperatively, biofeedback was reported to be effective in improving gait symmetry, reducing pain, and increasing activity levels in a systematic review [7].

Cryotherapy is initiated immediately postoperatively and is continued throughout the entire rehabilitation program as required for pain and swelling control [12]. This treatment may be accomplished with an ice bag, commercial cold pack, or motorized cooler unit. Motorized cooler units are empirically preferred by the patients because they maintain a constant temperature, thereby providing excellent pain control. Cryotherapy is used for 20 minutes at a time, from three to five times per day if required depending on the extent of pain and swelling. Vasopneumatic devices are another option for cryotherapy. The Game Ready device (CoolSystems, Concord, CA) allows the clinician to set the temperature as well as one of four different compression levels based on patient tolerance.

6.3 Range of Motion and Weight-Bearing

ROM exercises are initiated immediately postoperatively using passive and active-assisted exercises. We do not routinely use a continuous passive motion machine. A systematic review of 16 studies determined that this modality does not offer any benefit in improving ROM or functional outcomes [10], and the APTA position statement agreed with this recommendation [12]. Patients perform passive and active-assisted ROM exercises in a seated position for 10 minutes per session, approximately four to six times per day.

The ROM goals are shown in Table 6.5. If 0° of extension has not been reached by the end of the first postoperative week, an overpressure program is initiated with the use of hanging weights (Fig. 6.1). The goal is to produce a gradual stretching of posterior capsular tissues, but not to induce soft tissue tearing because this could lead to an inflammatory response. The foot and ankle are propped on a towel or other device to elevate the hamstrings and gastrocnemius that allows the knee to "drop" into full extension. This position is maintained for 10–15 minutes and repeated four to six times per day. Weight may be added to the distal thigh and knee to provide overpressure to stretch the posterior capsule. We begin with 10 pounds and may increase to 15–20 pounds if 0° has not been obtained by the end of the second postoperative week. An extension board may also be used at this time in the clinic. If these measures are not effective, a drop-out (bi-valved) cast is used for 24–36 hours to provide continuous overpressure. There is a possibility of continuing the use of the drop-out cast as a night splint for the following 1–2 weeks if full knee extension is not maintained.

Knee flexion of 90° must be obtained by the end of the first postoperative week and is slowly advanced, with the goal of 130° to be achieved by postoperative weeks 9–12. Passive flexion exercises are performed in the seated position using the opposite lower extremity to provide overpressure. Patients who do not achieve the goals shown in Table 6.5 use overpressure exercises, including a rolling-stool option (Fig. 6.2), wall slides (Fig. 6.3), and commercial knee flexion devices (Fig. 6.4)

Table 6.5 Noyes Knee Institute rehabilitation protocol for TKA (weeks 1–12)

	Postoperative weeks				
	1–2	3–4	5–6	7–8	9–12
Brace: long-leg postoperative: use in high risk patients with concurrent patellar realignment or medial collateral ligament repair, or lack of quadriceps control, difficulty with balance/coordination	X	X			
Modalities:					
Electrical muscle stimulation	X	X	X		
Pain/edema management (cryotherapy)	X	X	X	X	X
Range of motion minimum goals:					
0°–90°	X				
0°–110°		X			
0°–120°			X		
0°–125°				X	
0°–130°					X
Weight-bearing:					
Toe touch to 50% body weight	X				
100% body weight, wean from assistive devices		X			
Patella mobilization	X	X	X	X	
Muscle flexibility:					
Hamstring, gastrocnemius-soleus, gluteal	X	X	X	X	X
Iliotibial band, quadriceps			X	X	X
Strengthening:					
Ankle pumps (begin plantar flexion with resistance band at week 3)	X	X			
Quadriceps isometrics, straight leg raises	X	X	X	X	X
Knee extension quadriceps active assisted	X				
Closed-chain: wall sits		X	X	X	X
Closed-chain: toe/heel raises		X	X	X	X
Closed-chain: forward step-ups, mini-squats			X	X	X
Closed-chain: lateral step-ups, forward step-downs				X	X
Knee flexion hamstring curls (0°–90°)		X	X	X	X
Knee extension quadriceps (90°–0°)		X	X	X	X
Hip abduction-adduction, multi-hip			X	X	X
Leg press (80°–10°)			X	X	X
Upper body weight training			X	X	X
Core training			X	X	X
Balance/gait/proprioceptive training:					
Weight shifting, cup walking	X	X	X		
Balance board two-legged, tandem stance		X	X		
Single-leg stance (insert ball catch at week 7)			X	X	X
Band walking: forward, lateral			X	X	X
Band walking: diagonal, monster walk					X
Y-balance reaching					X
Conditioning:					
Upper body conditioner		X	X	X	X
Stationary bicycling (high seat, low resistance)		X	X	X	X
Aquatic program (water walking, depth at thigh or waist)			X	X	X
Stair machine (low resistance, low stroke)				X	X
Ski machine (short stride, level, low resistance)				X	X
Elliptical machine				X	X
Swimming (kicking)					X
Walking					X

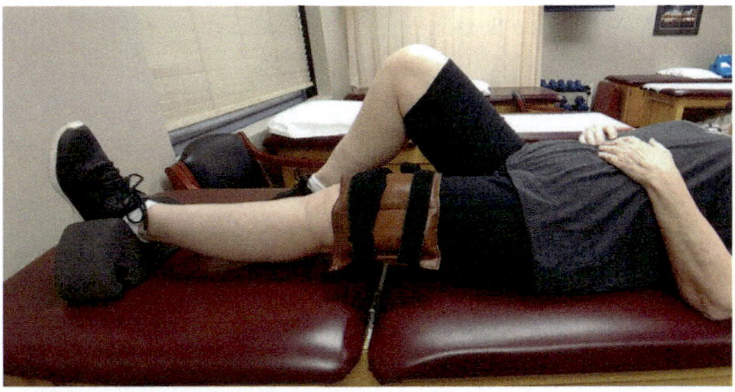

Fig. 6.1 Hanging weight extension overpressure exercise

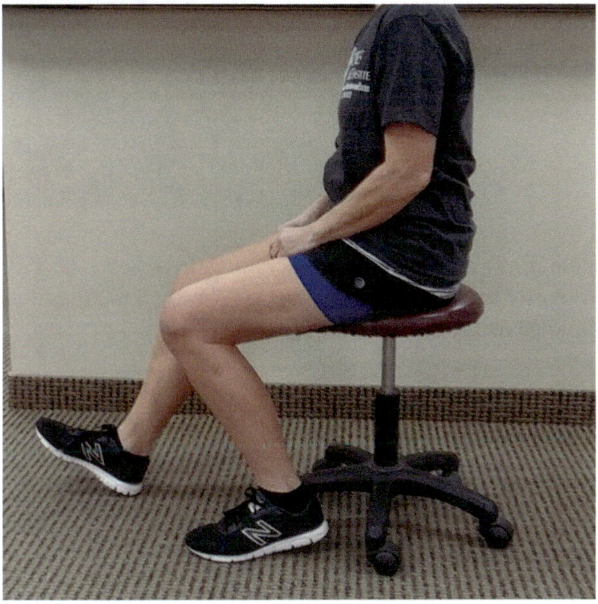

Fig. 6.2 Rolling-stool flexion overpressure exercise

[29]. At the end of the third to fourth postoperative week, the surgeon conducts a thorough examination and may recommend a gentle ranging of the knee under anesthesia for those who fail to reach 100° of flexion. Usually, the therapist can tell by the second to third week that the patient is only achieving 70°–80° of flexion, with no progression after the third week. Significant pain may occur with knee flexion that inhibits the therapist's ability to gently move the knee joint. This indicates early arthrofibrosis and may be accompanied by limited patella mobility. It is important to perform an early manipulation, well before six postoperative weeks, if the scar tissue is pronounced. This is not a forceful manipulation because no more than two to three fingers of pressure are used at the distal tibia to achieve knee flexion. If more force is required, this indicates that a peripatellar contracture is present that consists of more dense, resistant scar that, if untreated, may result in the need for an arthroscopic debridement. In our center, careful attention to these knee motion

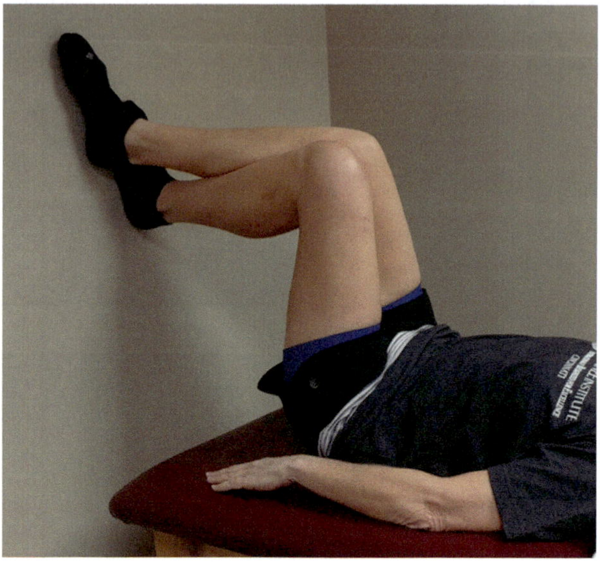

Fig. 6.3 Wall slide flexion overpressure exercise

guidelines and treatment procedures avoids the necessity for further surgery in the majority of cases. We previously described the diagnosis, prevention, and treatment of knee arthrofibrosis elsewhere [29].

6.4 Patellar Mobilization and Muscle Flexibility

Restoring normal patellar mobility is critical to regain normal ROM. The loss of patellar mobility is often associated with arthrofibrosis and, in extreme cases, the development of patella infera [30–32]. Patellar glides are initiated on the first post-operative day in all four planes (superior, inferior, medial, and lateral) with sustained pressure applied to the appropriate patellar border for at least 10 seconds (Fig. 6.5). This exercise is performed for 5 minutes before ROM exercises. Caution is warranted if an extensor lag is detected because this may be associated with poor superior migration of the patella, indicating the need for additional emphasis on this exercise. Patellar mobilization is performed for approximately 8 weeks postoperatively.

Hamstring and gastrocnemius-soleus flexibility exercises are also initiated on the first postoperative day. A sustained static stretch is held for 30 seconds and repeated five times. The most common hamstring stretch is the modified hurdler stretch, while the most common gastrocnemius-soleus stretch is the towel pull. These exercises help control pain owing to the reflex response created in the hamstrings when the knee is kept in the flexed position. In addition, the towel-pulling exercise can help lessen discomfort in the calf, Achilles tendon, and ankle. These stretches represent critical components of the knee extension ROM program because the ability to relax these two muscle groups is imperative to achieve full passive knee

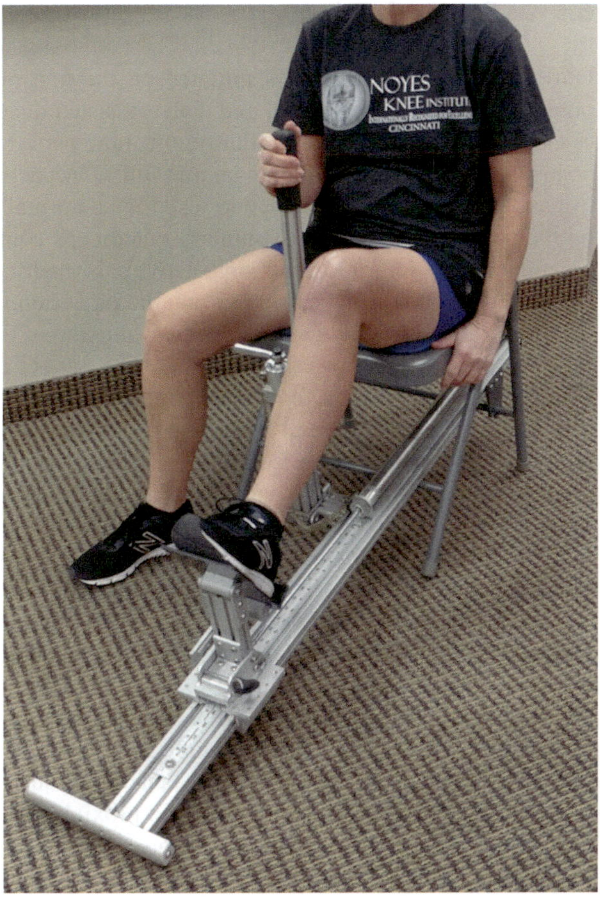

Fig. 6.4 Commercial flexion overpressure device (Knee Flexionater, ERMI, Atlanta, GA)

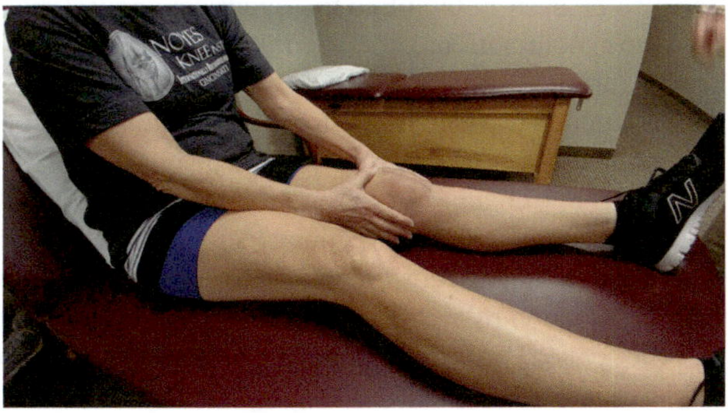

Fig. 6.5 Patellar mobilization performed by the patient

extension. Quadriceps and iliotibial band flexibility exercises are initiated 5 weeks postoperatively to assist in achieving full knee flexion and controlling lateral hip and thigh tightness.

6.5 Strengthening

Our strengthening program is initiated on the first postoperative day with ankle pumps, quadriceps isometrics, and active-assisted quadriceps knee extension exercises. These exercises are used during this time period when emphasis is placed on controlling pain and swelling, regaining full ROM, achieving early quadriceps control and proximal stabilization, and resuming a normal gait pattern. Early emphasis on the generation of a good voluntary quadriceps contraction is critical for a successful and safe return to functional activity. Isometric quadriceps contractions are completed on an hourly basis following the repetition rules of 10-second holds, ten repetitions, ten times per day. Adequate evaluation of the quadriceps contraction by both the therapist and patient is critical. The patient can monitor contractions by visual or manual means, comparing the quality of the contractions with those achieved by the contralateral limb. The patient can also assess the superior migration of the patella during the contraction, which should be approximately 1 cm, and the inferior migration of the patella during the initial relaxation of the contraction. The patient should not let the knee go into hyperextension during isometric contractions but hold the neutral knee flexion position throughout the exercise. If necessary, biofeedback can also be used to reinforce a good quadriceps contraction.

Straight leg raises are initiated at the first postoperative visit in hip flexion and then progressed in all four planes of hip movement once the quadriceps can control knee position. They are continued through the first 12 postoperative weeks. The adduction straight leg raise has been suggested to have a beneficial effect on the recruitment of the VMO. Supine straight leg raises must include a sufficient isometric quadriceps contraction in order to benefit the quadriceps. Straight leg raises in the other two planes are also important for proximal stabilization. As these exercises become easy to perform, ankle weights are added to progress muscle strengthening. Initially, 1–2 pounds of weight is used, and eventually, up to 10 pounds is added as long as this is not more than 10% of the patient's body weight. Active-assisted ROM can also be used to facilitate the quadriceps muscle if poor tone is observed during isometric contractions. Resisted knee extension is initiated with Velcro ankle weights from 90° to 0°.

Gastrocnemius-soleus strength is a key component for early ambulation. A resistance band is added to ankle pumps at postoperative week 2 for plantar flexion. Closed kinetic chain exercises are initiated during this time period, with toe and heel raises for further gastrocnemius-soleus strengthening and wall-sitting isometrics (Fig. 6.6) for quadriceps control. The goal of wall sitting is to improve the quadriceps contraction by performing the exercise to muscle fatigue. If anterior knee pain is experienced, the position may be modified by either altering the knee flexion angle of the sit or by subtly changing the toe-out/toe-in angle up to 10°. The exercise may also be modified to produce greater challenge to the quadriceps. The patient may voluntarily set the quadriceps muscle once he or she reaches the desired knee flexion angle, which is typically between 30° and 45°. This contraction and knee flexion position are held until muscle fatigue occurs and the exercise is repeated three to five times. The patient may squeeze a ball between the distal thighs, inducing a hip adduction contraction which can facilitate a stronger VMO contraction. In a third variation, the patient holds dumbbell weights in the hands to increase body weight, which promotes an even stronger quadriceps contraction. An additional variation includes the use of an elastic band placed proximal to the patella. The patient is encouraged to maintain a hip abduction contraction in addition to their quadriceps contraction to facilitate improved balance of quadriceps and hip abductor strength. Finally, the patient can shift the body weight over the involved side to stimulate a single-leg contraction. This exercise is promoted as an excellent one for the patient to perform at home four to six times per day to achieve quadriceps fatigue in a safe knee flexion angle that does not induce an abnormal anterior tibial translation.

Forward step-ups are initiated during postoperative week 5, while lateral step-ups and forward step-downs are initiated 2 weeks later. The height of the step is gradually increased based on patient tolerance (Fig. 6.7).

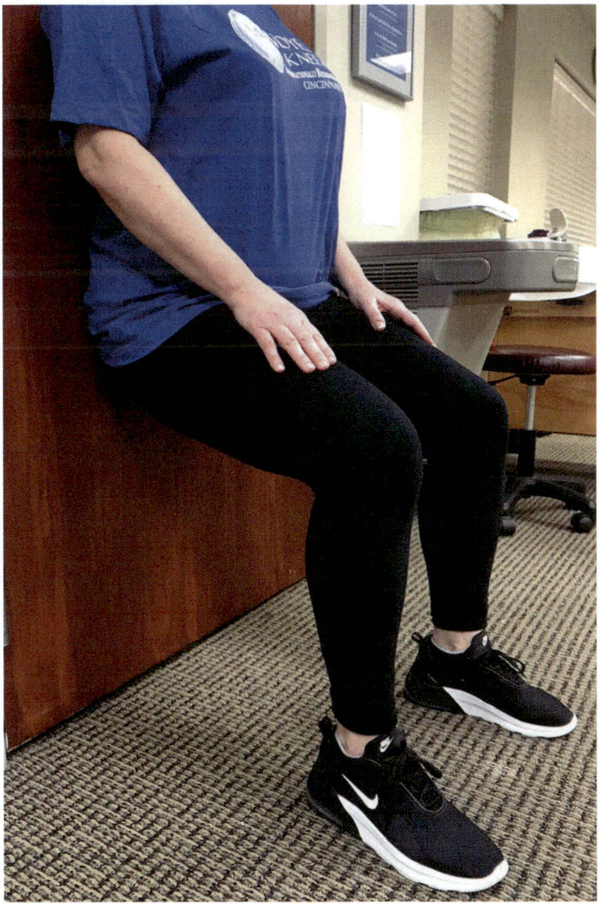

Fig. 6.6 Wall sit exercise

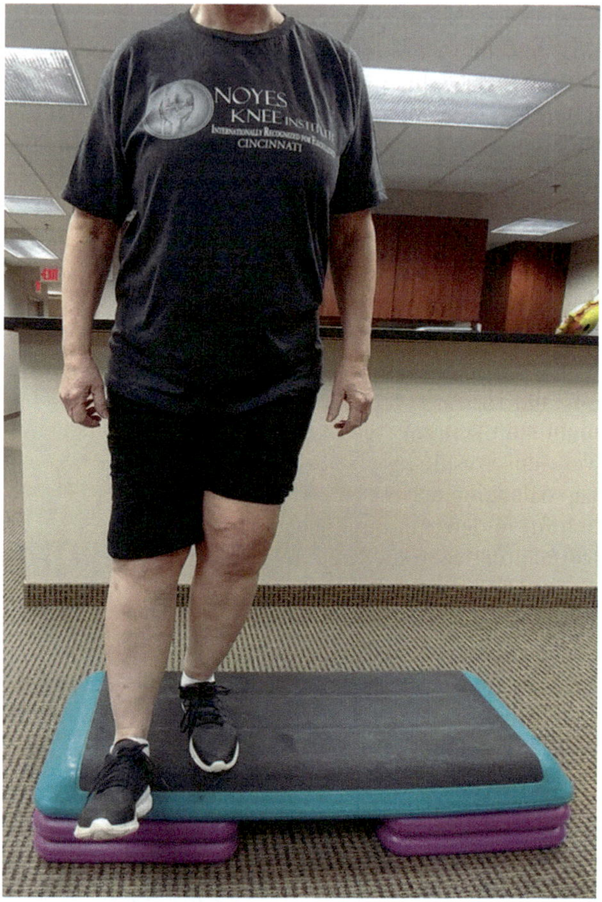

Fig. 6.7 Forward step-down exercise

A full lower extremity strengthening program is critical for early and long-term success of the rehabilitation program. Knee extension on a weight machine is initiated at postoperative week 4 from 90° to 0° (Fig. 6.8). Knee flexion curls are initiated with Velcro ankle weights at postoperative week 3 and eventually advanced to weight machines (Fig. 6.9). Weight machines are initiated at postoperative week 5 for hip abductors, hip adductors, hip flexors, and hip extensors. Leg press exercises are also initiated at postoperative weeks 5 to 6 from 80° to 10° (Fig. 6.10). Weight machines are advantageous owing to the muscle isolation obtained as the machine provides stability to the knee joint. The patient exercises the involved limb alone as well as both limbs together. If the lightest amount of weight on the machine is too heavy to be lifted by the involved limb alone, the exercise may be performed as an eccentric contraction in which the patient lifts the weight with both legs and lowers the weight with the involved side. Eccentric contractions may also be used in the advanced stages of strength training. In addition, upper extremity and core strength are important for a safe and effective return to work or physical activities.

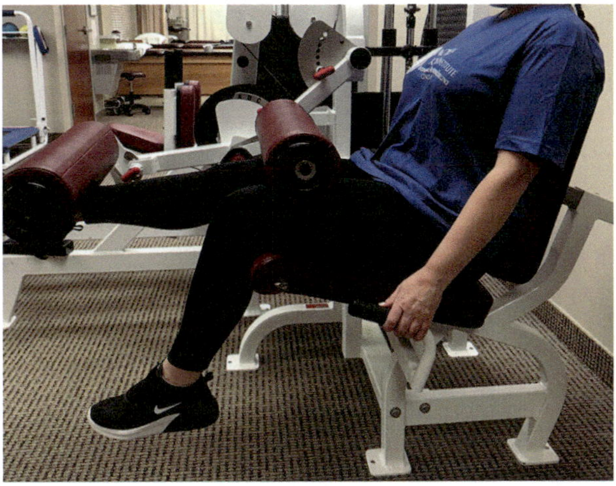

Fig. 6.8 Knee extensions performed from 90° to 0°

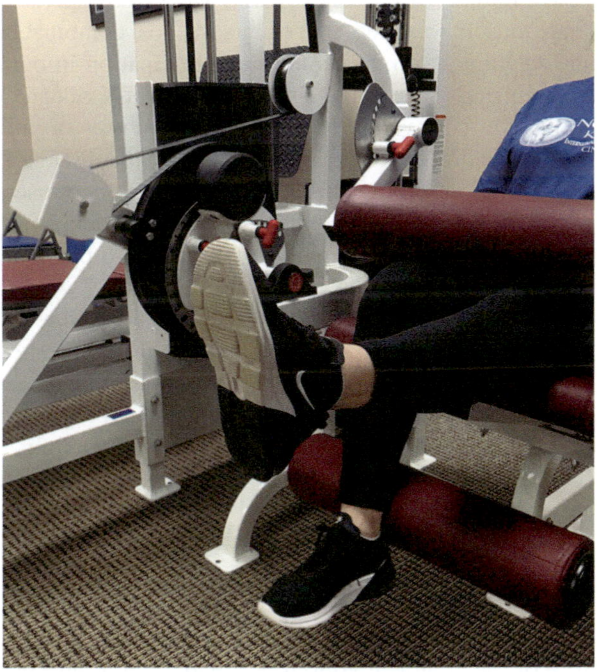

Fig. 6.9 Knee flexion curls performed from 0° to 90°

6.6 Blood Flow Restriction Training

Substantial evidence exists that many TKA patients suffer from persistent quadriceps and hamstrings strength deficits postoperatively [33, 34]. Blood flow restriction training (BFRT) with low-resistance loads (30% of 1-RM) has been advocated to lessen muscle atrophy after a variety of operative procedures [35–37]. Partial

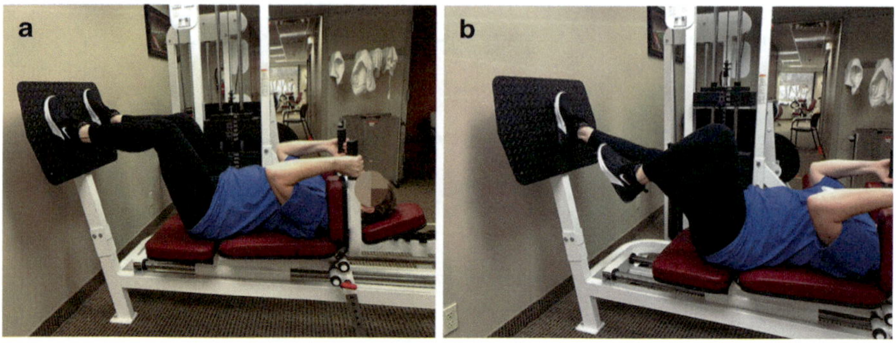

Fig. 6.10 Leg press machine may be performed either bilaterally (**a**) or unilaterally (**b**)

vascular occlusion is achieved with an extremity tourniquet and is combined with weight-bearing, non-weight-bearing, and resistance machine exercises [38, 39].

We initiate BFRT as early as 4 weeks postoperatively in patients who demonstrate muscle weakness that occurs due to a combination of postoperative knee pain and swelling that inhibits normal participation in our rehabilitation protocol. The incision must be completely healed and no evidence of the following: history or current varicose veins, deep venous thrombosis or pulmonary embolism, diabetes, neurological disease, peripheral vascular insufficiency, lower leg edema, myocardial infarction, stroke, unstable cardiac disease, or use of heart medications, as well as no hypertension (>140/90) or cardiac disorders of any type including tachycardia (>100 bpm) [40]. Patients must be willing to perform the program initially in the clinic, which entails three visits per week for 2 weeks. Then, the program may be done at home in addition to the other home-based rehabilitation exercises. Our data indicates that in this population, at least 18 training sessions (three times per week for 6 weeks) are required for strength gains to be achieved.

Patients are instructed to place the cuff around their upper thigh as close to the inguinal area as comfortable and tighten it snugly against their skin or shorts (Fig. 6.11). In patients who have adipose tissue, the cuff is instructed to be comfortably tight. Pressure is determined using a Doppler ultrasound in either the supine or 45° inclined position. Patients are instructed to inflate the cuff, and limb occlusion pressure is measured until there are no Doppler arterial pulses, indicating complete arterial occlusion. The limb muscles remain in a relaxed state during this process. The cuff pressures during the exercises are individualized and set between 60% and 80% of the complete arterial occlusion pressure to provide a minimum and maximum threshold for BFRT.

The exercise protocol consists of leg press (Fig. 6.12a), knee extension either with ankle weight (Fig. 6.12b) or on a weight machine, mini-squats, and hamstring curls (Table 6.6). Straight leg raises may be used as a substitute in the exercise protocol, depending on patient tolerance (Fig. 6.12c, d). The cuff is inflated for the duration of each of the four exercises. After the fourth set of repetitions for each exercise, the cuff is deflated for 2 minutes. We use a commercially available 10-cm

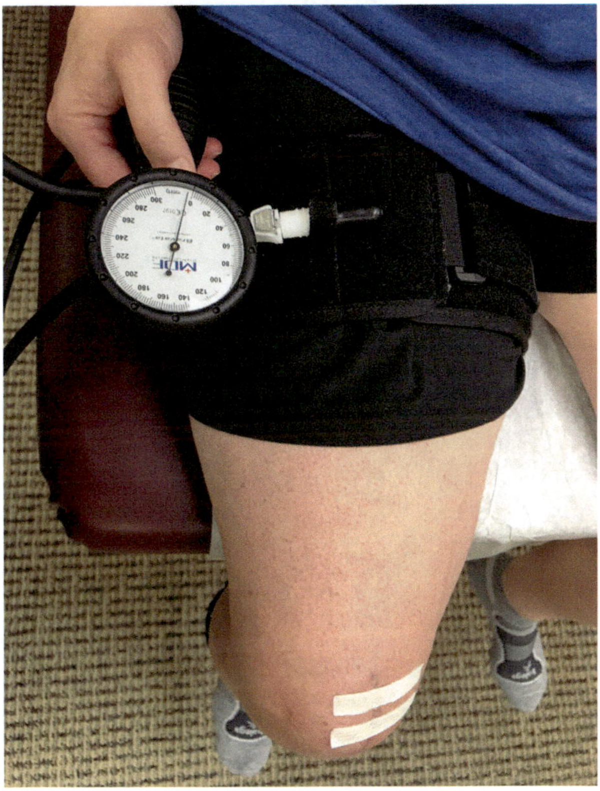

Fig. 6.11 Blood flow resistance training cuff setup

wide cuff (SmartCuffs, Strongsville, OH) because of better tolerance and less pressure required to achieve partial occlusion [41]. Total occlusion time for the exercise session is expected to be approximately 28–32 minutes.

Recent BFRT studies have evaluated safety and adverse events and concluded that this treatment modality is safe and no more likely to result in an adverse event when compared with standard exercises [38, 39, 42, 43]. Still, clinicians need to be aware of preexisting or risk factors before recommending BFRT. The most frequent patient complaints are delayed muscle soreness and fatigue, so close supervision is necessary to monitor cuff pressures, exercises, and patient safety.

6.7 Balance, Gait, and Proprioceptive Training

Restoration of normal balance and knee joint proprioception is an important element of neuromuscular function leading to a successful outcome [2, 4, 5, 12, 22]. Balance and proprioceptive training are initiated on the first postoperative week. Initially, the patient simply stands and shifts weight from side to side and front to back. This activity encourages confidence in the leg's ability to withstand the pressures of weight-bearing and initiates the stimulus to knee joint position sense. Cup

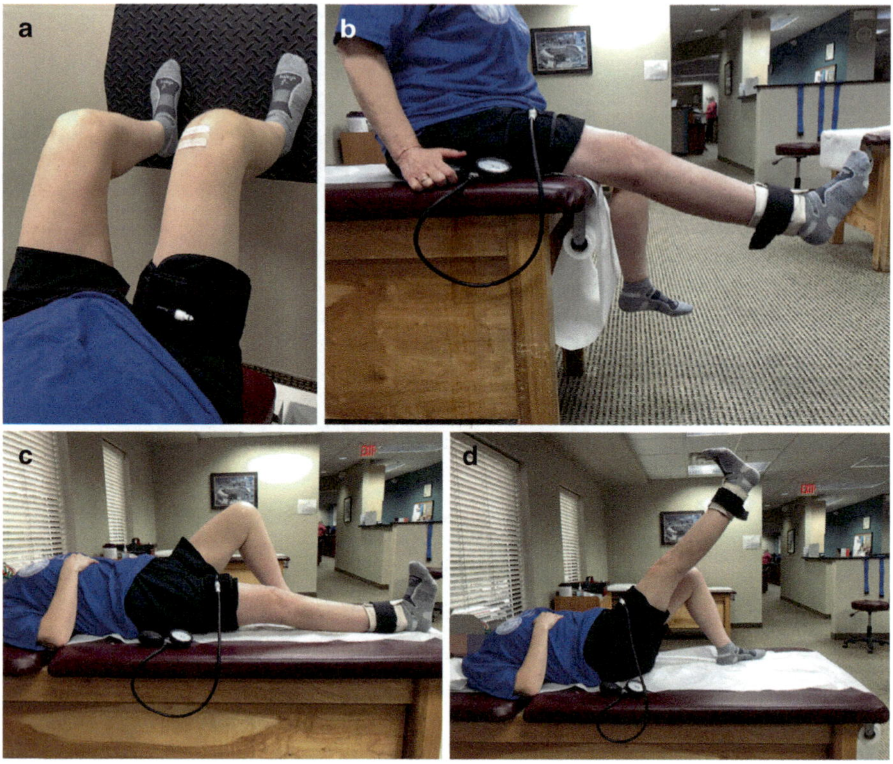

Fig. 6.12 Blood flow resistance training with a leg press (**a**), knee extension with ankle weight (**b**), and supine straight leg raise (**c**, **d**)

Table 6.6 Blood flow restriction training exercise protocol

Exercise	Repetitions	Rest	Repetitions	Rest	Repetitions	Rest	Repetitions	Rest
#1 Leg press machine, 30% 1-RM	30	1 min	15	1 min	15	1 min	15	2 min, cuff deflated
#2 Hamstring curl machine, 30% 1-RM	30	1 min	15	1 min	15	1 min	15	2 min, cuff deflated
#3 Leg extension machine, 30% 1-RM	30	1 min	15	1 min	15	1 min	15	2 min, cuff deflated
#4 Mini-squat	30	1 min	15	1 min	15	1 min	15	2 min, cuff deflated

1-RM 1 repetition maximum, *min* minute

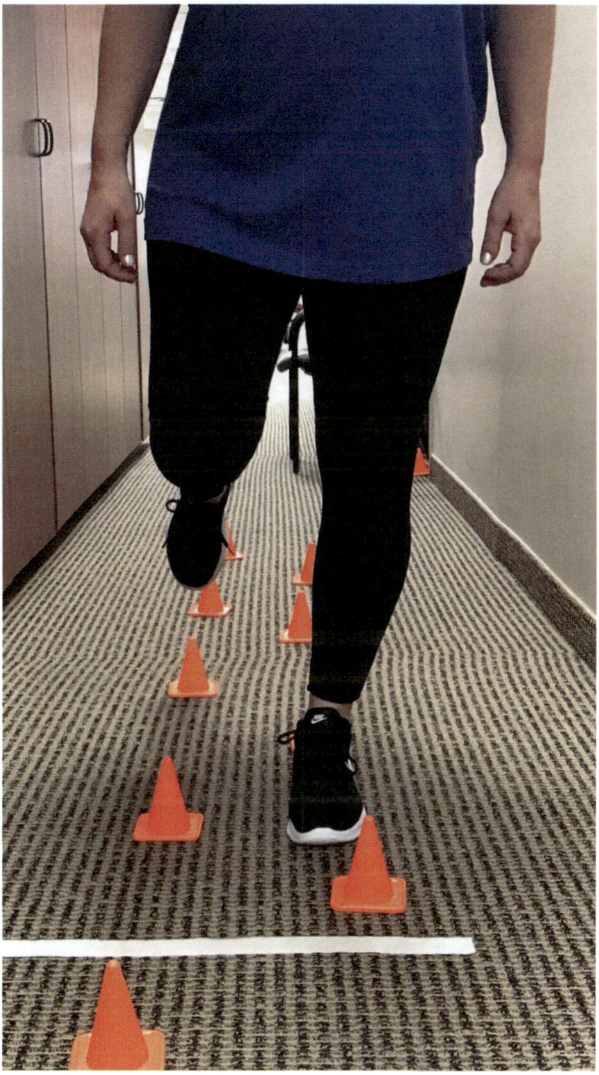

Fig. 6.13 Cup walking done to promote symmetry between the surgical and uninvolved limbs

walking is also initiated to promote symmetry between the surgical and uninvolved limbs (Fig. 6.13). This exercise helps develop hip and knee flexion, as well as quadriceps control during midstance of gait to prevent knee hyperextension. In addition, cup walking controls hip and pelvic motion during midstance, gastrocnemius-soleus activity during push-off, and excessive hip hiking.

Double-leg balance exercises in the stance position are highly beneficial and begin during postoperative weeks 3–4. These are advanced from tandem stance to single-leg stance, with the foot pointed straight ahead, the knee flexed 20°–30°, the arms extended outward to horizontal, and the torso positioned upright with the shoulders above the hips and the hips above the ankles. The objective is to remain

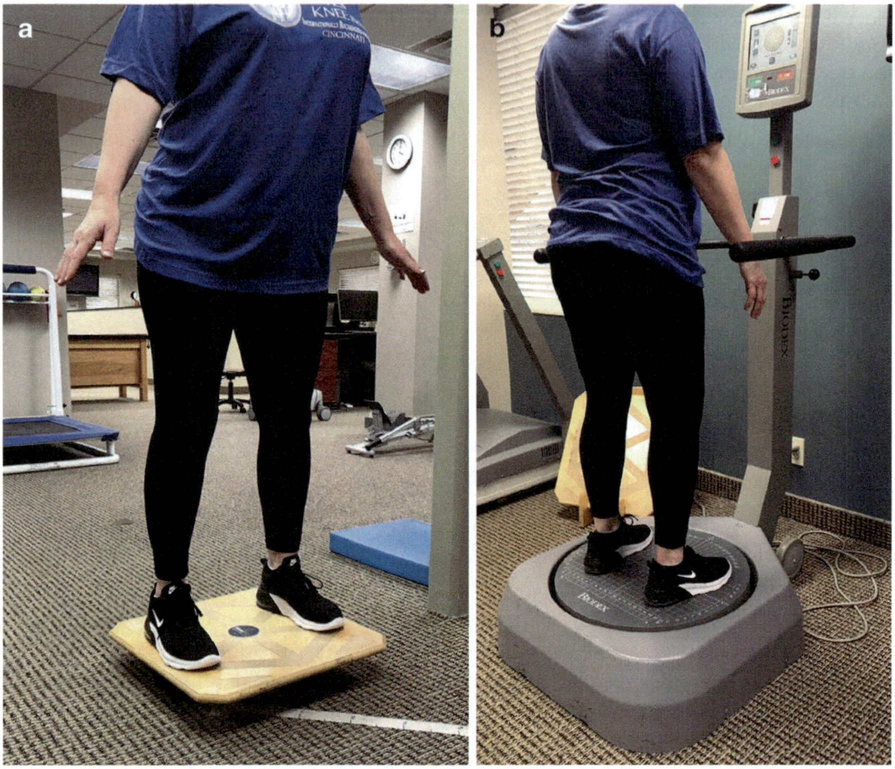

Fig. 6.14 Balance exercises using a balance board (**a**) or Biodex stability system (**b**)

in this position until balance is disturbed. A mini trampoline or unstable platform (Fig. 6.14a, b) may be used to make this exercise more challenging because these devices promote greater dynamic limb control than that required to stand on a stable surface. To provide a greater challenge, patients may assume the single-leg stance position and throw/catch a weighted ball against an inverted mini trampoline (pitch back) until fatigue occurs.

Half foam rolls are also used in this time frame as part of the gait retraining and balance program. This exercise helps the patient develop balance and dynamic muscular control required to maintain an upright position and to walk from one end of the roll to the other. Developing a center of balance, limb symmetry, quadriceps control in midstance, and postural positioning are benefits developed from this type of training. Resistance band walking in the forward and lateral positions (Fig. 6.15a, b) is initiated during postoperative week 5 and advanced to diagonal and monster walking (exaggerated walking) during postoperative week 9. At this time, the patient may also begin balance reaching using the Y-balance test setup (Fig. 6.16).

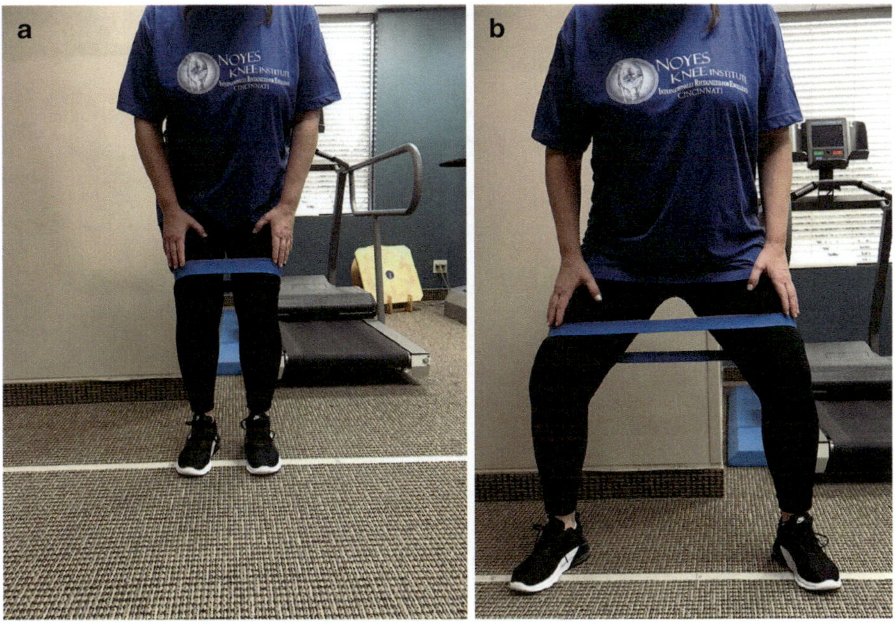

Fig. 6.15 Band walking in the lateral position (**a**, **b**)

6.8 Aerobic Conditioning

The primary consideration for a conditioning program throughout the rehabilitation period is to stress the cardiovascular system without compromising the knee joint. Early goals include facilitation of full ROM, gait retraining, and cardiovascular reconditioning. Depending on accessibility, an aerobic conditioning program is initiated with an upper extremity ergometer at postoperative week 3. The surgical limb should be elevated to minimize lower extremity swelling. This exercise is performed as tolerated. Stationary bicycling is also initiated at this time, with the seat height adjusted to its highest level based on patient body size and a low resistance level used initially. Patient access and tolerance may dictate the use of a recumbent style bicycle as opposed to a traditional upright bicycle. Water walking may be initiated during the fifth postoperative week for patients who have access to a pool and have complete wound closure.

Cross-country ski, stair climbing, and elliptical machines are permitted during the seventh to eighth postoperative weeks. Stair-climbing machines are adjusted to produce a short step and low resistance. In order to improve cardiovascular endurance, the program should be performed at least three times per week for 20–30 minutes, and the exercise performed to at least 60–85% of maximal heart rate. It is generally regarded that performing exercise in the higher percentage levels of maximal heart rate achieves greater cardiovascular efficiency and endurance. It is critical as the patient progresses on weight and conditioning exercises to monitor for knee

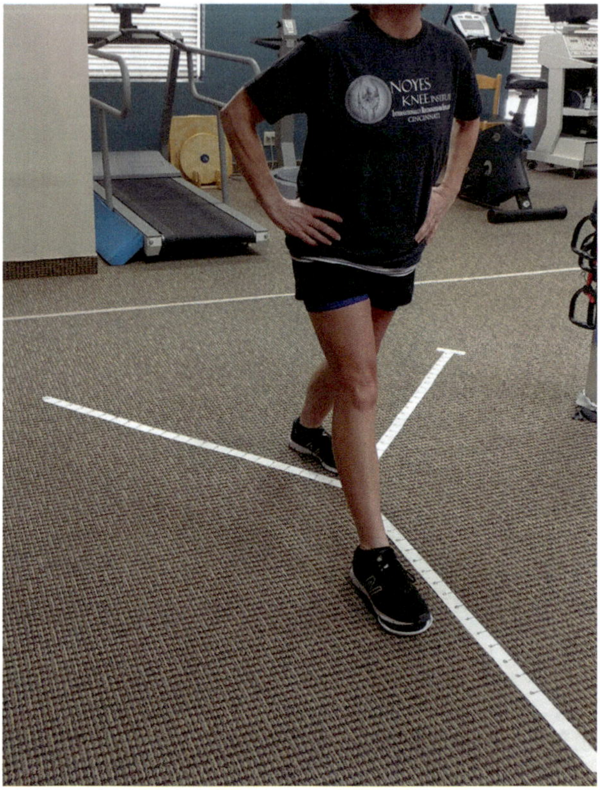

Fig. 6.16 Y-balance reach exercise

joint pain and swelling and to adjust the program as required. Swimming (lap work using freestyle or flutter kicking, water aerobics) and walking for exercise are permitted at 9–12 weeks postoperatively.

References

1. Buhagiar MA, Naylor JM, Harris IA, Xuan W, Adie S, Lewin A. Assessment of outcomes of inpatient or clinic-based vs home-based rehabilitation after total knee arthroplasty: a systematic review and meta-analysis. JAMA Netw Open. 2019;2(4):e192810. https://doi.org/10.1001/jamanetworkopen.2019.2810.
2. Bragonzoni L, Rovini E, Barone G, Cavallo F, Zaffagnini S, Benedetti MG. How proprioception changes before and after total knee arthroplasty: a systematic review. Gait Posture. 2019;72:1–11. https://doi.org/10.1016/j.gaitpost.2019.05.005.
3. Dávila Castrodad IM, Recai TM, Abraham MM, Etcheson JI, Mohamed NS, Edalatpour A, Delanois RE. Rehabilitation protocols following total knee arthroplasty: a review of study designs and outcome measures. Ann Transl Med. 2019;7(Suppl 7):S255. https://doi.org/10.21037/atm.2019.08.15.
4. Doma K, Grant A, Morris J. The effects of balance training on balance performance and functional outcome measures following total knee arthroplasty: a systematic review and

meta-analysis. Sports Med (Auckland, NZ). 2018;48(10):2367–85. https://doi.org/10.1007/s40279-018-0964-7.
5. Domínguez-Navarro F, Igual-Camacho C, Silvestre-Muñoz A, Roig-Casasús S, Blasco JM. Effects of balance and proprioceptive training on total hip and knee replacement rehabilitation: a systematic review and meta-analysis. Gait Posture. 2018;62:68–74.
6. Kuijer P, van Haeren MM, Daams JG, Frings-Dresen MHW. Better return to work and sports after knee arthroplasty rehabilitation? Occup Med (Lond). 2018;68(9):626–30. https://doi.org/10.1093/occmed/kqy131.
7. Pfeufer D, Gililland J, Böcker W, Kammerlander C, Anderson M, Krähenbühl N, Pelt C. Training with biofeedback devices improves clinical outcome compared to usual care in patients with unilateral TKA: a systematic review. Knee Surg Sports Traumatol Arthrosc. 2019;27(5):1611–20. https://doi.org/10.1007/s00167-018-5217-7.
8. Sattler LN, Hing WA, Vertullo CJ. What is the evidence to support early supervised exercise therapy after primary total knee replacement? A systematic review and meta-analysis. BMC Musculoskelet Disord. 2019;20(1):42. https://doi.org/10.1186/s12891-019-2415-5.
9. Wang X, Hunter DJ, Vesentini G, Pozzobon D, Ferreira ML. Technology-assisted rehabilitation following total knee or hip replacement for people with osteoarthritis: a systematic review and meta-analysis. BMC Musculoskelet Disord. 2019;20(1):506. https://doi.org/10.1186/s12891-019-2900-x.
10. Yang X, Li GH, Wang HJ, Wang CY. Continuous passive motion after total knee arthroplasty: a systematic review and meta-analysis of associated effects on clinical outcomes. Arch Phys Med Rehabil. 2019;100(9):1763–78. https://doi.org/10.1016/j.apmr.2019.02.001.
11. Yue C, Zhang X, Zhu Y, Jia Y, Wang H, Liu Y. Systematic review of three electrical stimulation techniques for rehabilitation after total knee arthroplasty. J Arthroplasty. 2018;33(7):2330–7. https://doi.org/10.1016/j.arth.2018.01.070.
12. Jette DU, Hunter SJ, Burkett L, Langham B, Logerstedt DS, Piuzzi NS, Poirier NM, Radach LJL, Ritter JE, Scalzitti DA, Stevens-Lapsley JE, Tompkins J, Zeni J Jr, American Physical Therapy A. Physical therapist management of total knee arthroplasty. Phys Ther. 2020;100(9):1603–31. https://doi.org/10.1093/ptj/pzaa099.
13. Bade MJ, Struessel T, Dayton M, Foran J, Kim RH, Miner T, Wolfe P, Kohrt WM, Dennis D, Stevens-Lapsley JE. Early high-intensity versus low-intensity rehabilitation after total knee arthroplasty: a randomized controlled trial. Arthritis Care Res. 2017;69(9):1360–8. https://doi.org/10.1002/acr.23139.
14. Bruun-Olsen V, Heiberg KE, Wahl AK, Mengshoel AM. The immediate and long-term effects of a walking-skill program compared to usual physiotherapy care in patients who have undergone total knee arthroplasty (TKA): a randomized controlled trial. Disabil Rehabil. 2013;35(23):2008–15. https://doi.org/10.3109/09638288.2013.770084.
15. Christiansen CL, Bade MJ, Davidson BS, Dayton MR, Stevens-Lapsley JE. Effects of weight-bearing biofeedback training on functional movement patterns following total knee arthroplasty: a randomized controlled trial. J Orthop Sports Phys Ther. 2015;45(9):647–55. https://doi.org/10.2519/jospt.2015.5593.
16. Hsu WH, Hsu WB, Shen WJ, Lin ZR, Chang SH, Hsu RW. Circuit training enhances function in patients undergoing total knee arthroplasty: a retrospective cohort study. J Orthop Surg Res. 2017;12(1):156. https://doi.org/10.1186/s13018-017-0654-4.
17. Hsu WH, Hsu WB, Shen WJ, Lin ZR, Chang SH, Hsu RW. Twenty-four-week hospital-based progressive resistance training on functional recovery in female patients post total knee arthroplasty. Knee. 2019;26(3):729–36. https://doi.org/10.1016/j.knee.2019.02.008.
18. Husby VS, Foss OA, Husby OS, Winther SB. Randomized controlled trial of maximal strength training vs. standard rehabilitation following total knee arthroplasty. Eur J Phys Rehabil Med. 2018;54(3):371–9. https://doi.org/10.23736/S1973-9087.17.04712-8.
19. Jakobsen TL, Kehlet H, Husted H, Petersen J, Bandholm T. Early progressive strength training to enhance recovery after fast-track total knee arthroplasty: a randomized controlled trial. Arthritis Care Res. 2014;66(12):1856–66. https://doi.org/10.1002/acr.22405.

20. Karaman A, Yuksel I, Kinikli GI, Caglar O. Do Pilates-based exercises following total knee arthroplasty improve postural control and quality of life? Physiother Theory Pract. 2017;33(4):289–95. https://doi.org/10.1080/09593985.2017.1289578.
21. Li L, Cheng S, Wang G, Duan G, Zhang Y. Tai chi chuan exercises improve functional outcomes and quality of life in patients with primary total knee arthroplasty due to knee osteoarthritis. Complement Ther Clin Pract. 2019;35:121–5. https://doi.org/10.1016/j.ctcp.2019.02.003.
22. Liao CD, Lin LF, Huang YC, Huang SW, Chou LC, Liou TH. Functional outcomes of outpatient balance training following total knee replacement in patients with knee osteoarthritis: a randomized controlled trial. Clin Rehabil. 2015;29(9):855–67. https://doi.org/10.1177/0269215514564086.
23. Molla RY, Sadeghi H, Kahlaee AH. The effect of early progressive resistive exercise therapy on balance control of patients with total knee arthroplasty: a randomized controlled trial. Topics Geriatr Rehab. 2017;33(4):286–94.
24. Piva SR, Schneider MJ, Moore CG, Catelani MB, Gil AB, Klatt BA, DiGioia AM, Almeida GJ, Khoja SS, Sowa G, Irrgang JJ. Effectiveness of later-stage exercise programs vs usual medical care on physical function and activity after total knee replacement: a randomized clinical trial. JAMA Netw Open. 2019;2(2):e190018. https://doi.org/10.1001/jamanetworkopen.2019.0018.
25. Sattler LN, Hing WA, Vertullo CJ. Pedaling-based protocol superior to a 10-exercise, non-pedaling protocol for postoperative rehabilitation after total knee replacement: a randomized controlled trial. J Bone Joint Surg Am. 2019;101(8):688–95. https://doi.org/10.2106/jbjs.18.00898.
26. Schache MB, McClelland JA, Webster KE. Incorporating hip abductor strengthening exercises into a rehabilitation program did not improve outcomes in people following total knee arthroplasty: a randomised trial. J Physiother. 2019;65(3):136–43. https://doi.org/10.1016/j.jphys.2019.05.008.
27. Stevens-Lapsley JE, Balter JE, Wolfe P, Eckhoff DG, Kohrt WM. Early neuromuscular electrical stimulation to improve quadriceps muscle strength after total knee arthroplasty: a randomized controlled trial. Phys Ther. 2012;92(2):210–26. https://doi.org/10.2522/ptj.20110124.
28. Yoshida Y, Ikuno K, Shomoto K. Comparison of the effect of sensory-level and conventional motor-level neuromuscular electrical stimulations on quadriceps strength after total knee arthroplasty: a prospective randomized single-blind trial. Arch Phys Med Rehabil. 2017;98(12):2364–70. https://doi.org/10.1016/j.apmr.2017.05.005.
29. Noyes FR, Barber-Westin SD. Prevention and treatment of knee arthrofibrosis. In: Noyes FR, Barber-Westin SD, editors. Noyes' knee disorders: surgery, rehabilitation, clinical outcomes. 2nd ed. Philadelphia: Elsevier; 2017. p. 1059–102. https://doi.org/10.1016/b978-0-323-2903-3.00038-x.
30. Noyes FR, Wojtys EM. The early recognition, diagnosis and treatment of the patella infera syndrome. In: Tullos HS, editor. Instructional course lectures, vol. XL. Rosemont: AAOS; 1991. p. 233–47.
31. Noyes FR, Wojtys EM, Marshall MT. The early diagnosis and treatment of developmental patella infera syndrome. Clin Orthop Relat Res. 1991;265:241–52.
32. Paulos LE, Rosenberg TD, Drawbert J, Manning J, Abbott P. Infrapatellar contracture syndrome. An unrecognized cause of knee stiffness with patella entrapment and patella infera. Am J Sports Med. 1987;15(4):331–41.
33. Schache MB, McClelland JA, Webster KE. Lower limb strength following total knee arthroplasty: a systematic review. Knee. 2014;21(1):12–20. https://doi.org/10.1016/j.knee.2013.08.002.
34. Moon YW, Kim HJ, Ahn HS, Lee DH. Serial changes of quadriceps and hamstring muscle strength following total knee arthroplasty: a meta-analysis. PLoS One. 2016;11(2):e0148193. https://doi.org/10.1371/journal.pone.0148193.
35. Gaunder CL, Hawkinson MP, Tennent DJ, Tubb CC. Occlusion training: pilot study for post-operative lower extremity rehabilitation following primary total knee arthroplasty. US Army Med Dep J. 2017;(2-17):39–43.

36. Kilgas MA, Lytle LLM, Drum SN, Elmer SJ. Exercise with blood flow restriction to improve quadriceps function long after ACL reconstruction. Int J Sports Med. 2019;40(10):650–6. https://doi.org/10.1055/a-0961-1434.
37. Tennent DJ, Hylden CM, Johnson AE, Burns TC, Wilken JM, Owens JG. Blood flow restriction training after knee arthroscopy: a randomized controlled pilot study. Clin J Sport Med. 2017;27(3):245–52. https://doi.org/10.1097/JSM.0000000000000377.
38. Barber-Westin S, Noyes FR. Blood flow-restricted training for lower extremity muscle weakness due to knee pathology: a systematic review. Sports Health. 2019;11(1):69–83. https://doi.org/10.1177/1941738118811337.
39. Hughes L, Paton B, Rosenblatt B, Gissane C, Patterson SD. Blood flow restriction training in clinical musculoskeletal rehabilitation: a systematic review and meta-analysis. Br J Sports Med. 2017;51(13):1003–11. https://doi.org/10.1136/bjsports-2016-097071.
40. Mattocks KT, Jessee MB, Mouser JG, Dankel SJ, Buckner SL, Bell ZW, Owens JG, Abe T, Loenneke JP. The application of blood flow restriction: lessons from the laboratory. Curr Sports Med Rep. 2018;17(4):129–34. https://doi.org/10.1249/jsr.0000000000000473.
41. Patterson SD, Hughes L, Warmington S, Burr JF, Scott BR, Owens J, Abe T, Nielsen J, Libardi CA, Laurentino GC. Blood flow restriction exercise position stand: considerations of methodology, application and safety. Front Physiol. 2019;10:533.
42. Minniti MC, Statkevich AP, Kelly RL, Rigsby VP, Exline MM, Rhon DI, Clewley D. The safety of blood flow restriction training as a therapeutic intervention for patients with musculoskeletal disorders: a systematic review. Am J Sports Med. 2019:363546519882652. https://doi.org/10.1177/0363546519882652.
43. DePhillipo NN, Kennedy MI, Aman ZS, Bernhardson AS, O'Brien LT, LaPrade RF. The role of blood flow restriction therapy following knee surgery: expert opinion. Arthroscopy. 2018;34(8):2506–10. https://doi.org/10.1016/j.arthro.2018.05.038.
44. Paravlic AH, Pisot R, Marusic U. Specific and general adaptations following motor imagery practice focused on muscle strength in total knee arthroplasty rehabilitation: a randomized controlled trial. PLoS One. 2019;14(8):e0221089. https://doi.org/10.1371/journal.pone.0221089.
45. Piva SR, Almeida GJ, Gil AB, DiGioia AM, Helsel DL, Sowa GA. Effect of comprehensive behavioral and exercise intervention on physical function and activity participation after Total knee replacement: a pilot randomized study. Arthritis Care Res. 2017;69(12):1855–62. https://doi.org/10.1002/acr.23227.

Postoperative Rehabilitation Part II: Strategies for Successful Return to Physical Activities and Athletics in Postoperative Weeks 13–52

7

Frank R. Noyes, Timothy Heckmann, and Sue Barber-Westin

7.1 Introduction

This is the second of two chapters that detail our total knee arthroplasty (TKA) postoperative rehabilitation program, whose overall goal is to return patients to an active lifestyle to enhance their overall quality of life. Chapter 6 discusses the protocol for the first 12 postoperative weeks and includes important concepts to avoid complications, such as limitations in range of motion (ROM) and severe muscle strength deficits. At the end of this time period, patients should be pain-free with activities of daily living and preparing to return to light work and low-impact aerobic activities such as walking, bicycling, and swimming over the course of the next few months. Because TKA is performed in many younger patients, the desire to return to more strenuous activities is important to these individuals. These patients have high preoperative expectations [1–3] that correlate strongly with postoperative patient satisfaction [2, 4, 5], as detailed in Chap. 12. In our experience, additional strengthening and conditioning exercises are usually required in order to safely prepare them to participate in activities such as doubles tennis, light jogging, hiking, and skiing.

We conducted a systematic review of studies published from 2005 through 2015 to determine what routine sports and physical activities patients participated in after TKA [6]. The review also determined if participation in these activities caused knee symptoms such as pain and swelling. In addition, the effect of postoperative rehabilitation on achieving fitness and sports goals was analyzed. Nineteen studies met the study criteria. There were 5179 knees (mean age, 67.5 years) followed a mean

F. R. Noyes
Cincinnati SportsMedicine and Orthopaedic Center, The Noyes Knee Institute, Cincinnati, OH, USA

T. Heckmann · S. Barber-Westin (✉)
Noyes Knee Institute, Cincinnati, OH, USA
e-mail: tpheckmann@mercy.com; sbwestin@csmref.org

F. R. Noyes, S. Barber-Westin (eds.), *Critical Rehabilitation for Partial and Total Knee Arthroplasty*, https://doi.org/10.1007/978-3-030-87003-4_7

of 4.8 years postoperatively. Marked variability was found in the percent of patients who resumed recreational activities (34% to 100%). A low range (0–16.5%) of patients met American Heart Association (AHA) guidelines for aerobic physical activity (see also Chap. 10). Few studies determined if symptoms or limitations were experienced, and none described rehabilitation exercises or factors that would influence patients' ability to return to recreational or fitness activities.

Kuijet et al. [7] conducted a review of studies published from the inception of several databases to March 2017 to determine the effect of exercise-based rehabilitation on return to work and sports after TKA. The search resulted in 3788 studies, none of which evaluated the study purpose. These authors stated the same concerns that we expressed in this near complete lack of information and noted that most published rehabilitation programs lasted no longer than 6–12 weeks postoperatively. This indicates that many patients may not receive additional support for the safe and successful return to recreational activities. In addition, the lack of additional strengthening and conditioning measures could play a major role in the high rate of variability of patients who return to physical activities and who have later complaints of knee pain or instability, and in the very low rate of patients who meet AHA physical activity guidelines.

7.2 Strengthening and Conditioning

Our rehabilitation program for postoperative weeks 13–26 (3–6 months) is shown in Table 7.1. In our experience, patients require this program during this time period to prepare them for return to recreational sports and other more strenuous activities. Return to sports is then usually accomplished 6–12 months postoperatively, provided the patient passes our criteria (which is detailed in the next section of this chapter), and there are no symptoms of pain or swelling with activity.

Progression of weight and the amount of time spent in aerobic conditioning is individualized and based on the final activity (or activities) the patient desires to return to and if recurrent pain or joint effusion occurs. Symptoms necessitate modification of the program until the problems are resolved. Fitness center training is eventually recommended two to three times per week and includes 20 minutes of strengthening, 30 minutes of cardiovascular exercise, and 10 minutes of flexibility. This is a realistic goal for our TKA patients and provides a reasonable level of fitness. There is a higher goal for more active patients, recommended by the AHA guidelines, to achieve up to 150 minutes of moderate-intensity or 75 minutes of vigorous-intensity physical activity per week, or an equivalent combination of moderate- and vigorous-intensity activity [8, 9]. For aerobic fitness, the patient is instructed on the options available, including the exercise bicycle. Rowing or eclipse machines are ideal because both the upper and lower extremities are exercised. A program of brisk walking on the treadmill is an option; however, jogging activities involve impact loads that may increase prosthetic loosening over the long term and are not recommended. At the time of writing, the most recent activity recommendations following TKA by the American Association of Hip and Knee Surgeons were

Table 7.1 Noyes Knee Institute rehabilitation protocol for total knee arthroplasty (postoperative weeks 13–26)

Modalities: Pain/edema management (cryotherapy)
Stretching: hamstring, gastrocnemius-soleus, gluteal, iliotibial band, quadriceps
Strengthening:
Straight leg raises
Closed chain: wall sits, mini squats
Closed chain: toe/heel raises
Knee flexion hamstring curls (0°–90°)
Knee extension quadriceps (90°–0°)
Hip abduction-adduction, multi-hip
Leg press (80°–10°)
Upper body weight training
Core training
Balance/gait/proprioceptive training:
Band walking (diagonal, monster walk), Y-balance reaching, perturbation training
Conditioning:
Stationary bicycling (high seat, low resistance)
Aquatic program (water walking, depth at thigh or waist)
Stair machine (low resistance, low stroke)
Ski machine (short stride, level, low resistance)
Elliptical machine
Swimming (kicking)
Walking
Fitness center training (2–3 ×/week):
25 minutes strengthening, 25 minutes cardiovascular training, 10 minutes flexibility
Achieve AHA guidelines.[a] Monitor for swelling, pain

[a]American Heart Association guidelines: physical activity per week: 150–300 minutes moderate intensity or 75–150 minutes vigorous intensity. Strengthening all major muscle groups ≥2 days/week

Table 7.2 Activity recommendations after TKA from the American Association of Hip and Knee Surgeons[a]

Activities allowed	Activities not allowed
Walking	Jogging
Climbing	Sprinting
Bicycling on level surfaces	Skiing on difficult terrain
Swimming	Singles tennis
Doubles tennis	
Golfing	

[a]From Swanson et al. [10]

published in 2009 (Table 7.2) [10]. Based on the results of 139 completed surveys from the 2007 annual meeting, consensus was reached for low-impact activities such as walking, climbing stairs, bicycling on level surfaces, swimming, doubles tennis, and golfing. Activities that were consistently discouraged included jogging, sprinting, skiing on difficult terrain, and singles tennis.

In addition, muscle-strengthening exercises of moderate or greater intensity that involve all major muscle groups should be performed at least 2 days per week. This strength program should be inclusive of the lower extremity, torso, core, and upper extremity muscle groups.

Our experience has found that the preoperative review of patient goals and prior athletic participation are important in order to establish realistic expectations regarding postoperative activities. For instance, if a patient played doubles tennis or cross-country skied before surgery, they potentially will be more successful in returning to these activities postoperatively than if they did not participate. There exists the problem that active younger patients recall, prior to the onset of knee arthritis, the ability to perform strenuous recreational activities such as singles tennis, jogging, softball, and other running sports. After TKA, these activities are not advised, and modification of athletic activities and realistic patient expectations need to be established in preoperative counseling.

Once patients satisfy our Biodex strength and function testing goals (described in the next section), progression to light agility and sports-specific drills may begin. Discussion, planning, and implementation of exercises and drills should be included as a component of functional progression to return to full activity. For example, a person returning to light doubles tennis may begin short-distance light jogging in a straight line and lateral directions. This may be followed by four-square surface agility moves in straight planar directions, then multidirectional patterns, and, finally, train with the racket on ground strokes. If the patient demonstrates apprehension or difficulty with any of these activities, remedial rehabilitation exercises using elastic resistance bands could be implemented to progress muscle strength and functional pattern simulations.

7.3 Recommended Testing for Return to Sports Training

As our patients begin training for recreational sports, they must pass specific criteria shown in Table 7.3. There must be no pain or swelling with the strengthening and fitness training program or in any other activities the patient is performing. The patient must demonstrate good patellar mobility and symmetrical gait. Muscle strength may be tested according to the equipment available. In our center, a Biodex test of isometric quadriceps and hamstring strength is performed (Fig. 7.1). Test scores are evaluated for bilateral comparisons, quadriceps peak torque-to-body weight ratios (adjusted based on age and sex), and agonist-to-antagonist ratios. Males aged 55–65 are expected to generate ≥60% of their body weight, and those aged >65 are expected to generate ≥50% of their body weight. Females aged ≥55 are expected to generate ≥50% of their body weight. For both genders, hamstring-to-quadriceps ratios are expected to be approximately 60%. These test scores relate to this higher functioning patient population and represent the strength component of the evaluation process. We established goals based on peak torque comparisons with the contralateral side for quadriceps and hamstrings of 70% to begin interval running, 80% to begin light agility work, and 90% for return to activity. Hip abductor strength may be tested either manually or with a handheld dynamometer.

Table 7.3 Noyes Knee Institute criteria for return to recreational sports training after total knee arthroplasty

Criteria/test	Goal
Pain	None, ≥6 Cincinnati Knee Rating Pain scale
Swelling	None visible and ≥6 Cincinnati Knee Rating Pain scale
Patellar mobility	Good
Gait	Symmetrical
Muscle strength	Manual test: 5/5
Quadriceps, hamstrings	Isometric handheld dynamometer: ≥80% of opposite side
	Isometric peak torque on Biodex: goals compared with opposite side are 70% for interval running, 80% for light agility work, and 90% for return to activity
Muscle strength	Manual test: 5/5
Hip abductors	Isometric handheld dynamometer: ≥80% of opposite side
Single-leg squat test	No knee valgus, medial-lateral movement, or pelvic tilt
Stair-climbing test	10 steps, up and down, can use rail: <13 secs
6-minute walk test	Aged 60–69 years: male ≥521 meters (0.32 mile), female ≥497 meters (0.31 mile)
	Aged 70–79 years: male ≥478 meters (0.29 mile), female ≥440 meters (0.27 mile)
	Aged 80–89 years: male ≥356 meters (0.22 mile), female ≥345 meters (0.21 mile)
Y-balance test	Anterior, posterolateral, posteromedial: ≥90% of opposite side. Normalize each distance by patient's leg length
Fitness training	Can be performed with no pain or swelling
PT/MD	Cleared for initiation of recreational sports

Several well-known objective clinic tests are also conducted (see also Chap. 9). A single-leg squat test is conducted in which the patient is instructed to squat down to 45° and return to single-leg stance without losing their balance (Fig. 7.2a, b). The head and eyes should remain focused straight ahead. The patient performs five consecutive trials, and the clinician notes the overall trunk control and the position of the hip, knee, and foot throughout the test. A stair-climbing test is performed using ten steps, with the goal of ascending and descending the flight in less than 13 seconds. The 6-minute walk test is done on a treadmill. The goals for this test according to gender and age are shown in Table 7.3.

The Y-balance test is performed in the anterior, posterolateral, and posteromedial directions (Fig. 7.3). This is a simplified version of the Star Excursion Balance test that requires the subject to maintain a stable base by balancing on one leg while reaching out with the other leg to push a block as far as possible in the anterior, posteromedial, and posterolateral directions. A detailed description of this test is provided in Chap. 9.

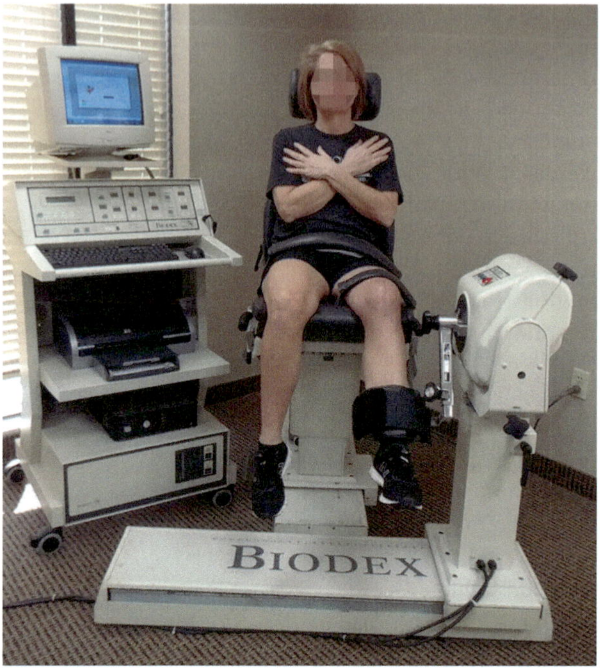

Fig. 7.1 Biodex test setup for isometric evaluation of quadriceps and hamstring muscle strength

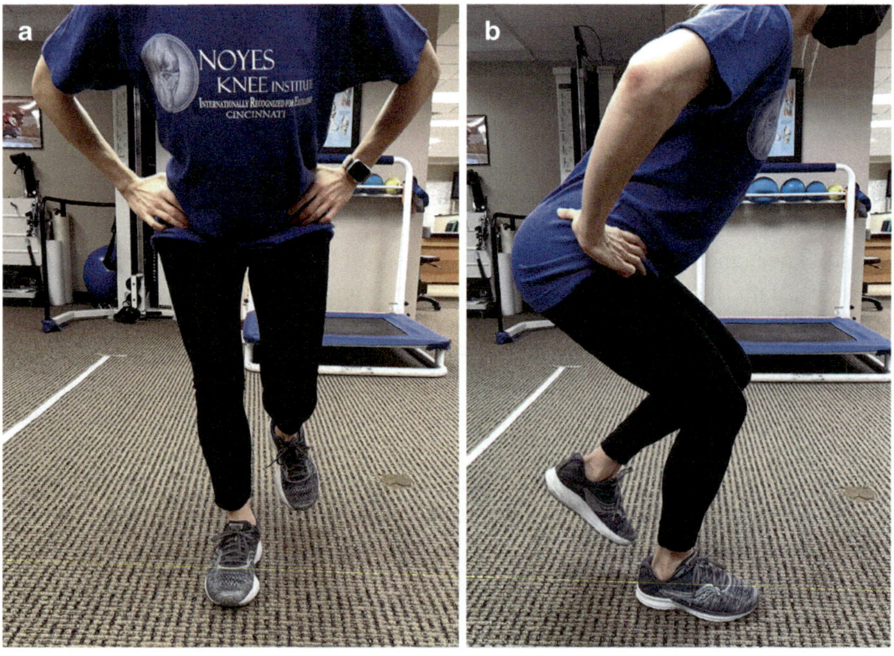

Fig. 7.2 Single-leg squat test as viewed from the front (**a**) and side (**b**)

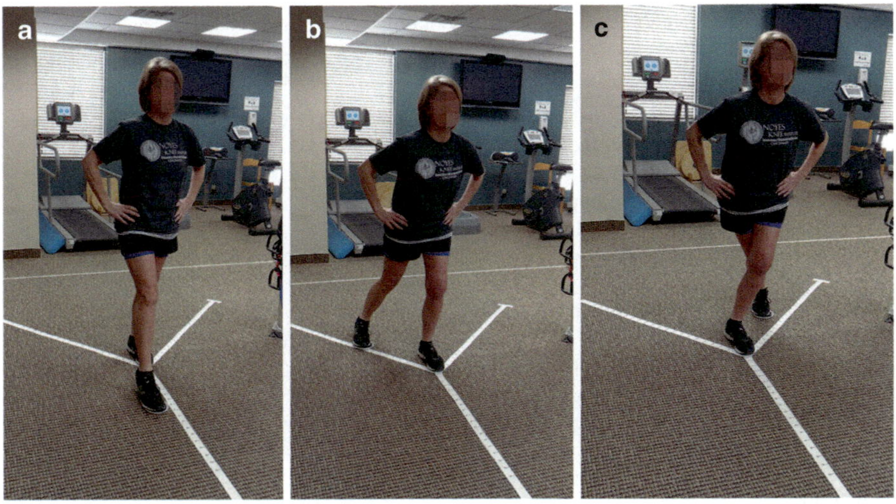

Fig. 7.3 The Y-balance test is performed in the (**a**) anterior, (**b**) posterolateral, and (**c**) posteromedial directions

7.4 Results of Studies From the Authors' Clinic

In 2016, we initiated an ongoing prospective study at our center in patients 65 years of age or younger who expressed the desire to return to recreational sports and/or work activities. Serial objective testing is conducted at 3, 6, 12, and 24 months after TKA. Several patient-reported outcomes are collected at 12 and 24 months postoperatively. The objective test battery includes the single-leg squat test, 6-minute walk test, stair-climb test (ten steps), Biodex isometric testing of quadriceps and hamstring strength, and Y-balance test. This study was devised based on the hypothesis that noteworthy deficits in strength and function are present at 3 months postoperatively, which is the time period the majority of TKA rehabilitation programs conclude. This problem demonstrates the necessity for extending the program to correct muscle weakness and conditioning deficits and allow patients to return to a physically active lifestyle.

Data on the results of objective testing for 50 patients (mean age at TKA, 57.5 ± 6.5; range, 45–69) are shown in Table 7.4. At 3 months postoperatively, less than 50% of the patients passed test goals for the single-leg squat test, 6-minute walk test, quadriceps strength, and Y-balance posteromedial test. In addition, only 21% had at least 130° of knee flexion. These individuals had undergone a mean of 21 ± 8 postoperative physical therapy visits in addition to their home exercise program. All were counseled to continue with the home and fitness center program as detailed in this chapter. At 6 months postoperatively, major improvements were noted in the percent that passed all of the tests with the exception of the single-leg squat.

Table 7.4 Results of authors' prospective study of objective testing after TKA

Test	Goal	3 months po		6 months po		12 months po	
		N tested	% Passed	N tested	% Passed	N tested	% Passed
6-minute walk	See Table 7.2	50	22%	44	39%	37	49%
Stair-climb test	<13 secs	50	64%	44	79%	36	94%
Biodex quads	≥70% of opposite side	48	54%	43	81%	28	78%
Biodex hams	≥70% of opposite side	48	85%	43	88%	28	86%
Both quads and hams	≥70% of opposite side	48	46%	43	74%	28	75%
Y-balance: anterior	≥90% of opposite side	50	60%	44	70%	35	74%
Y-balance: posterolateral	≥90% of opposite side	49	77%	44	66%	35	86%
Y-balance: posteromedial	≥90% of opposite side	50	28%	44	91%	35	86%
Single-leg squat	"Good" rating	48	10%	42	2%	34	32%
ROM active extension	0° or hyperextension	33	91%	38	92%	37	97%
ROM active flexion	≥130°	33	21%	38	74%	37	81%

ROM range of motion

We conducted a study to determine, in a historical younger group of patients (TKA 2013–2015) with high physical activity expectations after TKA, the ability to return to recreational sports and work activities without symptoms or functional limitations. A second purpose was to determine the ability of these patients to achieve aerobic fitness guidelines. There were 51 patients (54 knees, mean age of 58 ± 7 years) who were evaluated in a mean of 4.4 ± 0.5 years (range, 3.4–5.6 years) after TKA. Our TKA registry included the patient-reported outcome measures (PROMs) of the Knee Injury and Osteoarthritis Outcome Joint Replacement Survey (KOOS JR) seven-item score; questions from the Cincinnati Knee Rating System related to the overall knee condition, pain, and swelling [11]; selected questions from the VR-12 Health Survey [12]; questions about general fitness level; and questions regarding patient expectations before and after surgery. Patients were also asked to list all physical, recreational, and work activities they participated in after surgery.

The patients underwent a mean of 14 ± 6 supervised postoperative physical therapy sessions (range, 4–28) in additional to a home exercise program. There were no significant complications, pulmonary embolism, infection, or prosthetic loosening. The final physical examination showed no evidence of knee instability or knee arthrofibrosis. There were no significant differences between genders for any of the outcome factors analyzed. The mean KOOS JR score improved from 43 ± 18 points preoperatively to 87 ± 18 postoperatively ($p < 0.0001$). The mean change was

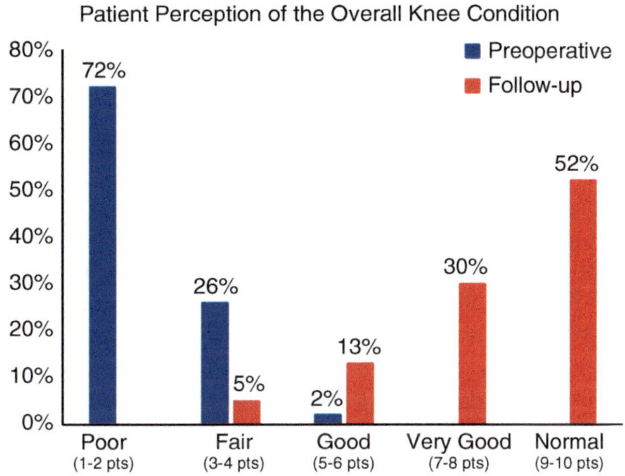

Fig. 7.4 The improvement in the patient-reported outcome of their overall knee condition is before and after TKA and was statistically significant ($p < 0.0001$). Pts points

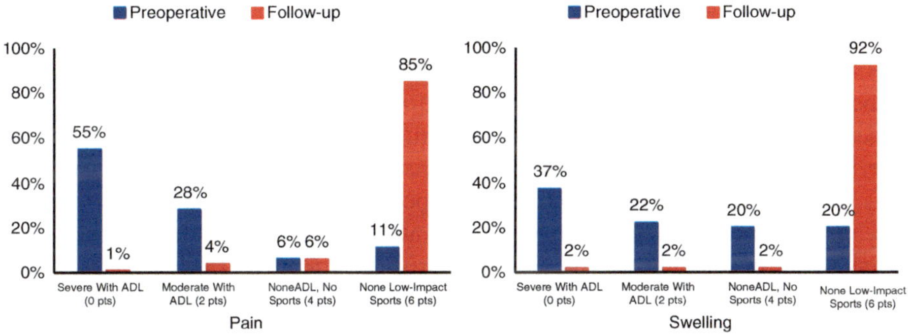

Fig. 7.5 The improvements in patient-reported pain and swelling scores related to patient activity between the preoperative and follow-up time periods are shown ($p < 0.0001$). Pts points

44 ± 24 points, and 48 knees (89%) achieved a minimal clinically important change in this score of ≥14 points [13]. There were significant improvements from preoperative to follow-up in the Cincinnati Knee Rating scores for the patient perception of the overall knee condition (2.0 ± 1.1 and 8.2 ± 1.9 points, respectively; $p < 0.0001$, Fig. 7.4), pain (1.4 ± 2.0 and 5.4 ± 1.6 points, respectively; $p < 0.0001$), and swelling (2.5 ± 2.3 and 5.7 ± 1.1 points, respectively; $p < 0.0001$, Fig. 7.5).

Overall, 44 of 51 patients (86%) were able to resume physical activity and work with no or only minor symptoms or limitations. Participation in sports and recreational activities was determined in 41 patients, of whom 91% resumed low-impact activities and 9% returned to higher-impact athletics. Only three patients had symptoms; one had occasional pain after scuba diving, and two complained of mild tightness after high-impact activities that were not recommended. Before surgery, 33 of the 51 patients were working (six were disabled, 11 were retired, and one did not work). At follow-up, 28 patients were employed, including seven patients who had retired before surgery and returned to the workforce. Only three patients reported symptoms and limitations with work.

There were significant improvements in the patient responses to the aerobic fitness level (Fig. 7.6a). Before surgery, 15 patients (28%) were able to take a brisk 20-minute walk 5 days per week, while at follow-up, 46 (85%) were able to do this activity ($p < 0.0001$). Before surgery, 18 patients (34%) were able to perform 20 minutes of vigorous activity 3 days per week, while at follow-up, 46 patients (85%) were able to do so ($p < 0.0001$; Fig. 7.6b).

Before surgery, 91% of patients expected a normal or almost normal ability to do activities of daily living (ADL), and 76% expected the same for recreational activities (Table 7.5). At follow-up, 24% indicated their expectations had not been met for ADL, and 22% expressed the same for recreational activities. Still, 96% were satisfied and expressed that the operation was worthwhile, and 85% believed their overall knee condition was a great deal improved compared with their preoperative symptoms (Fig. 7.7).

In conclusion, active younger patients who desire a return to recreational activities first require realistic expectations and goals established preoperatively. Otherwise, patients may express dissatisfaction after surgery because they expected a nearly normal knee and ability to perform unrealistic activities such as impact sports that involve running and turning or twisting. Even with preoperative counselling, patients may maintain unrealistic expectations after TKA. The disuse and strength deficits that patients have going into surgery may be pronounced after many years of declining activity, particularly in patients that delayed TKA until even walking activities up to 30–60 minutes became limited. After TKA, there exists a minimum of 6 months to restore adequate muscle strength and conditioning, and most patients require up to 12 months to achieve the ability to perform recreational activities without symptoms. The team approach is required of the surgeon and therapist working with the patients in an individualized manner, with encouragement and understanding of the patients' goals. Often it is necessary to substitute or modify athletic pursuits to achieve patient satisfaction of the final clinical outcome. The objective tests provided in this chapter establish light posts for the patient to achieve these gains and the ability to return to activities in a safe manner without symptoms.

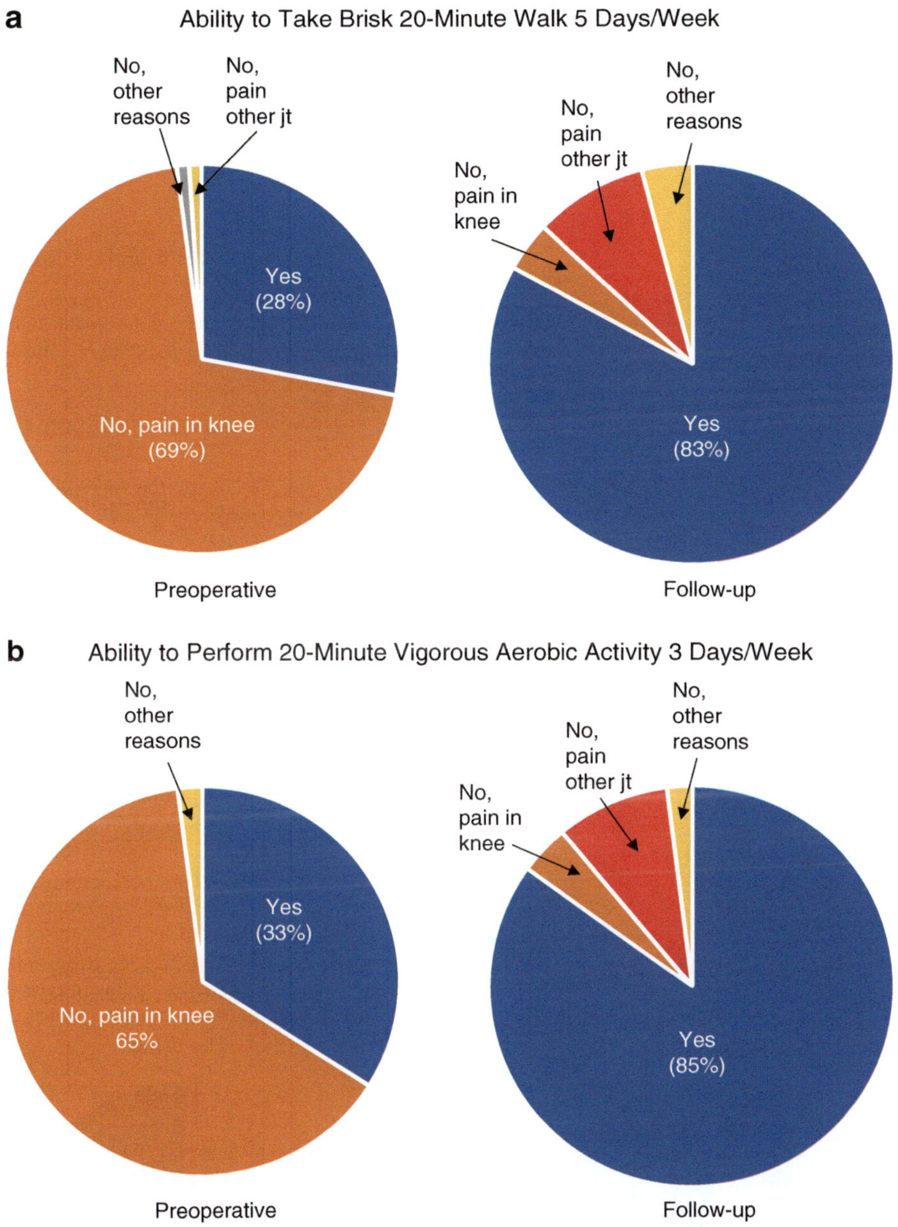

Fig. 7.6 (**a**) Significant improvements were reported in (**a**) the ability to take a brisk 20-minute walk 5 days per week ($p < 0.0001$) and in (**b**) the ability to perform 20 minutes of vigorous aerobic activity 3 days per week ($p < 0.0001$). Jt, joint

Table 7.5 Patient expectations

	Normal, no limitations	*Almost normal, some limitations*	*Improved, some problems*	*Improved, but bothersome problems*	*Not possible or not interested*
Preoperative					
I expect that after surgery, activities such as walking, stairs, and kneeling to be:	22 (41%)	27 (50%)	5 (9%)	0	NA
I expect that after surgery, my recreational activities such as bicycling, hiking, golf, and light tennis to be:	19 (35%)	22 (41%)	6 (11%)	0	7 (13%)
Postoperative					
	Just right, my expectations were met	*Too low, I'm a lot better than I thought*	*Too low, I'm somewhat better than I thought*	*Too high, I'm somewhat worse than I thought*	*Too high, I'm a lot worse than I thought*
My expectations for being able to do my normal activities of daily living after surgery were:	31 (57%)	8 (15%)	2 (4%)	12 (22%)	1 (2%)
My expectations for being able to do my leisure, recreational, or sports activities after surgery activities were:	31 (57%)	8 (15%)	3 (5%)	11 (20%)	1 (2%)

NA not applicable

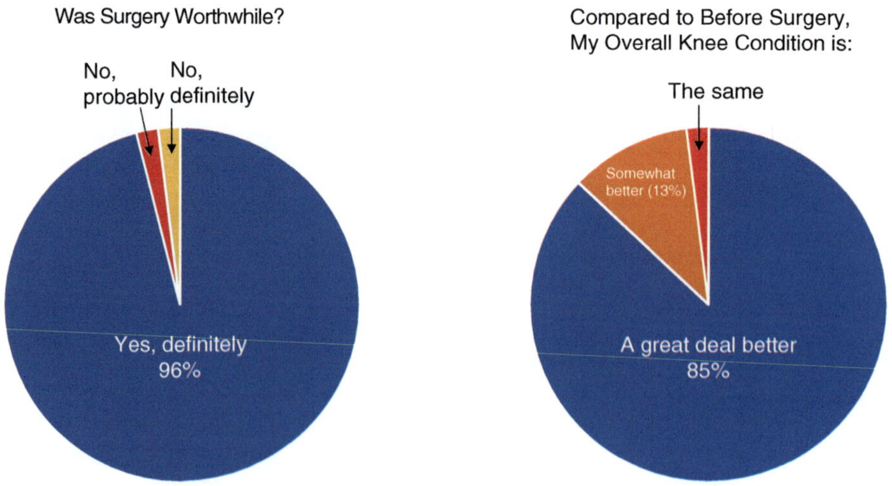

Fig. 7.7 The patient-reported overall opinion as to the surgery being worthwhile and compared to the preoperative state of the amount of improvement. Jt joint

References

1. Deakin AH, Smith MA, Wallace DT, Smith EJ, Sarungi M. Fulfilment of preoperative expectations and postoperative patient satisfaction after total knee replacement. A prospective analysis of 200 patients. Knee. 2019;26(6):1403–12. https://doi.org/10.1016/j.knee.2019.07.018.
2. Jain D, Nguyen LL, Bendich I, Nguyen LL, Lewis CG, Huddleston JI, Duwelius PJ, Feeley BT, Bozic KJ. Higher patient expectations predict higher patient-reported outcomes, but not satisfaction, in total knee arthroplasty patients: a prospective multicenter study. J Arthroplasty. 2017;32(9S):S166–70. https://doi.org/10.1016/j.arth.2017.01.008.
3. Jassim SS, Douglas SL, Haddad FS. Athletic activity after lower limb arthroplasty: a systematic review of current evidence. Bone Joint J. 2014;96-B(7):923–7. https://doi.org/10.1302/0301-620X.96B7.31585.
4. Lützner C, Postler A, Beyer F, Kirschner S, Lützner J. Fulfillment of expectations influence patient satisfaction 5 years after total knee arthroplasty. Knee Surg Sports Traumatol Arthrosc. 2019;27(7):2061–70. https://doi.org/10.1007/s00167-018-5320-9.
5. Husain A, Lee GC. Establishing realistic patient expectations following total knee arthroplasty. J Am Acad Orthop Surg. 2015;23(12):707–13. https://doi.org/10.5435/JAAOS-D-14-00049.
6. Barber-Westin SD, Noyes FR. Aerobic physical fitness and recreational sports participation after Total knee arthroplasty. Sports Health. 2016;8(6):553–60. https://doi.org/10.1177/1941738116670090.
7. Kuijer PPFM, Kievit AJ, Pahlplatz TMJ, Hooiveld T, Hoozemans MJM, Blankevoort L, Schafroth MU, van Geenen RCI, Frings-Dresen MHW. Which patients do not return to work after total knee arthroplasty? Rheumatol Int. 2016;36(9):1249–54. https://doi.org/10.1007/s00296-016-3512-5.
8. Piercy KL, Troiano RP, Ballard RM, Carlson SA, Fulton JE, Galuska DA, George SM, Olson RD. The physical activity guidelines for Americans. JAMA. 2018;320(19):2020–8.
9. Piercy KL, Troiano RP. Physical activity guidelines for Americans from the US department of health and human services: cardiovascular benefits and recommendations. Circ Cardiovasc Qual Outcomes. 2018;11(11):e005263.
10. Swanson EA, Schmalzried TP, Dorey FJ. Activity recommendations after total hip and knee arthroplasty: a survey of the American Association for Hip and Knee Surgeons. J Arthroplasty. 2009;24(6 Suppl):120–6. https://doi.org/10.1016/j.arth.2009.05.014.
11. Barber-Westin SD, Noyes FR, McCloskey JW. Rigorous statistical reliability, validity, and responsiveness testing of the Cincinnati knee rating system in 350 subjects with uninjured, injured, or anterior cruciate ligament-reconstructed knees. Am J Sports Med. 1999;27(4):402–16.
12. Selim AJ, Rogers W, Fleishman JA, Qian SX, Fincke BG, Rothendler JA, Kazis LE. Updated U.S. population standard for the Veterans RAND 12-item Health Survey (VR-12). Qual Life Res. 2009;18(1):43–52. https://doi.org/10.1007/s11136-008-9418-2.
13. Lyman S, Lee YY, McLawhorn AS, Islam W, MacLean CH. What are the minimal and substantial improvements in the HOOS and KOOS and JR versions after total joint replacement? Clin Orthop Relat Res. 2018;476(12):2432–41. https://doi.org/10.1097/CORR.0000000000000456.

8 Common Patient-Reported Outcome Measures for Knee Arthroplasty Patients

Sue Barber-Westin and Frank R. Noyes

8.1 Introduction

The determination of outcome after knee arthroplasty requires assessment of both patient-reported outcome measures (PROMs) and objective parameters that measure strength, balance, and functional performance. In 2018, Lovelock et al. [1] determined the most frequently used outcome measures in clinical trials on knee arthroplasty from 452 randomized controlled trials (RCT) and 184 clinical trials registries (CTR). The top ten measures included eight PROMs and two performance-based measures. The Knee Society Score (KSS, also known as the American Knee Society score) was the most frequently used PROM (57% in RCT and 41% in CTR), followed by the Western Ontario and McMaster Universities Osteoarthritis Index (WOMAC), as shown in Table 8.1. The majority of studies used more than one outcome measure (64% in RCT and 79% in CTR). The authors cautioned that the KSS and Hospital for Special Surgery instruments have significant ceiling effects and may potentially overestimate actual patient results. That same year, Siljander et al. [2] reviewed PROMs used in four major orthopedic journals in 644 studies. The most frequently used instruments for total knee arthroplasty studies were the KSS, WOMAC, SF-36, Oxford Knee Score (OKS), visual analogue scale (VAS), and Knee Injury and Osteoarthritis Outcome Score (KOOS). The number of articles using more than one PROM from 2004 to 2016 increased 48%.

In 2016, Theodoulou et al. [3] identified 438 publications in the knee arthroplasty literature, of which 59% used the original KSS, followed by the WOMAC (24%), OKS (19%), VAS for pain (~15%), and Short Form-36 (~15%). Another

S. Barber-Westin (✉)
Noyes Knee Institute, Cincinnati, OH, USA
e-mail: sbwestin@csmref.org

F. R. Noyes
Cincinnati SportsMedicine and Orthopaedic Center, The Noyes Knee Institute,
Cincinnati, OH, USA

F. R. Noyes, S. Barber-Westin (eds.), *Critical Rehabilitation for Partial and Total Knee Arthroplasty*, https://doi.org/10.1007/978-3-030-87003-4_8

Table 8.1 Most frequently used outcome measures after total knee arthroplasty in 452 randomized controlled trials and 184 clinical trials registries[a]

Instrument	Type	RCT % of studies	CTR % of studies
KSS	Disease specific-hybrid	57%	41%
WOMAC	Disease specific-PROM	33%	26%
Oxford Knee Score	Disease specific-PROM	15%	33%
Visual analogue pain scale	Generic	15%	18%
HSS	Disease specific-PROM	14%	1%
SF-36	Generic	13%	11%
SF-12	Generic	8%	14%
Stair-climbing test	Performance-based	7%	8%
KOOS	Disease specific-PROM	6%	30%
6-Minute walk test	Performance-based	4%	9%

CTR clinical trials registries, *HSS* Hospital for Special Surgery, *KSS* Knee Society Score, *KOOS* Knee Injury and Osteoarthritis Outcome Score, *PROM* patient-reported outcome measure, *RCT* randomized controlled trials, *WOMAC* Western Ontario and McMaster Universities Osteoarthritis Index

[a]From Lovelock et al. [1]

publication of a survey of 41 members of the International Society of Arthroplasty Registries (SAR) determined that the most common disease-specific instruments used after knee arthroplasty were the KOOS, pain VAS, and WOMAC. The most common generic instruments were the EuroQol five-dimension health outcome survey and the Short Form-12 health survey (SF-12) [4].

It is important to acknowledge that there are many other factors that influence the outcome of knee arthroplasty, including the patient's mental status, hospital experience, socioeconomic status, social support, and body mass index [5]. Commonly used measures for strength, balance, and function are discussed in Chap. 9. This chapter details the most commonly used PROMs and provides reliability, validity, responsiveness, minimal clinically important difference (MCID), and minimally important change (MIC) when possible to assist users in understanding these instruments.

8.2 Mandated Collection of PROMS in the USA

In April 2016, the Centers for Medicare and Medicaid Services (CMS) in the USA adopted the Comprehensive Care for Joint Replacement (CJR) model to provide episode and value-based reimbursement for total joint procedures [6]. This 5-year model initially involved 800 hospitals within 67 metropolitan areas that had populations ≥50,000 during the first 2 years, which was then reduced to 465 hospitals for years 3 through 5. The model, which ran through December 31, 2020, held participant hospitals financially accountable for the quality and cost of total joint procedures. Three measures are used to determine a hospital's composite quality score: complication rates (50%), Health Consumer Assessment of Healthcare Providers and Systems survey results (40%), and voluntary completion of PROMs (10%). The composite quality score places hospitals in one of four categories, and those in excellent or good receive reimbursement payments per the CMS pay-for-performance methodology [7].

The CJR requires an improvement for one global quality-of-life measure, obtained from either the Patient-Reported Outcomes Measurement Information System (PROMIS) ten-item survey for functional and global health status or VR-12 (Veterans RAND 12-Item Survey) instruments, and one joint-specific measure (KOOS or KOOS Joint Replacement Survey [KOOS JR]). Data is collected preoperatively (90–0 days before the procedure) and postoperatively (270–365 days). The percent of required preoperative and postoperative PROM data increases from 50% in year 1 to 80% in year 5. As of mid-2020, the percentage of patient PROM data that had been completed in participating hospitals preoperatively and postoperatively was unknown [7].

The CJR program increased the number of hospitals participating in bundled payments from CMS and is not associated with changes in volume of procedures, complications, patient satisfaction, or readmission [8–11]. Molloy et al. [7] conducted a study that reported completion rates of PROM in the CJR postoperative period (270–365 days) in an established practice that had been collecting these data for 6 years prior to the implementation of the CJR model. Patients could complete the PROMIS-10 in person at the office, online through electronic health record portal, or through a hyperlink emailed to them. There were 725 patients, in whom only 215 (30%) completed surveys within the CJR postoperative timeline. The percentage increased to 46% when the postoperative time period was increased to 396 days. The authors suggested that the CJR consider extending the postoperative data collection period beyond 365 days.

Finch et al. [10] conducted a study to compare function, general health, and pain after joint arthroplasty between patients undergoing surgery in bundle (n = 1984) and nonbundle (n = 4490) hospitals. There were significant improvements in KOOS JR, PROMIS-10 physical health, and numeric pain rating scores in both groups from pre-surgery to 6 months post-surgery. There was a small but significant decrease in adjusted KOOS JR scores in bundle hospital patients compared with nonbundle (1.8 points, P = 0.01). There were no differences in the percentage of patients who achieved an MCID in these scores in this short-term follow-up study. The authors concluded that continued evaluation of PROMs is required to ensure that cost savings measures in bundled payment programs do not result in inferior outcomes.

8.3 Knee Society Score

The original KSS was published in 1989 and consisted of two separate assessments for knee rating (pain, range of motion, and stability) and function (walking, stairs) (Table 8.2) [12]. Twenty-three years later (2012), the KSS underwent a major revision to consist of an objective knee score (seven items), a satisfaction score (five items), an expectation score (three items), and a functional activity score (19 items) [13]. The developers published adequate validity and reliability assessments for the

Table 8.2 History of items in the Knee Society Scoring System

Original Knee Society Scoring System [12]		2012 New Knee Society Long-Form [13, 61]		2016 Knee Society Short-Form [16]	
Item	Points	Item	Points	Item	Points
Knee rating	100 possible	Objective knee score	100 possible	Total score	100 possible
				Walking distance	20
				Standard activities:	
		Alignment	25		
Pain	50	Stability	25	Walking on uneven surface	15
Stability	25	ROM	25		
ROM	25	Symptoms	25	Stair climbing/ descending	15
Knee function	100 possible	Satisfaction score	40 possible	Getting up from chair without arms	15
		Pain while sitting	8		
		Pain lying in bed	8	Running	20
Walking	50	Knee function getting out of bed	8	Discretionary activity	15
Stairs	50				
		Knee function light household duties	8		
		Knee function recreational activities	8		
		Expectation score	15 possible		
		Pain relief	5		
		Ability to carry out ADL	5		
		Ability to perform leisure, recreational, or sport activities	5		
		Functional activity score	100 possible		
		Walking and standing (5 items)	30		
		Standard activities (6 items)	30		
		Advanced activities (5 items)	25		
		Discretionary activities (3 items)	15		

subscales [13]. Others reported that this instrument had superior responsiveness 12 months after total knee arthroplasty (TKA; ES 3.38) compared with the WOMAC, SF-12, and OKS scales, with no noteworthy floor or ceiling effects [14]. A minimal detectable change value of 34.5 points was reported for the function score by Jacobs and Christensen [15].

Although comprehensive, the long-form KSS was cumbersome, time-consuming, and office resource intensive. In 2016, the KSS short form was introduced for use in clinics and practices not involved in TKA research [16]. The form consists of ten questions and a list of discretionary activities. Six of the questions are scored. The

Table 8.3 Knee Society Short-Form: psychometric properties and correlations with other instruments at 1 year postoperatively[a]

	KSS short-form	KSS long-form	WOMAC	SF-12
Responsiveness	ES 3.58, SRM 2.92	ES 3.39, SRM 2.68	ES -1.43, SRM −1.16	ES 1.11, SRM 0.77
Ceiling effect (scores ≥90%)	4.7%	5.4%	31.8%	NA
Correlation with KSS short-form	---	$r = 0.9$, $P < 0.001$	$r = -0.60$, $P < 0.001$	$r = 0.60$, $P < 0.001$
Correlation with KSS of changes of scores from preoperative to 1 year postoperatively	---	$r = 0.9$, $P < 0.001$	$r = -0.60$, $P < 0.001$	$r = 0.50$, $P < 0.001$

ES effect size, *KSS* Knee Society Score, *SRM* standardized response mean
[a]From Maniar et al. [17]

five satisfaction scores in the 2012 long form were reduced to one item in the short form, which correlated highly with the five-item subscale score ($r = 0.81$; effect size [ES] difference pre- to postoperatively, 3.24). The 17 items related to function in the long form were reduced to six items, and the subscales showed strong linear associations ($r = 0.97$, $P < 0.01$). The KSS short form was responsive to change after TKA (ES 2.19, $P < 0.01$). In an independent investigation not conducted by the KSS developers, Maniar et al. [17] reported excellent responsiveness (ES 3.58) and no floor or ceiling effects in 148 TKA patients (Table 8.3). The KSS short form was found to be more responsive, with higher ES than the KSS long form, WOMAC, and SF-12 instruments. There was a strong correlation between the scores of the short form and the long form ($r = 0.90$, $P < 0.001$) 1 year after surgery, indicating the two instruments may be used interchangeably. MCID data was not available at the time of writing for the KSS short form.

8.4 Western Ontario and McMaster Universities Osteoarthritis Index

The WOMAC instrument was first introduced in 1988 as a multidimensional health status instrument for patients with knee or hip osteoarthritis [18, 19]. There are three dimensions: function (17 questions), pain (five questions), and stiffness (two questions, Table 8.4). Each question is rated on a Likert scale from 0 (best) to 4 (worst), and the total score is transformed into a 0–100 scale. Roos et al. [20] reported adequate internal consistency, reliability (intraclass correlation coefficient [ICC], 0.58–0.92), and responsiveness of the Swedish version in 32 patients who underwent arthroscopy for knee osteoarthritis. Escobar et al. [21] reported excellent responsiveness at 6 months postoperatively, with ES ranging from 1.13 to 1.71 and standardized response means (SRM) ranging from 0.90 to 1.46. The MCID at

Table 8.4 WOMAC items[a]

Pain	Stiffness	Function
Walking on flat surface	After first wakening in the morning	Descending stairs
Going up or down stairs	After sitting, lying or resting later in the day	Ascending stairs
At night while in bed		Rising from sitting
Sitting or lying		Standing
Standing upright		Bending to floor
		Walking on flat surface
		Getting in/out of car
		Going shopping
		Putting on socks/stockings
		Rising from bed
		Taking off socks/stockings
		Lying in bed
		Getting in/out of bath
		Sitting
		Getting on/off toilet
		Heavy domestic duties
		Light domestic duties

[a]From Bellamy et al. [18]. Each question is rated on a 0–4 scale where 0 = none, 1 = slight, 2 = moderate, 3 = very, and 4 = extremely. Total score 0 (best)–100 (worst) points

Table 8.5 Thresholds for treatment success after total knee arthroplasty[a]

WOMAC dimension	Postoperative time point	Threshold points to predict success	Sensitivity	Specificity
Pain	2 months	17.5	0.65	0.75
	12 months	7.5	0.83	0.74
Stiffness	2 months	31.5	0.76	0.58
	12 months	18.5	0.72	0.61
Function	2 months	33.5	0.82	0.53
	12 months	16.5	0.84	0.67
Total	2 months	29.5	0.80	0.57
	12 months	16.5	0.85	0.68

[a]From Giesinger et al. [5]

12 months postoperatively was determined to be 15 points for the total score, 25–29 points for pain, and 22–27 points for function.

Giesinger et al. [5] found that the WOMAC pain score and the total score were highly predictive of TKA success at 2 and 12 months postoperatively. In this study, treatment success was defined by the responses to four questions: (1) how satisfied are you with your knee arthroplasty (must respond very highly or highly satisfied), (2) would you undergo the procedure again (must respond yes), (3) did the surgery increase your functional capacity (must respond yes), and (4) did the surgery relieve your pain (must respond yes)? The study provided thresholds for scores (and sensitivity and specificity data) that would be expected to predict high patient satisfaction (Table 8.5).

8.5 Oxford Knee Score

In 1998, Dawson et al. [22], within the Public Health and Primary Health Care at the University of Oxford, developed the OKS, a 12-item questionnaire that was designed to assess pain and function after TKA. There are five factors that assess pain and seven that determine function. The recommendations for item scoring are to score each question from 0 to 4, with 4 being the best outcome (Table 8.6). This produces a possible total of 0 (worse score) to 48 (best score) [23]. This is slightly different than the original proposed scoring system in which each question was scored from 1 to 5, with 1 (or an overall score of 12) representing the best outcome. The OKS is available at http://www.orthopaedicscore.com/scorepages/oxford_knee_score.html. A scoring manual and licensing information may be obtained at https://innovation.ox.ac.uk/outcome-measures/oxford-knee-score-oks. The OKS is used by the United Kingdom Department of Health for the assessment of TKA performed each year in National Health Service hospitals.

Dawson et al. [22] found that TKA patients completed the OKS at a higher rate than the SF-36, the original KSS, and the Stanford Health Assessment Questionnaire. These investigators reported the OKS had adequate reliability, internal consistency, and responsiveness for this patient cohort. Other authors have confirmed these findings [24–28]. The OKS is predictive of patient satisfaction postoperatively [29]. A study of 101,036 patients found no floor or ceiling effects 6 months post-TKA [30].

Beard et al. [24] determined the minimally important change (MIC) value for the OKS score using a reference question that compared the knee condition now (6 months postoperatively) to its condition before the procedure with five possible responses (much better, little better, about the same, little worse, much worse). A receiver operating characteristic (ROC) analysis was performed to differentiate between patients who responded they were a little better versus the same. The authors reported that 7 points was the MIC for an individual patient, 9 points represented the MIC value for a single group, and 5 points was the MIC to detect a relevant difference between groups. In addition, a minimal detectable change value of 4.15 points was provided, which can be interpreted to mean that in 90% of the cases, patients will have experienced real change (beyond measurement error) if their score changed by 4.15 points.

8.6 Knee Injury and Osteoarthritis Outcome Score (KOOS)

The KOOS was first presented by Roos et al. [31] in 1989 as a knee joint-specific instrument consisting of 42 items. It was originally validated in patients undergoing anterior cruciate ligament reconstruction and has since been validated in TKA and knee osteoarthritis patients [20, 32–36] There are five subscales: pain (nine items), symptoms (five items), activities of daily living (17 items), sports and recreation (five items), and quality of life (four items). Each subscale is calculated separately from 0 (worst) to 100 (best) points. There are also two questions related to knee

Table 8.6 Oxford Knee Score: all responses are based on symptoms in the preceding 4 weeks

Question	Possible Responses	Points
1. How would you describe the pain you usually have from your knee?	None	4
	Very mild	3
	Mild	2
	Moderate	1
	Severe	0
2. Have you had any trouble with washing and drying yourself (all over) because of your knee?	No trouble at all	4
	Very little trouble	3
	Moderate trouble	2
	Extreme trouble	1
	Impossible to do	0
3. Have you had any trouble getting in and out of a car or using public transport because of your knee? (whichever you tend to use)	No trouble at all	4
	Very little trouble	3
	Moderate trouble	2
	Extreme trouble	1
	Impossible to do	0
4. For how long have you been able to walk before the pain in your knee becomes severe? (with or without a stick)	No pain/>30 min	4
	16–30 min	3
	5–15 min	2
	Around the house only	1
	Not at all – severe on walking	0
5. After a meal (sat at a table), how painful has it been for you to stand up from a chair because of your knee?	Not at all painful	4
	Slightly painful	3
	Moderately painful	2
	Very painful	1
	Unbearable	0
6. Have you been limping when walking because of your knee?	Rarely/never	4
	Sometimes or just at first	3
	Often, not just at first	2
	Most of the time	1
	All of the time	0
7. Could you kneel down and get back up again afterward?	Yes, easily	4
	With little difficulty	3
	With moderate difficulty	2
	With extreme difficulty	1
	No, impossible	0
8. Have you been troubled by pain from your knee in bed at night?	No nights	4
	Only 1 or 2 nights	3
	Some nights	2
	Most nights	1
	Every night	0
9. How much has pain from your knee interfered with your usual work (including housework)?	Not at all	4
	A little bit	3
	Moderately	2
	Greatly	1
	Totally	0

(continued)

Table 8.6 (continued)

Question	Possible Responses	Points
10. Have you felt that your knee might suddenly "give way" or let you down?	Rarely/never	4
	Sometimes or just at first	3
	Often, not just at first	2
	Most of the time	1
	All of the time	0
11. Could you do the household shopping on your own?	Yes, easily	4
	With little difficulty	3
	With moderate difficulty	2
	With extreme difficulty	1
	No, impossible	0
12. Could you walk down a flight of stairs?	Yes, easily	4
	With little difficulty	3
	With moderate difficulty	2
	With extreme difficulty	1
	No, impossible	0

Table 8.7 Patient acceptable symptom state thresholds for KOOS subscales after TKA[a]

KOOS subscale	Threshold score		Sensitivity		Specificity	
	1 year p.o.	3 years p.o.	1 year p.o.	3 years p.o.	1 year p.o.	3 years p.o.
Pain	84.5	87.5	0.74	0.71	0.81	0.81
Symptoms	80.5	84.0	0.74	0.69	0.86	0.81
Activities of daily living	83.0	87.5	0.76	0.72	0.84	0.83
Quality of life	66.0	66.0	0.74	0.75	0.89	0.81

[a]From Connelly et al. [37]

joint stiffness, for a total of 42 items. A total score has not been validated and is not recommended. The instrument and scoring calculators are available at http://www.koos.nu.

In 2019, Connelly et al. [37] determined patient acceptable symptom state (PASS) thresholds for the KOOS subscales 1 and 3 years after TKA in a group of 383 patients (Table 8.7). The PASS was determined based on an anchor question of patient satisfaction. The study found that the subscales were predictive of satisfaction at 1 year ($r = 0.46$ to 0.52, $P < 0.001$) and 3 years postoperatively ($r = 0.44$ to 0.48, $P < 0.001$). Scores were significantly lower in unsatisfied patients compared with satisfied patients at both time periods ($P < 0.05$).

In 2018, Lyman et al. [38] calculated minimal clinically important change (MCIC) and substantial clinical benefit (SCB) data for the subscales of the KOOS instrument (Table 8.8). In their cohort of 2630 TKA patients, the MCIC for the subscales was achieved in 76% to 81% and the SCB was achieved in 60–78% at

Table 8.8 KOOS minimal clinically important change and substantial clinical benefit after TKA[a]

KOOS subscale	Minimal clinically important change (points)	Substantial clinical benefit (points)
Pain	18	22
Symptoms	7	21
Activities of daily living	16	15
Quality of life	17	23

[a]From Lyman et al. [38]

Table 8.9 Responsiveness and floor/ceiling effects of KOOS subscales 6 months after TKA[a]

KOOS subscale	Responsiveness		% Floor effect		% Ceiling effect	
	ES	SRM	Preop	Follow-up	Preop	Follow-up
Pain	1.80	1.51	1.3	0	0.5	13.7
Symptoms	1.25	1.10	0.7	0	0.3	3.6
Activities of daily living	1.53	1.49	0.7	0	0.3	9.4
Quality of life	1.99	1.46	14.5	0.6	0.1	8.2
Sport	1.49	1.07	28.8	4.1	0.9	3.9

[a]From Gandek and Ware [40]

2 years postoperatively. Using these data, Haydel et al. [39] reported the MCIC was achieved in 68–79% and the SCB was achieved in 61–73% in their cohort of 159 TKA patients analyzed 6 months postoperatively. The authors believed the overall 30% failure rate to achieve an adequate outcome (according to the KOOS scale) was attributed to their population that had a high rate of comorbidities (2–3 in 52% and >3 in 38%) and markedly poor preoperative pain and ADL scores.

Gandek and Ware [40] reported that the KOOS subscales were highly responsive to change from preoperative to 6 months post-TKA in a cohort of 820 patients (Table 8.9). There were no noteworthy floor or ceiling effects postoperatively. Before surgery, nearly 29% of the patients had a floor effect on the sport subscale. These authors also reported acceptable convergent validity. Peer et al. [33] reported that the KOOS subscales had moderate to high validity with existing instruments, acceptable reliability, and large responsiveness, with the exception of the sport and recreation subscale that had low construct validity and reliability values (ICC, 0.45–0.65).

8.7 KOOS Joint Replacement Survey (KOOS JR)

In 2016, Lyman et al. [41] conducted a validation study of the KOOS JR in response to the CMS mandate for PROM data. The goal was to devise a shorter instrument than the KOOS or WOMAC that would be appropriate for TKA patients. In a study of 2291 patients, the seven-item PROM was found to have high internal consistency, excellent responsiveness (SRM 1.79), high construct validity, but a concerning 20% ceiling effect. The authors recommended also using the KOOS sports and recreation domain (five items) for younger active patients. The KOOS JR has a raw score that ranges from 0 to 28 points, which is converted to an interval score on a 0–100 scale, with 0 indicating complete disability and 100 perfect knee health. In 2018, Lyman et al. [38] provided MCIC and SCB change data for the KOOS JR, which were 14 and 20 points, respectively. In their cohort of 2630 TKA patients, 81% achieved the MCIC and 68% achieved the SCB 2 years postoperatively. The instrument and online scoring are available at https://www.orthotoolkit.com/koos-jr. In 2020, the American Physical Therapy Association's clinical practice guideline included the use of the KOOS JR, in addition to the 30-second sit-to-stand and timed-up-and-go tests, to determine outcomes [42].

8.8 Short Form-36 and Short Form-12

In 1992, Ware et al. [43] introduced the Short Form-36 Health Survey, a generic measure of health status. The original SF-36 stemmed from the Medical Outcome Study, conducted by the RAND Corporation. Since then, a free commercial version became available, which is available at https://www.rand.org/health-care/surveys_tools/mos/36-item-short-form.html. The SF-36 consists of eight subscales—vitality, physical functioning, bodily pain, general health perceptions, physical role functioning, emotional role functioning, social role functioning, and mental health—and takes approximately 6–9 minutes to complete. Each scale is directly transformed into a 0–100-point scale, with lower scores indicating greater disability. There are two distinct concepts measured by the SF-36: a physical dimension, represented by a Physical Component Summary score (PCS-36), and a mental dimension, represented by the Mental Component Summary score (MCS-36). Reliability, validity, and responsiveness of the SF-36 have been reported by numerous studies [44–47].

In 1996, Ware et al. described the construction and initial tests of reliability and validity for the SF-12 [46], which takes approximately 2 minutes to complete (Table 8.10). Significant association was found with the scoring of this instrument in the prediction of the PCS-36 ($R^2 = 0.91$) and MCS-36 ($R^2 = 0.92$) in 2474 individuals from the general US population. Gandek et al. [48] reported similar findings from 9151 individuals in nine European countries. The SF-12 has adequate psychometric properties as reported by multiple studies [49–53]. The questionnaire, scoring, and downloadable reports are available at no cost at https://www.orthotoolkit.com/sf-12/.

8.9 PROMIS Global-10 Short Form

The PROMIS Global-10 Short Form consists of ten items that assess general domains of health and functioning including overall physical health, mental health, social health, pain, fatigue, and overall perceived quality of life (Table 8.11). There are two four-item summary scores: a global physical health (GPH) score and a global mental health (GMH) score [54]. These scores may be used to determine an overall summary of health and mental status. In addition, one may estimate an

Table 8.10 SF-12

Patient instruction: This survey asks for your views about your health. This information will help keep track of how you feel and how well you are able to do your usual activities. Answer each question by choosing just one answer. If you are unsure how to answer a question, please give the best answer you can.

1. In general, would you say your health is:

☐ Excellent ☐ Very Good ☐ Good ☐ Fair ☐ Poor

The following questions are about activities you might do during a typical day. Does **your health now limit you** in these activities? If so, how much?

	YES, limited a lot	YES, limited a little	No, not limited at all
2. **Moderate activities** such as moving a table, pushing a vacuum cleaner, bowling, and playing light golf	☐	☐	☐
3. Climbing **several** flights of stairs	☐	☐	☐

During the **past 4 weeks**, have you had any of the following problems with your work or other regular daily activities **as a result of your physical health?**

	YES	NO
4. **Accomplished less** than you would like	☐	☐
5. Were limited in the **kind** of work or other activities	☐	☐

During the **past 4 weeks**, have you had any of the following problems with your work or other regular daily activities **as a result of any emotional problems** (such as feeling depressed or anxious)?

	YES	NO
6. **Accomplished less** than you would like	☐	☐
7. Did work or activities **less carefully than usual**	☐	☐

During the **past 4 weeks**, how much **did pain interfere** with your normal work (including work outside the home and housework)?

☐ Not at all ☐ A little bit ☐ Moderately ☐ Quite a bit ☐ Extremely

These questions are about how you feel and how things have been with you during the past 4 weeks.
For each question, please give the ONE answer that comes closest to the way you have been feeling.

How much time during the past 4 weeks....

	All of the time	Most of the time	A good bit of the time	Some of the time	A little of the time	None of the time
9. Have you felt calm and peaceful?	☐	☐	☐	☐	☐	☐
10. Did you have a lot of energy?	☐	☐	☐	☐	☐	☐
11. Have you felt downhearted and blue?	☐	☐	☐	☐	☐	☐

12. During the **past 4 weeks**, how much of the time has your **physical health or emotional problems** interfered with your social activities (like visiting friends, relatives, etc.)?

☐ All of the time ☐ Most of the time ☐ Some of the time ☐ A little of the time ☐ None of the time

EQ-5D score from a combination of eight Global-10 items. There are a variety of data collection and scoring tools available online at http://www.healthmeasures.net/index.php?option=com_content&view=category&layout=blog&id=135&Itemid=935. Developed by the National Institutes of Health, scores are compared with normative values calculated in US populations. A study of 21,000 patients in the USA demonstrated adequate reliability and construct validity for the GPH and GMH subscales [55].

Table 8.11 PROMIS Global-10 Health Scale items[a]

Question	Responses
1. In general, would you say your health is:	Excellent, very good, good, fair, poor
2. In general, would you say your quality of life is:	Excellent, very good, good, fair, poor
3. In general, how would you rate your physical health?	Excellent, very good, good, fair, poor
4. In general, how would you rate your mental health, including your mood and ability to think?	Excellent, very good, good, fair, poor
5. In general, how would you rate your satisfaction with your social activities and relationships?	Excellent, very good, good, fair, poor
6. In general, please rate how well you carry out your usual social activities and roles	Excellent, very good, good, fair, poor
7. To what extent are you able to carry out your everyday physical activities such as walking, climbing stairs, carrying groceries, and moving a chair?	Completely, mostly, moderately, a little, not at all
8. How often have you been bothered by emotional problems such as feeling anxious, depressed, or irritable?	Never, rarely, sometimes, often, always
9. How would you rate your fatigue on average?	Never, rarely, sometimes, often, always
10. How would you rate your pain on average	0–10, where 0 = no pain and 10 = worst pain imaginable

[a]2010–2018 PROMIS Health Organization, Version 1.2

Shim and Hamilton [56] compared the responsiveness of the PROMIS Global-10 GPH and GMH subscales with the EQ-5D and the OKS. A cohort of 721 patients who underwent TKA was followed for 1 year after surgery. SRM and ES calculated from 3 to 12 months postoperatively demonstrated excellent responsiveness of all scales except the GMH subscale. The GPH subscale and EQ-5D measures correlated with the OKS ($r = 0.57$ and 0.51, respectively, $P < 0.01$), and these outcome measures were able to discriminate between patients who achieved the OKS MCID (>5) and those who did not. The GPH subscale was also reported to have adequate responsiveness after meniscectomy and ACL reconstruction [57].

8.10 Activity Rating Scoring Systems

Introduced in 1984, the University of California Los Angeles (UCLA) activity rating score is frequently used to determine overall levels after TKA (see Chap. 10) [58]. The 1–10 scale includes impact sports, very active events, active events, moderate activities, mild activities, and inactive states (Table 8.12). Naal et al. [59] reported that this score had adequate reliability, feasibility, and floor and ceiling effects after total joint arthroplasty in 205 patients. It was found to be superior to the Tegner scale and the Activity Rating Scale. The main criticism was that it does not assess frequency, duration, and intensity of activities.

The Lower Extremity Activity Scale (LEAS) was published in 2005 by Saleh et al. [60]. This scale includes 18 levels that range from complete bed confinement

Table 8.12 UCLA activity rating[a]

Level	Activity
10	Regularly participate in *impact sports* such as jogging, tennis, skiing, aerobatics, ballet, heavy labor, and backpacking
9	Sometimes participate in *impact sports*
8	Regularly participate in *very active* events, such as bowling and golf
7	Regularly participate in *active* events, such as bicycling
6	Regularly participate in *moderate activities*, such as swimming and unlimited housework or shopping
5	Sometimes participate in *moderate activities*
4	Regularly participate in *mild activities*, such as walking, limited housework, and limited shopping
3	Sometimes participate in *mild activities*
2	Mostly *inactive*; restricted to minimal activities of daily living
1	Wholly *inactive*; dependent on others; cannot leave residence

[a]From Amstutz et al. [58]

Table 8.13 The Lower Extremity Activity Scale[a]

Points	Description
1	I am confined to bed all day
2	I am confined to bed most of the day except for minimal transfer activities (going to the bathroom, etc.)
3	I am either in bed or sitting in a chair most of the day
4	I sit most of the day, except for minimal transfer activities, no walking or standing
5	I sit most of the day, but I stand occasionally and walk a minimal amount in my house (I may rarely leave the house for an appointment and may require the use of a wheelchair or scooter for transportation)
6	I walk around my house to a moderate degree but I don't leave the house on a regular basis. I may leave the house occasionally for an appointment
7	I walk around my house and go outside at will, walking one or two blocks at a time
8	I walk around my house, go outside at will, and walk several blocks at a time without any assistance (weather permitting)
9	I am up and about at will in my house and can go out and walk as much as I would like with no restrictions (weather permitting)
10	I am up and about at will in my house and outside. I also work outside the house in a minimally active job
11	I am up and about at will in my house and outside. I also work outside the house in a moderately active job
12	I am up and about at will in my house and outside. I also work outside the house in an extremely active job
13	I am up and about at will in my house and outside. I also participate in relaxed physical activities such as jogging, dancing, cycling, and swimming occasionally (2–3 times per month)
14	I am up and about at will in my house and outside. I also participate in relaxed physical activities such as jogging, dancing, cycling, and swimming 2–3 times per week
15	I am up and about at will in my house and outside. I also participate in relaxed physical activities such as jogging, dancing, cycling, and swimming daily
16	I am up and about at will in my house and outside. I also participate in vigorous physical activities such as competitive level sports occasionally (2–3 times per month)
17	I am up and about at will in my house and outside. I also participate in vigorous physical activities such as competitive level sports (2–3 times per week)
18	I am up and about at will in my house and outside. I also participate in vigorous physical activities such as competitive level sports daily

[a]From Saleh et al. [60]

to participation in vigorous physical activity including competitive sports (Table 8.13). In a study of revision TKA patients, this scale correlated with pedometer readings ($R = 0.79$). The authors also reported adequate reliability (ICC = 0.9), responsiveness, and validity. The scale correlated with the WOMAC function and pain scores ($P < 0.001$).

References

1. Lovelock TM, Broughton NS, Williams CM. The popularity of outcome measures for hip and knee arthroplasties. J Arthroplasty. 2018;33(1):273–6. https://doi.org/10.1016/j.arth.2017.08.024.
2. Siljander MP, McQuivey KS, Fahs AM, Galasso LA, Serdahely KJ, Karadsheh MS. Current trends in patient-reported outcome measures in total joint arthroplasty: a study of 4 major orthopaedic journals. J Arthroplasty. 2018;33(11):3416–21. https://doi.org/10.1016/j.arth.2018.06.034.
3. Theodoulou A, Bramwell DC, Spiteri AC, Kim SW, Krishnan J. The use of scoring systems in knee arthroplasty: a systematic review of the literature. J Arthroplasty. 2016;31(10):2364–2370 e2368. https://doi.org/10.1016/j.arth.2016.05.055.
4. Rolfson O, Eresian Chenok K, Bohm E, Lubbeke A, Denissen G, Dunn J, Lyman S, Franklin P, Dunbar M, Overgaard S, Garellick G, Dawson J, Patient-Reported Outcome Measures Working Group of the International Society of Arthroplasty R. Patient-reported outcome measures in arthroplasty registries. Acta Orthop. 2016;87(Suppl 1):3–8. https://doi.org/10.1080/17453674.2016.1181815.
5. Giesinger JM, Hamilton DF, Jost B, Behrend H, Giesinger K. WOMAC, EQ-5D and knee society score thresholds for treatment success after total knee arthroplasty. J Arthroplasty. 2015. https://doi.org/10.1016/j.arth.2015.06.012.
6. Services CfMM. Comprehensive care for joint replacement model. 2020. https://innovation.cms.gov/innovation-models/cjr. Accessed 31 Mar 2020.
7. Molloy IB, Yong TM, Keswani A, Keeney BJ, Moschetti WE, Lucas AP, Jevsevar DS. Do medicare's patient-reported outcome measures collection windows accurately reflect academic clinical practice? J Arthroplasty. 2020;35(4):911–7. https://doi.org/10.1016/j.arth.2019.11.006.
8. Dummit LA, Kahvecioglu D, Marrufo G, Rajkumar R, Marshall J, Tan E, Press MJ, Flood S, Muldoon LD, Gu Q, Hassol A, Bott DM, Bassano A, Conway PH. Association between hospital participation in a medicare bundled payment initiative and payments and quality outcomes for lower extremity joint replacement episodes. JAMA. 2016;316(12):1267–78. https://doi.org/10.1001/jama.2016.12717.
9. Finkelstein A, Ji Y, Mahoney N, Skinner J. Mandatory medicare bundled payment program for lower extremity joint replacement and discharge to institutional Postacute care: interim analysis of the first year of a 5-year randomized trial. JAMA. 2018;320(9):892–900. https://doi.org/10.1001/jama.2018.12346.
10. Finch DJ, Pellegrini VD Jr, Franklin PD, Magder LS, Pelt CE, Martin BI, Investigators P. The effects of bundled payment programs for hip and knee arthroplasty on patient-reported outcomes. J Arthroplasty. 2020;35(4):918–925 e917. https://doi.org/10.1016/j.arth.2019.11.028.
11. Navathe AS, Liao JM, Dykstra SE, Wang E, Lyon ZM, Shah Y, Martinez J, Small DS, Werner RM, Dinh C, Ma X, Emanuel EJ. Association of hospital participation in a medicare bundled payment program with volume and case mix of lower extremity joint replacement episodes. JAMA. 2018;320(9):901–10. https://doi.org/10.1001/jama.2018.12345.
12. Insall JN, Dorr LD, Scott RD, Scott WN. Rationale of the knee society clinical rating system. Clin Orthop Relat Res. 1989;248:13–4.

13. Noble PC, Scuderi GR, Brekke AC, Sikorskii A, Benjamin JB, Lonner JH, Chadha P, Daylamani DA, Scott WN, Bourne RB. Development of a new knee society scoring system. Clin Orthop Relat Res. 2012;470(1):20–32. https://doi.org/10.1007/s11999-011-2152-z.
14. Maniar RN, Maniar PR, Chanda D, Gajbhare D, Chouhan T. What is the responsiveness and respondent burden of the new knee society score? Clin Orthop Relat Res. 2017;475(9):2218–27. https://doi.org/10.1007/s11999-017-5338-1.
15. Jacobs CA, Christensen CP. Correlations between knee society function scores and functional force measures. Clin Orthop Relat Res. 2009;467(9):2414–9. https://doi.org/10.1007/s11999-009-0811-0.
16. Scuderi GR, Sikorskii A, Bourne RB, Lonner JH, Benjamin JB, Noble PC. The knee society short form reduces respondent burden in the assessment of patient-reported outcomes. Clin Orthop Relat Res. 2016;474(1):134–42. https://doi.org/10.1007/s11999-015-4370-2.
17. Maniar RN, Maniar PR, Chanda D, Gajbhare D, Chouhan T. Short-form new knee society score: what is its responsiveness and convergent validity with other scores? J Knee Surg. 2020. https://doi.org/10.1055/s-0040-1702190.
18. Bellamy N, Buchanan WW, Goldsmith CH, Campbell J, Stitt LW. Validation study of WOMAC: a health status instrument for measuring clinically important patient relevant outcomes to antirheumatic drug therapy in patients with osteoarthritis of the hip or knee. J Rheumatol. 1988;15(12):1833–40.
19. Bellamy N. Pain assessment in osteoarthritis: experience with the WOMAC osteoarthritis index. Semin Arthritis Rheum. 1989;18(4 Suppl 2):14–7. https://doi.org/10.1016/0049-0172(89)90010-3.
20. Roos EM, Klassbo M, Lohmander LS. WOMAC osteoarthritis index. Reliability, validity, and responsiveness in patients with arthroscopically assessed osteoarthritis. Western Ontario and MacMaster Universities. Scand J Rheumatol. 1999;28(4):210–5.
21. Escobar A, Quintana JM, Bilbao A, Arostegui I, Lafuente I, Vidaurreta I. Responsiveness and clinically important differences for the WOMAC and SF-36 after total knee replacement. Osteoarthr Cartil. 2007;15(3):273–80. https://doi.org/10.1016/j.joca.2006.09.001.
22. Dawson J, Fitzpatrick R, Murray D, Carr A. Questionnaire on the perceptions of patients about total knee replacement. J Bone Joint Surg. 1998;80(1):63–9.
23. Murray DW, Fitzpatrick R, Rogers K, Pandit H, Beard DJ, Carr AJ, Dawson J. The use of the Oxford hip and knee scores. J Bone Joint Surg. 2007;89(8):1010–4. https://doi.org/10.1302/0301-620X.89B8.19424.
24. Beard DJ, Harris K, Dawson J, Doll H, Murray DW, Carr AJ, Price AJ. Meaningful changes for the Oxford hip and knee scores after joint replacement surgery. J Clin Epidemiol. 2015;68(1):73–9. https://doi.org/10.1016/j.jclinepi.2014.08.009.
25. Jenny JY, Diesinger Y. The Oxford Knee Score: compared performance before and after knee replacement. Orthop Traumatol Surg Res. 2012;98(4):409–12. https://doi.org/10.1016/j.otsr.2012.03.004.
26. Harris K, Dawson J, Doll H, Field RE, Murray DW, Fitzpatrick R, Jenkinson C, Price AJ, Beard DJ. Can pain and function be distinguished in the Oxford Knee Score in a meaningful way? An exploratory and confirmatory factor analysis. Qual Life Res. 2013;22(9):2561–8. https://doi.org/10.1007/s11136-013-0393-x.
27. Harris K, Dawson J, Gibbons E, Lim CR, Beard DJ, Fitzpatrick R, Price AJ. Systematic review of measurement properties of patient-reported outcome measures used in patients undergoing hip and knee arthroplasty. Patient Relat Outcome Meas. 2016;7:101–8. https://doi.org/10.2147/PROM.S97774.
28. Xie F, Ye H, Zhang Y, Liu X, Lei T, Li SC. Extension from inpatients to outpatients: validity and reliability of the Oxford Knee Score in measuring health outcomes in patients with knee osteoarthritis. Int J Rheum Dis. 2011;14(2):206–10. https://doi.org/10.1111/j.1756-185X.2010.01580.x.
29. Clemente CD. Anatomy: a regional atlas of the human body. 5th ed. Baltimore: Lippincott, Williams and Wilkins; 2007.

30. Harris K, Lim CR, Dawson J, Fitzpatrick R, Beard DJ, Price AJ. The Oxford knee score and its subscales do not exhibit a ceiling or a floor effect in knee arthroplasty patients: an analysis of the National Health Service PROMs data set. Knee Surg Sports Traumatol Arthrosc. 2017;25(9):2736–42. https://doi.org/10.1007/s00167-015-3788-0.
31. Roos EM, Roos HP, Lohmander LS, Ekdahl C, Beynnon BD. Knee injury and Osteoarthritis Outcome Score (KOOS)--development of a self-administered outcome measure. J Orthop Sports Phys Ther. 1998;28(2):88–96.
32. Bekkers JE, de Windt TS, Raijmakers NJ, Dhert WJ, Saris DB. Validation of the Knee Injury and Osteoarthritis Outcome Score (KOOS) for the treatment of focal cartilage lesions. Osteoarthr Cartil. 2009;17(11):1434–9. https://doi.org/10.1016/j.joca.2009.04.019.
33. Peer MA, Lane J. The Knee Injury and Osteoarthritis Outcome Score (KOOS): a review of its psychometric properties in people undergoing total knee arthroplasty. J Orthop Sports Phys Ther. 2013;43(1):20–8. https://doi.org/10.2519/jospt.2013.4057.
34. Roos EM, Engelhart L, Ranstam J, Anderson AF, Irrgang JJ, Marx RG, Tegner Y, Davis AM. ICRS recommendation document: patient-reported outcome instruments for use in patients with articular cartilage defects. Cartilage. 2011;2(2):122–36. https://doi.org/10.1177/1947603510391084.
35. Roos EM, Lohmander LS. The Knee injury and Osteoarthritis Outcome Score (KOOS): from joint injury to osteoarthritis. Health Qual Life Outcomes. 2003;1(1):64.
36. Roos EM, Toksvig-Larsen S. Knee injury and Osteoarthritis Outcome Score (KOOS) - validation and comparison to the WOMAC in total knee replacement. Health Qual Life Outcomes. 2003;1(1):17.
37. Connelly JW, Galea VP, Rojanasopondist P, Matuszak SJ, Ingelsrud LH, Nielsen CS, Bragdon CR, Huddleston JI 3rd, Malchau H, Troelsen A. Patient acceptable symptom state at 1 and 3 years after total knee arthroplasty: thresholds for the Knee Injury and Osteoarthritis Outcome Score (KOOS). J Bone Joint Surg Am. 2019;101(11):995–1003. https://doi.org/10.2106/jbjs.18.00233.
38. Lyman S, Lee YY, McLawhorn AS, Islam W, MacLean CH. What are the minimal and substantial improvements in the HOOS and KOOS and JR versions after total joint replacement? Clin Orthop Relat Res. 2018;476(12):2432–41. https://doi.org/10.1097/CORR.0000000000000456.
39. Haydel A, Guilbeau S, Roubion R, Leonardi C, Bronstone A, Dasa V. Achieving validated thresholds for clinically meaningful change on the knee injury and osteoarthritis outcome score after Total knee arthroplasty: findings from a university-based orthopaedic tertiary care safety net practice. J Am Acad Orthop Surg Glob Res Rev. 2019;3(11):e00142. https://doi.org/10.5435/JAAOSGlobal-D-19-00142.
40. Gandek B, Ware JE Jr. Validity and responsiveness of the knee injury and osteoarthritis outcome score: a comparative study among total knee replacement patients. Arthritis Care Res. 2017;69(6):817–25. https://doi.org/10.1002/acr.23193.
41. Lyman S, Lee YY, Franklin PD, Li W, Cross MB, Padgett DE. Validation of the KOOS, JR: a Short-form Knee Arthroplasty Outcomes Survey. Clin Orthop Relat Res. 2016. https://doi.org/10.1007/s11999-016-4719-1.
42. Jette DU, Hunter SJ, Burkett L, Langham B, Logerstedt DS, Piuzzi NS, Poirier NM, Radach LJL, Ritter JE, Scalzitti DA, Stevens-Lapsley JE, Tompkins J, Zeni J Jr, American Physical Therapy A. Physical therapist management of total knee arthroplasty. Phys Ther. 2020;100(9):1603–31. https://doi.org/10.1093/ptj/pzaa099.
43. Ware JE Jr, Sherbourne CD. The MOS 36-item short-form health survey (SF-36). I. Conceptual framework and item selection. Med Care. 1992;30(6):473–83.
44. Ruta D, Hurst N, Kind P, Hunter M, Stubbings A. Measuring health status in British patients with rheumatoid arthritis: reliability, validity and responsiveness of the short form 36-item health survey (SF-36). Br J Rheumatol. 1998;37(4):425–36.
45. Linde L, Sørensen J, Østergaard M, Hørslev-Petersen K, Hetland ML. Health-related quality of life: validity, reliability, and responsiveness of SF-36, EQ-15D, EQ-5D, RAQoL, and HAQ in patients with rheumatoid arthritis. J Rheumatol. 2008;35(8):1528–37.

46. Ware J Jr, Kosinski M, Keller SD. A 12-Item Short-Form Health Survey: construction of scales and preliminary tests of reliability and validity. Med Care. 1996;34(3):220–33.
47. McHorney CA, Ware JE, Rachel JF, Sherbourne CD. The MOS 36-item short-form health survey (SF-36): III. Tests of data quality, scaling assumptions, and reliability across diverse patient groups. Med Care. 1994;32(1):40–66.
48. Gandek B, Ware JE, Aaronson NK, Apolone G, Bjorner JB, Brazier JE, Bullinger M, Kaasa S, Leplege A, Prieto L, Sullivan M. Cross-validation of item selection and scoring for the SF-12 Health Survey in nine countries: results from the IQOLA Project. International Quality of Life Assessment. J Clin Epidemiol. 1998;51(11):1171–8.
49. Jenkinson C, Layte R, Jenkinson D, Lawrence K, Petersen S, Paice C, Stradling J. A shorter form health survey: can the SF-12 replicate results from the SF-36 in longitudinal studies? J Public Health Med. 1997;19(2):179–86.
50. Gandhi SK, Salmon JW, Zhao SZ, Lambert BL, Gore PR, Conrad K. Psychometric evaluation of the 12-item short-form health survey (SF-12) in osteoarthritis and rheumatoid arthritis clinical trials. Clin Ther. 2001;23(7):1080–98.
51. Resnick B, Nahm ES. Reliability and validity testing of the revised 12-item Short-Form Health Survey in older adults. J Nurs Meas. 2001;9(2):151–61.
52. Schofield MJ, Mishra G. Validity of the SF-12 compared with the SF-36 Health Survey in pilot studies of the Australian Longitudinal Study on Women's Health. J Health Psychol. 1998;3(2):259–71.
53. Cheak-Zamora NC, Wyrwich KW, McBride TD. Reliability and validity of the SF-12v2 in the medical expenditure panel survey. Qual Life Res. 2009;18(6):727–35.
54. Hays RD, Bjorner JB, Revicki DA, Spritzer KL, Cella D. Development of physical and mental health summary scores from the patient-reported outcomes measurement information system (PROMIS) global items. Qual Life Res. 2009;18(7):873–80. https://doi.org/10.1007/s11136-009-9496-9.
55. Cella D, Riley W, Stone A, Rothrock N, Reeve B, Yount S, Amtmann D, Bode R, Buysse D, Choi S, Cook K, Devellis R, DeWalt D, Fries JF, Gershon R, Hahn EA, Lai JS, Pilkonis P, Revicki D, Rose M, Weinfurt K, Hays R, Group PC. The Patient-Reported Outcomes Measurement Information System (PROMIS) developed and tested its first wave of adult self-reported health outcome item banks: 2005–2008. J Clin Epidemiol. 2010;63(11):1179–94. https://doi.org/10.1016/j.jclinepi.2010.04.011.
56. Shim J, Hamilton DF. Comparative responsiveness of the PROMIS-10 global health and EQ-5D questionnaires in patients undergoing total knee arthroplasty. Bone Joint J. 2019;101-b(7):832–7. https://doi.org/10.1302/0301-620x.101b7.Bjj-2018-1543.R1.
57. Oak SR, Strnad GJ, Bena J, Farrow LD, Parker RD, Jones MH, Spindler KP. Responsiveness comparison of the EQ-5D, PROMIS global health, and VR-12 questionnaires in knee arthroscopy. Orthop J Sports Med. 2016;4(12):2325967116674714. https://doi.org/10.1177/2325967116674714.
58. Amstutz HC, Thomas BJ, Jinnah R, Kim W, Grogan T, Yale C. Treatment of primary osteoarthritis of the hip. A comparison of total joint and surface replacement arthroplasty. J Bone Joint Surg Am. 1984;66(2):228–41.
59. Naal FD, Impellizzeri FM, Leunig M. Which is the best activity rating scale for patients undergoing total joint arthroplasty? Clin Orthop Relat Res. 2009;467(4):958–65. https://doi.org/10.1007/s11999-008-0358-5.
60. Saleh KJ, Mulhall KJ, Bershadsky B, Ghomrawi HM, White LE, Buyea CM, Krackow KA. Development and validation of a lower-extremity activity scale. Use for patients treated with revision total knee arthroplasty. J Bone Joint Surg Am. 2005;87(9):1985–94. https://doi.org/10.2106/JBJS.D.02564.
61. Scuderi GR, Bourne RB, Noble PC, Benjamin JB, Lonner JH, Scott WN. The new knee society knee scoring system. Clin Orthop Relat Res. 2012;470(1):3–19. https://doi.org/10.1007/s11999-011-2135-0.

Common Objective Measurements for Strength, Balance, and Function in the Arthroplasty Patient

9

Frank R. Noyes and Sue Barber-Westin

9.1 Introduction

The determination of outcome after total knee arthroplasty (TKA) requires assessment of both patient-reported outcome measures (PROMs) and objective parameters that measure strength, balance, and functional performance. This chapter details the most common objective assessments used postoperatively in the standard clinic setting. Commonly used and recommended PROMs are discussed in Chap. 8.

Multiple investigations have sought to determine relationships between various objective measures using the tests described in this chapter (Table 9.1) [1–8]. For instance, Aalund et al. [1] reported significant associations between isometric knee extension strength and the 30-second chair-stand test ($r = 0.40$, $P = 0.01$) and 10-meter fast speed walk test ($r = 0.51$, $P = 0.001$). Almeida et al. [2] found a significant relationship between performance on the stair-climb test and isometric knee extension strength ($r = 0.58$; $P < 0.01$) and hip abduction strength ($r = 0.60$, $P < 0.001$) in patients tested 2–6 months postoperatively. Mizner et al. [9] found quadriceps weakness was associated with decreased performance in the timed up and go test (TUG) ($r = 0.64$, $P < 0.05$) and the stair-climb test ($r = 0.63$; $P < 0.05$) over the first postoperative year. Others such as Loyd et al. [10] used validated strength and function assessments to determine if correlations existed with postoperative symptoms such as swelling. These authors reported that swelling significantly contributed to lower quadriceps strength and slower up-and-go test times

F. R. Noyes
Cincinnati SportsMedicine and Orthopaedic Center, The Noyes Knee Institute, Cincinnati, OH, USA

S. Barber-Westin (✉)
Noyes Knee Institute, Cincinnati, OH, USA
e-mail: sbwestin@csmref.org

F. R. Noyes, S. Barber-Westin (eds.), *Critical Rehabilitation for Partial and Total Knee Arthroplasty*, https://doi.org/10.1007/978-3-030-87003-4_9

Table 9.1 Correlations between isometric quadriceps strength and physical function after TKA

Study	Time postoperative (mos)	30-s chair stand test	10-m fast speed walk	Timed-up-and-go test	Stair-climb test	6-minute walk test
Aalund [1]	1	$r = 0.40$ $P = 0.01$	$r = 0.51$ $P = 0.001$			
Yoshida [95]	3			$r = 0.59$ $P = 0.04$	$r = 0.79$ $P = 0.002$	$r = 0.76$ $P = 0.004$
	12			$r = 0.79$ $P = 0.002$	$r = 0.79$ $P = 0.002$	$r = 0.90$ $P < 0.01$
Mizner [9]	6			$r = 0.64$ $P < 0.05$	$r = 0.63$ $P < 0.05$	
Mizner [96]	1			$r = 0.40$ $P < 0.05$	$r = 0.36$ $P < 0.05$	$r = 0.44$ $P < 0.05$
	12			$r = 0.48$ $P < 0.05$	$r = 0.45$ $P < 0.05$	$r = 0.58$ $P < 0.05$
Farquhar [5]	12				$r = 0.49$ $P < 0.001$	$r = 0.55$ $P < 0.001$
	24				$r = 0.45$ $P < 0.001$	$r = 0.43$ $P < 0.001$
	36				$r = 0.15$ $P =$ NS	$r = 0.50$ $P = 0.003$
Almeida [2]	2–6				$r = 0.58$ $P < 0.01$	

NS not significant

6 weeks after surgery. Fleeton et al. [11] reported that knee instability symptoms 6 months postoperatively were associated with reduced muscle power in the stair-climb test conducted 6 weeks postsurgery. Graff et al. [12] found significant relationships a mean of 2 years postoperatively between the TUG and scores on the Knee Society Score, Knee Injury and Osteoarthritis Outcome Score, and the Oxford Knee Score ($r = 0.51$–0.77; $P < 0.05$).

In 2013, the Osteoarthritis Research Society International advisory group formed a consensus of physical function tests for use in patients with hip or knee osteoarthritis or after joint replacement [13]. The tests recommended were the 30-s chair stand, 40-m fast-paced walk, TUG, and 6-minute walk. In addition, a stair-climb test was recommended; however, due to the lack of consistency with stair negotiation tests in the literature, a specific test could not be recommended. In 2020, the American Physical Therapy Association's clinical practice guideline included the use of the 30-s sit-to-stand and the TUG tests, in addition to the Knee Injury and Osteoarthritis Outcome Score Joint Replacement Survey (KOOS JR), to determine outcomes [14].

9.2 Common Measurements for Strength

9.2.1 Isometric Tests

9.2.1.1 Knee Flexion and Extension

Quadriceps and hamstrings strength may be measured as a maximum voluntary isometric contraction using a handheld dynamometer (HHD). Protocols typically involve the following:

1. Make sure no test contraindications are present such as knee joint pain, swelling, limited knee range of motion, and patellar instability.
2. Have the patient warm up for 5 minutes on a stationary bicycle.
3. Properly position the patient. Use stabilizing straps to ensure an isometric contraction is measured.
4. Educate the patient regarding the requirements of the test.
5. Test the noninvolved extremity first.
6. Knee extensors are typically tested with the patient seated, knee flexed to 90°, with the dynamometer placed on the anterior aspect of the shank, proximal to the ankle joint.
7. Knee flexors are usually tested with the patient seated, knee flexed to 90°, with the dynamometer placed on the posterior aspect of the shank, proximal to the ankle joint.
8. Perform three maximal repetitions, with 1-minute rest between tests. Use either the average of the three repetitions or take the highest value.
9. Use verbal encouragement throughout the test such as "push as hard as possible."
10. Convert to Nm and normalize to body weight.

Isometric strength testing with an HHD is a reliable measure in patients with knee osteoarthritis (ICC, 0.98) [15] and after TKA (ICC, 0.95–0.96) [6, 16].

Isometric testing may also be performed with an isokinetic dynamometer. Protocols typically involve the following:

1. Make sure no test contraindications are present such as knee joint pain, swelling, limited knee range of motion, and patellar instability.
2. Have the patient warm up for 5 minutes on a stationary bicycle.
3. Properly position the patient on the test equipment.
4. Educate the patient regarding the requirements of the test.
5. Test the noninvolved extremity first.
6. Set the knee flexion angle at 90° for quadriceps, 60° or 90° for hamstrings.
7. Perform three maximal repetitions; use either the mean value or highest value for test interpretation.
8. Use verbal encouragement throughout the test, such as "push as hard as possible."
9. Normalize the maximal force generated (peak torque, measured in Newton-meters) to the patient's body weight (Nm/kg).

9.2.1.2 Hip Abduction

A HHD may be used to measure hip abduction strength. Protocols typically involve the following:

1. Make sure no test contraindications are present such as knee joint pain, swelling, limited knee range of motion, and patellar instability.
2. Have the patient warm up for 5 minutes on a stationary bicycle.
3. Place the patient in a side-lying position with the limb to be tested facing up. The tested hip is in neutral flexion/extension and neutral rotation. The knee of the tested limb is in full extension. The dynamometer is positioned on the lateral aspect of the tested limb just proximal to the lateral femoral epicondyle, and a stabilization strap is used to secure the dynamometer against the leg and provide resistance to hip abduction.
4. Educate the patient regarding the requirements of the test.
5. Test the noninvolved extremity first.
6. Instruct the patient to push as hard as possible against the dynamometer for 5 seconds. Three trials are performed on each side.
7. Convert to Nm and normalize to body weight.

This test has been shown to be valid and reliable in patients with osteoarthritis (ICC, 0.94) [17] and in those who have undergone TKA (ICC, 0.82–0.95) [3, 18].

9.2.2 Isokinetic Testing Knee Flexion and Extension

Although not as commonly available as other strength measures, isokinetic testing with a dynamometer at varying velocities may be used later in the postoperative course to measure quadriceps and hamstring strength. Isokinetic strength after TKA is usually measured at 60°/s and 180°/s [19]. The protocol typically involves:

1. Make sure no test contraindications are present such as knee joint pain, swelling, limited knee range of motion, and patellar instability.
2. Have the patient warm up for 5 minutes on a stationary bicycle.
3. Properly position the patient on the test equipment (Fig. 9.1).
4. Educate the patient regarding the requirements of the test.
5. Test the noninvolved extremity first.
6. Perform three maximal continuous flexion-extension trials at 60°/s and five trials at 180°/s.
7. Use verbal encouragement throughout the test, such as "push as hard as possible."
8. Normalize the maximal force generated (peak torque, measured in Nm) to the patient's body weight (Nm/kg).

Devices such as the Biodex System 3 have well-known reliability (ICC, 0.93–0.99) [6, 15, 20, 21] and validity (ICC, 0.99) [20].

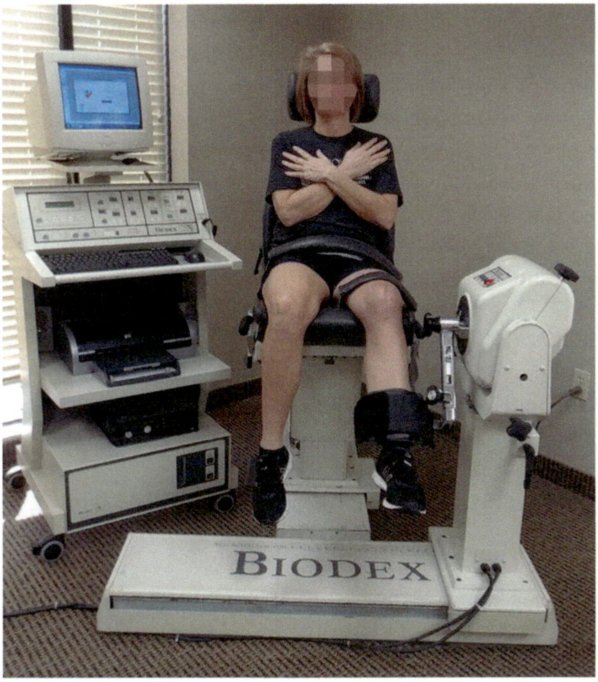

Fig. 9.1 Proper position of the patient in the Biodex dynamometer

9.2.3 1-Rep Max Leg Press and Knee Extension

If isokinetic or isometric equipment is not available, a 1-repetition maximum (1-RM) leg press is recommended if weight room equipment, an experienced test administrator, and a sufficient amount of time to safely conduct the test are available. The protocol typically involves:

1. A 5-minute warmup on a stationary bicycle, followed by 1 minute of rest.
2. Eight to ten repetitions of a light load, ~50% of predicted 1-RM, followed by 1 minute of rest.
3. One load of ~80% of predicted 1-RM through full ROM, followed by 1 minute of rest. After each successful performance, the weight is increased until a failed attempt occurs. A 1-minute rest period is given between attempts.
4. The 1-RM will usually be attained within five attempts.

9.3 Common Measurements for Balance

9.3.1 Balance Evaluation Systems Test (BESTest)

Developed by Horak et al. [22], the Balance Evaluation Systems Test (BESTest) is a clinical assessment tool that targets six different balance control systems: (1)

biomechanical constraints (such as ankle or hip weakness and flexed postural alignment), (2) stability limits (how far the body's center of mass can be moved over its base of support) and verticality (representation of gravitational upright), (3) anticipatory postural adjustments, (4) postural responses, (5) sensory integration for spatial orientation, and (6) dynamic balance during gait (Table 9.2). The ICC for the entire test in a group of 12 subjects was 0.91, with the six section ICCs ranging from 0.79 to 0.96. Subsequent studies demonstrated the test's validity and reliability in patients with bilateral cerebral palsy [23], fibromyalgia [24], chronic obstructive pulmonary disease [25], multiple sclerosis [26], and Parkinson's disease [27]. Chan et al. [28] reported, for the overall score and six categories, excellent inter-rater reliability (ICCs, 0.99–1.00), intra-rater reliability (ICCs, 0.76–1.00), and internal consistency (Cronbach's alpha, 0.86–1.00) in a group of 92 patients who were at least 6 months post-TKA. There were no significant floor or ceiling effects. In a later study, Chan et al. [29] longitudinally tested 134 individuals on five separate

Table 9.2 Balance Evaluation Systems Test (BESTest) items[a]

Biomechanical constraints	Stability limits, verticality	Anticipatory postural adjustments	Postural responses	Sensory orientation	Stability in gait
1. Base of support	6. Sitting vertically (left and right) and lateral lean (left and right)	9. Sit to stand	14. In-place response, forward	19. Sensory integration for balance (modified CRSIB) Stance on firm surface, EO Stance on firm surface, EC Stance on foam, EO Stance on foam, EC	21. Gait, level surface
2. CoM alignment	7. Functional reach forward	10. Rise to toes	15. In-place response, backward		22. Change in gait speed
3. Ankle strength and ROM	8. Functional reach lateral (left and right)	11. Stand on one leg (left and right)	16. Compensatory stepping correction, forward		23. Walk with head turns, horizontal
4. Hip/trunk lateral strength		12. Alternate stair touching	17. Compensatory stepping correction, backward	20. Incline, EC	24. Walk with pivot turns
5. Sit on floor and stand up		13. Standing arm raise	18. Compensatory stepping correction, lateral (left and right)		25. Step over obstacles
					26. Timed TUG
					27. Timed TUG with dual task

[a]From Horak et al. [22]

occasions after TKA (2–24 weeks after surgery). Compared with the Mini-BESTest, the Brief-BESTest, and the Berg Balance Scale, the BESTest demonstrated the highest internal and external responsiveness to change over time. The problem is that the test consists of 36 tasks and takes approximately 30 minutes to administer. In an effort to reduce the duration and redundancy of the BESTest, researchers developed two shortened versions, which will be discussed next.

9.3.2 Mini-BESTest

Franchignoni et al. [30] developed the Mini-BESTest, which consists of 16 items that may be administered in approximately 15 minutes (Table 9.3). In a group of 115 patients with a variety of balance disorders, this test showed high content validity and internal construct validity. In a group of 92 patients who were at least 6 months post-TKA, Chan et al. [28] reported excellent inter-rater reliability (ICC, 0.96), intra-rater reliability (ICC, 0.92), internal consistency (Cronbach's alpha, 0.96), and no significant floor or ceiling effects. Di Carlo et al. [31] reported on the available reliability, validity, and responsiveness from 24 studies. Test-retest reliability was excellent, with ICCs ranging between 0.92 and 0.98, as was inter-rater reliability (ICCs, 0.86–0.99). Criterion validity was excellent with significant associations with other established balance measures such as the Berg Balance Scale ($r = 0.79$–0.94). Construct validity was also adequate with the TUG ($r = 0.66$–0.89). No evidence of a floor or ceiling effect was reported and responsiveness was adequate. In the study by Chan et al. [29] discussed previously, the Mini-BESTest was suggested as a "reasonable option if time constraints are a concern."

9.3.3 Brief-BESTest

Padgett et al. [32] proposed the Brief-BESTest (Table 9.4) which consists of eight items and takes approximately 10 minutes to administer. These authors reported excellent inter-rater reliability (ICC, 0.99), internal consistency (Cronbach's alpha, >0.85), and high specificity and accuracy identifying patients with and without a fall history in the previous 3 months and patients with and without a neurological disorder. Shah Mital et al. [33] evaluated the reliability of this test in 30 patients 1 month after TKA. Intra-rater reliability and inter-rater reliability were high for the total test score (ICCs 0.98), as well as the six components (ICCs, 0.67–0.96). Chan et al. [28] reported excellent inter-rater reliability (ICC, 0.97), intra-rater reliability (ICC, 0.94), internal consistency (Cronbach's alpha, 0.97), and no significant floor or ceiling effects. These authors compared the BESTest, Mini-BESTest, and Brief-BESTest and concluded that although all had adequate psychometric properties, the Brief-BESTest was the least time-consuming and was particularly useful for clinicians.

Table 9.3 Mini-BESTest items[a]

Item	Rating criteria	Points
1. Sit to stand	Normal: stable for 3 s with maximum height	2
	Moderate: comes to stand with the use of hands on first attempt	1
	Severe: impossible to stand up from chair without assistance or several attempts with the use of hands	0
2. Rise to toes	Normal: stable for 3 s with maximum height	2
	Moderate: heels up, but no full range (smaller than when holding hands) or noticeable instability for 3 s	1
	Severe: ≤3 s	0
3. Stand on one leg, right side	Normal: 20 s	2
	Moderate: <20 s	1
	Severe: unable	0
4. Stand on one leg, left side	Normal: 20 s	2
	Moderate: <20 s	1
	Severe: unable	0
5. Compensatory stepping correction: forward	Normal: recovers independently a single, large step (second realignment step is allowed)	2
	Moderate: more than one step used to recover equilibrium	1
	Severe: no step or would fall if not caught or falls spontaneously	0
6. Compensatory stepping correction: backward	Normal: recovers independently a single, large step	2
	Moderate: more than one step used to recover equilibrium	1
	Severe: no step or would fall if not caught or falls spontaneously	0
7. Compensatory stepping correction: lateral, left side	Normal: recovers independently with 1 step (crossover or lateral OK)	2
	Moderate: several steps to recover equilibrium	1
	Severe: falls or cannot step	0
8. Compensatory stepping correction: lateral, right side	Normal: recovers independently with 1 step (crossover or lateral OK)	2
	Moderate: several steps to recover equilibrium	1
	Severe: falls or cannot step	0
9. Stance eyes open, firm surface, feet together	Normal: 30 s	2
	Moderate: <30 s	1
	Severe: unable	0
10. Stance eyes closed, foam surface, feet together	Normal: 30 s	2
	Moderate: <30 s	1
	Severe: unable	0
11. Incline, eyes closed	Normal: stands independently 30 s and aligns with gravity	2
	Moderate: stands independently <30 s or aligns with surface	1
	Severe: unable	0
12. Change in gait speed	Normal: significantly changes walking speed without imbalance	2
	Moderate: unable to change walking speed or imbalance	1
	Severe: unable to achieve significant change in speed and signs of imbalance	0

(continued)

Table 9.3 (continued)

Item	Rating criteria	Points
13. Walk with head turns, horizontal	Normal: performs head turns with no change in gait speed and good balance	2
	Moderate: performs head turns with reduction in gait speed	1
	Severe: performs head turns with imbalance	0
14. Walk with pivot turns	Normal: turns with feet close, fast (≤3 steps) with good balance	2
	Moderate: turns with feet close slow (≥4 steps) with good balance	1
	Severe: cannot turn with feet close at any speed without imbalance	0
15. Step over obstacles	Normal: able to step over box with minimal change of speed and with good balance	2
	Moderate: steps over shoe boxes but touches box or displays cautious behavior by slowing gait	1
	Severe: cannot step over shoe boxes or hesitates or steps around box	0
16. TUG and cognitive TUG with dual task TUG: ____ s Dual task TUG: ____ s	Normal: no noticeable change between sitting and standing in backward counting and no change in gait speed compared with TUG with dual task	2
	Moderate: dual task affects either counting or walking	1
	Severe: stops counting while walking or stops walking while counting	

TUG timed up and go
[a]From Franchignoni et al. [30]

9.3.4 Berg Balance Scale (BBS)

Berg et al. [34] introduced the Berg Balance Scale (BBS) in 1989 (Table 9.5). The BBS consists of 14 five-level items and takes approximately 20 minutes to complete. Scoring criteria varies from item to item, and concern was raised regarding item redundancy and intra-rater reliability, especially for raters with little training [35]. Chou et al. [35] developed a shortened version of the BBS that consisted of seven items (seven-item BBS) that are scored on a three-level gradient and requires approximately 10 minutes to complete. The seven items included are #1, 2, 6, 9, 10, 13, and 14 in Table 9.5. The reliability of the seven-item BBS, measured in 226 stroke subjects, was high (ICC, 0.97), as was concurrent and convergent validity (random-effects model ICC, 0.99 and 0.86, respectively). However, there was a noteworthy increase in the floor effect (43% versus 25%) which the authors attributed to the removal of the sitting balance item #3 in Table 9.5. The responsiveness to change was adequate (effect size, 0.75), and there was no notable trend between the difference and average scores between this instrument and the original BBS. Jorgi et al. [36] further studied the psychometric properties of the seven-item BBS in patients who had undergone TKA or total hip arthroplasty and found high correlations with the BBS ($r = 0.92–0.97$) and highly responsive to change (standardized response mean [SRM], 1.8). Finally, Kim et al. [37] evaluated the seven-item BBS

Table 9.4 Brief-BESTest items[a]

Item	Rating criteria	Points
1. Hip/trunk lateral strength	Normal: 10 s with trunk vertical	3
	Mild: 10 s without trunk vertical	2
	Moderate: 1 hip abducts with trunk vertical	1
	Severe: neither hip, 10 s and vertical or not vertical	0
2. Functional reach forward	>32 cm	3
	16.5–32 cm	2
	<16.5 cm	1
	No measurable lean (or must be caught)	0
3. Stand on one leg, left side	Normal (stable >20 s)	3
	Trunk motion or 10–20 s	2
	Stand 2–10 s	1
	Unable	0
4. Stand on one leg, right side	Normal (stable >20 s)	3
	Trunk motion or 10–20 s	2
	Stand 2–10 s	1
	Unable	0
5. Compensatory stepping, lateral, left side	Recovers with 1 side/crossover step	3
	Several steps to recover independently	2
	Steps but needs assistance to prevent fall	1
	No step or falls	0
6. Compensatory stepping, lateral, right side	Recovers with 1 side/crossover step	3
	Several steps to recover independently	2
	Steps but needs assistance to prevent fall	1
	No step or falls	0
7. Stance with eyes closed, on foam surface	30 s stable	3
	30 s unstable	2
	<30 s	1
	Unable	0
8. Timed up and go	Fast, <11 s, good balance	3
	Slow, >11 s, good balance	2
	Fast, <11 s, imbalance	1
	Slow, >11 s, imbalance	0

[a]From Padgett et al. [32]

in 255 stroke patients and reported high concurrent validity with the 10-minute walk test ($r = 0.75$) and the TUG test ($r = 0.77$).

9.3.5 Y-Balance Test

The Y-balance test, a simplified version of the Star Excursion Balance Test (SEBT), has been used extensively in various populations to determine dynamic postural control [38–46]. The test requires the subject to maintain a stable base by balancing on one leg while reaching out with the other leg to push a block as far as possible in the anterior, posteromedial, and posterolateral directions. The original SEBT included a total of eight reach directions that measure similar functional factors, leading to redundancy. The Y-balance test is appropriate for TKA patients who wish

Table 9.5 Berg Balance Scale, full version[a]

Item	Rating criteria	Points
1. Sit to stand	Able to stand without using hands and stabilize independently	4
	Able to stand independently using hands	3
	Able to stand using hands after several tries	2
	Needs minimal aid to stand or to stabilize	1
	Needs moderate or maximal assistance to stand	0
2. Standing unsupported with outstretched arms	Able to stand safely for 2 minutes	4
	Able to stand 2 minutes with supervision	3
	Able to stand 30 seconds unsupported	2
	Needs several tries to stand 30 seconds unsupported	1
	Unable to stand 30 seconds unassisted	0
3. Sit with back unsupported but feet supported on floor or on a stool	Able to sit safely and securely for 2 minutes	4
	Able to sit 2 minutes under supervision	3
	Able to sit 30 seconds	2
	Able to sit 10 seconds	1
	Unable to sit without support 10 seconds	0
4. Stand to sit	Sits safely with minimal use of hands	4
	Controls descent by using hands	3
	Uses back of legs against chair to control descent	2
	Sits independently but has uncontrolled descent	1
	Needs assistance to sit	0
5. Transfers: to one chair with armrest and then to one chair without armrest	Able to transfer safely with minor use of hands	4
	Able to transfer safely with definite need of hands	3
	Able to transfer with verbal cueing and/or supervision	2
	Needs one person to assist	1
	Needs two people to assist or supervise to be safe	0
6. Standing unsupported with eyes closed	Able to stand 10 seconds safely	4
	Able to stand 10 seconds with supervision	3
	Able to stand 3 seconds	2
	Unable to keep eyes closed 3 seconds but stays steady	1
	Needs help to keep from falling	0
7. Standing unsupported with feet together	Able to place feet together independently and stand 1 minute safely	4
	Able to place feet together independently and stand 1 minute with supervision	3
	Able to place feet together independently but unable to hold for 30 seconds	2
	Needs help to attain position but able to stand 15 seconds with feet together	1
	Needs help to attain position and unable to hold for 15 seconds	0

(continued)

Table 9.5 (continued)

Item	Rating criteria	Points
8. Reaching forward with outstretched arm while standing	Can reach forward confidently >25 cm	4
	Can reach forward >12 cm safely	3
	Can reach forward >5 cm safely	2
	Reaches forward but needs supervision	1
	Loses balance while trying/requires external support	0
9. Pick up object from the floor from a standing position	Able to pick up slipper safely and easily	4
	Able to pick up slipper but needs supervision	3
	Unable to pick up but reaches 2–5 cm from slipper and keeps balance independently	2
	Unable to pick up and needs supervision while trying	1
	Unable to try/needs assistance to keep from losing balance or falling	0
10. Turn to look behind over left and right shoulders while standing	Looks behind from both sides and weight shifts well	4
	Looks behind one side only, other side shows less weight shift	3
	Turns sideways only but maintains balance	2
	Needs supervision when turning	1
	Needs assistance to keep from losing balance or falling	0
11. Turn 360°	Able to turn 360° safely in 4 seconds or less	4
	Able to turn 360° safely one side only in 4 seconds or less	3
	Able to turn 360° safely but slowly	2
	Needs close supervision or verbal cueing	1
	Needs assistance while turning	0
12. Placing alternate foot on step or stool while standing unsupported	Able to stand independently and safely and complete 8 steps in 20 seconds	4
	Able to stand independently and complete 8 steps in >20 seconds	3
	Able to complete 4 steps without aid with supervision	2
	Able to complete >2 steps, needs minimal assistance	1
	Needs assistance to keep from falling/unable to try	0
13. Standing unsupported one foot in front	Able to place foot tandem independently and hold 30 seconds	4
	Able to place foot ahead of other independently and hold 30 seconds	3
	Able to take small step independently and hold 30 seconds	2
	Needs help to step but can hold 15 seconds	1
	Loses balance while stepping or standing	0

(continued)

Table 9.5 (continued)

Item	Rating criteria	Points
14. Standing on one leg	Able to lift leg independently and hold >10 seconds	4
	Able to lift leg independently and hold 5–10 seconds	3
	Able to lift leg independently and hold ≥3 seconds	2
	Tries to lift leg, unable to hold 3 seconds but remains standing independently	1
	Unable to try or needs assistance to prevent fall	0

Maximal score 56
[a]From Berg et al. [97]

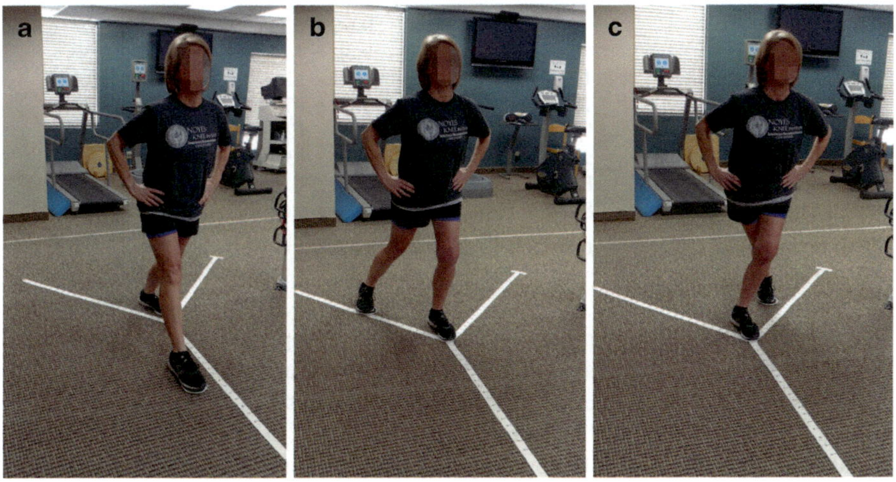

Fig. 9.2 The Y-balance test in the (**a**) anterior, (**b**) posteromedial, and (**c**) posterolateral directions

to resume recreational and athletic activities as it requires strength, neuromuscular control, and adequate range of motion at the hip, knee, and ankle joints.

The test should be conducted on a firm hard surface, such as concrete or a gymnastics floor. Either a commercially available kit may be purchased to conduct the test (Move2Perform, Evansville, IN), or the clinician can easily make a grid on the floor using tape measures (Fig. 9.2) consisting of three lines extending at 45° angles from the center of the grid. The lines are designated as anterior, posterolateral, and posteromedial. The subject stands on one foot and pushes a target with the other foot in the anterior directional. The athlete then returns to bilateral stance. The target remains over the tape measure after the test, making the determination of reach distance precise to the nearest 0.5 cm. Four practice trials are conducted, followed by three test trials in each direction. A 1-min rest period is allowed between

Table 9.6 Normalized Y-balance test distance in healthy adult women[a]

	Aged 45–60		Aged 70–80	
Direction	Mean ± SD	95% CI	Mean ± SD	95% CI
Anterior, right leg	78.2 ± 4.6	0.71–0.93	62.4 ± 5.8	0.76–0.94
Anterior, left leg	77.0 ± 4.9	0.84–0.96	63.1 ± 5.8	0.67–0.92
Posteromedial, right leg	120.9 ± 7.3	0.69–0.92	98.2 ± 8.9	0.78–0.95
Posteromedial, left leg	119.0 ± 7.3	0.65–0.91	97.8 ± 9.5	0.72–0.93
Posterolateral, right leg	117.7 ± 8.7	0.83–0.96	93.4 ± 10.2	0.76–0.94
Posterolateral, left leg	118.6 ± 8.6	0.80–0.95	95.0 ± 10.3	0.72–0.93
Composite, both legs	105.2 ± 5.5	NA	85.0 ± 6.9	NA

NA not available
[a]From Lee et al. [40], used original plastic Y-balance test kit

Table 9.7 Normalized Y-balance test distance in healthy adult women[a]

Direction	Aged 50–59	Aged 60–69	Aged 70–79
Anterior, right leg	64.28 ± 5.13	59.66 ± 7.29	58.33 ± 6.02
Anterior, left leg	62.63 ± 5.45	59.39 ± 7.16	57.92 ± 6.30
Posteromedial, right leg	102.75 ± 11.57	92.83 ± 11.39	89.70 ± 10.10
Posteromedial, left leg	101.35 ± 9.74	93.62 ± 10.54	91.60 ± 8.70
Posterolateral, right leg	97.64 ± 9.83	86.68 ± 12.89	78.24 ± 21.88
Posterolateral, left leg	97.04 ± 9.34	88.50 ± 13.40	79.80 ± 14.07
Composite, right leg	88.22 ± 7.96	79.72 ± 10.06	75.42 ± 11.04
Composite, left leg	87.01 ± 7.18	80.50 ± 9.68	76.44 ± 8.75

[a]From Freund et al. [38], used professional model wooden test kit. Data shown are mean ± standard deviation

directions. Then, the same process is repeated on the opposite leg. The average of the three test trials is calculated for each leg in each direction.

For normalization, the patient's leg lengths are measured in the supine position from the anterior superior iliac spine to the distal tip of the medial malleolus using a standard tape measure. The leg length is used to normalize reach distances by dividing the distance reached by the leg length and then multiplying by 100 [41].

Lee et al. [40] conducted this test in 20 healthy women aged 45–60 years and 20 women aged 70–80 years and reported normative values (Table 9.6) and excellent intra-rater reliability (ICC, 0.92–0.97). Women in the 45–60 years group had significantly greater normalized reach distances compared with those in the 70–80 years group ($P < 0.01$). Freund et al. [38] determined reliability and normative values of this test in women aged 50–79 years (Table 9.7). Inter-rater and test-retest ICCs were excellent, ranging from 0.75 to 1.00. There were significant differences in all of the normalized reach distances between subjects in the 50–59 years group compared with those in the 60–69 years group and those in the 70–79 years group ($P < 0.05$). Sipe et al. [44] conducted a trial of 15 males and 15 females whose mean age was 66.8 ± 5.4 years to determine correlations between the Y-balance and the standard TUG test, an 8-foot TUG test, and a 30-second chair-stand test. Significant associations were found for all measures ($P < 0.001$–0.03; $r = 0.50$–0.72). Lee et al. [39] reported significant correlations in women aged 45–80 years between Y-balance reach distances and hip extensor ($r = 0.70$–0.75) and knee flexor ($r = 0.71$–0.83)

isometric strength. Knee extensor strength only moderately correlated with reach distances ($r = 0.56$–0.62). As of the time of writing, no normative data had been published for normalized reach distances for adult males.

9.3.6 Static Postural Control on Force Platform

Double- or single-leg stance may be measured on a force platform (such as the Biodex Balance System) if available to assess static postural control [47, 48]. Reliability of the overall stability index of this system in the elderly has been reported to range from an ICC of 0.79 [49] to 0.69 [50, 51]. Parraca et al. [51] reported that the reliability using the Bland-Altman method showed that the mean difference between test and retest was nearly zero and the 95% limits of agreement were narrow, indicating good reliability of the system.

9.4 Common Measurements for Function (Table 9.8)

9.4.1 6-Minute Walk Test

The 6-minute walk measures the distance a patient can walk on a level surface in 6 minutes [52]. The ICC for this test has been reported to range from 0.84 to 0.97 [53–57], and it has been found to be responsive to improvements over time after TKA [58, 59]. Ko et al. [60] reported significant differences in the performance of this test between 32 TKA patients who were 12–18 months postoperative and a group of 43 control patients (423.5 and 582.1 meters, respectively; $P < 0.001$). This study found that the 6-minute walk strongly correlated with ($r = 0.97$, $P < 0.001$) and predicted the outcome of a 30-minute walk test, allowing its use clinically. Another study found that this test moderately correlated with the repeated chair-stand test ($r = 0.67$, $P < 0.05$) and tandem balance ($r = 0.52$, $P < 0.05$).

9.4.2 10-Meter Walk Test

The 10-m walk test measures the time required to complete this distance. This test has excellent reliability (ICC, 0.90–0.95) [61, 62].

9.4.3 Timed Up and Go (TUG) Test

First described by Podsiadio and Richardson [63], the TUG test measures the time required for a patient to rise from an arm chair (seat height of 46 cm), walk 3 meters, turn, and return to sitting in the same chair without assistance. This test has excellent validity and reliability (ICCs, 0.95–0.99) [57, 61, 63–66]. Doll et al. [65] reported a clinically meaningful change value of 1.62 seconds when this test is

Table 9.8 Age and gender-related normative values (means and standard deviations)

Age range (y)	Gender	6-minute walk test (m)	Timed up and go test (secs)	Berg balance scale (scores)	Sit-to-stand test (5 rep, secs)	30-second chair-stand (no.)	Stair-climb test (9 steps, sec)
60–69	Male ($n = 15$)	572 ± 92[a]	8 ± 2[a]	55 ± 1[a]			
	Female ($n = 22$)	538 ± 92[a]	8 ± 2[a]	55 ± 2[a]			
	Male ($n = 21$)	448 ± 57[b]					
	Both ($n = 25$)		8.0 ± 1.0[c]				
	Both ($n = 32$)					14.0 ± 2.4[d]	
	Both ($n = 150$, preop)	412 ± 123[e]	9.8 ± 3[e]				17.1 ± 8.2[e]
	Both ($n = 85$, preop)	429 ± 116[f]	9.6 ± 2.9[f]				
70–79	Male ($n = 14$)	527 ± 85[a]	9 ± 3[a]	54 ± 3[a]			
	Female ($n = 22$)	471 ± 75[a]	9 ± 2[a]	53 ± 4[a]			
	Both ($n = 96$)					12.9 ± 3.0[d]	
80–89	Male ($n = 8$)	417 ± 73[a]	10 ± 1[a]	53 ± 2[a]			
	Female ($n = 15$)	392 ± 85[a]	11 ± 3[a]	50 ± 3[a]			
	Both ($n = 62$)					11.9 ± 3.6[d]	
71–79	Both ($n = 51$)	497 ± 95[g]					
	Male ($n = 1239$)				13.2[h]		
	Female ($n = 2033$)				14.4[h]		
≥80	Male ($n = 547$)				15.0[h]		
	Female ($n = 1287$)				16.1[h]		

[a]Steffen [57]
[b]Parent [98]
[c]Piva [66]
[d]Jones [68]
[e]Kennedy [54]
[f]Stratford [89]
[g]Harada [99]
[h]Gurainik [92]

performed preoperatively and then 12 weeks postoperatively. Unnanuntana et al. [67] measured the responsiveness of the TUG in a group of 157 patients at 1 year postoperatively and reported a moderate effect size (0.58).

9.4.4 30-Second Chair-Stand Test

The 30-second chair-stand test measures how many times a patient can rise from a chair with a seat height of 43.2 cm and sit down again in 30 seconds. The patient's arms are crossed at the wrists and held against the chest. The patient sits in the middle of the chair, back straight, feet approximately shoulder width apart and placed on the floor at an angle slightly back from the knees, with one foot slightly in front of the other to help maintain balance when standing. No personal assistance is given. The patient rises to a full stand, with the body erect and straight, and then returns to the seated position. This test has been shown to be reliable in older adults (mean age, 70.5 years), with ICCs of 0.84 for men and 0.92 for women [68] and in patients awaiting TKA (ICC, 0.95–0.98) [69]. Moderate correlations were reported between chair-stand test performance and 1-RM (leg press) for older men ($r = 0.78$) and women ($r = 0.71$) [68].

9.4.5 Stair-Climb Test

Many versions of the stair-climb test have been published [70]. In short, this test may be conducted in less than 1 minute and requires only access to a flight of stairs and a stopwatch. The test may either be interpreted based on time alone, or leg power may be calculated based on the number of stairs, stair height, ascent time, and body weight. Power is calculated as *force times velocity*. Stair-climb time and vertical height of the stairs are used to calculate velocity (distance/time), and body mass and acceleration due to gravity are used to calculate force. The examiner and patient begin at the bottom of a flight of stairs. The patient is instructed to ascend the flight as fast as possible and may use the handrail if deemed necessary for safety purposes. The examiner times the test, with the time stopped when both feet of the patient reach the top step.

Test-retest of the stair-climb test is excellent for nine steps (ICC, 0.90) [54], 11 steps (ICC, 0.94) [2], and 12 steps (ICC, 0.92–0.93) [56, 65].

9.4.6 Sit-to-Stand (Repeated Chair-Stand) Test

This test measures the amount of time required to rise from a chair to a full stand and return. The amount of repetitions reported in the literature has varied from three to ten. Reliability for this test with five repetitions has ranged from ICC 0.80 [53] to 0.96 [61]. The ten-repetition test ICC was reported to be 0.84–0.82 [53, 71]. Patients may either rise from a chair with their arms folded on their chest or use the chair armrests.

9.4.7 Single-Leg Squat

The single-leg squat test is a useful and reliable clinical tool that assesses frontal plane lower extremity motion and may identify weakness or poor control of the core and hip musculature with the observation of hip adduction and internal rotation, poor knee flexion, and knee abduction. This test is valid for the arthroplasty patient who wishes to resume more challenging recreational or sports activities such as tennis. The single-leg squat is conducted by asking the patient to stand on one leg with their hands placed on their hips. The opposite leg should be maintained in approximately 45° of knee flexion during the entire test. The head and eyes should remain focused straight ahead. The patient is instructed to squat down to 45° and return to single-leg stance without losing their balance (Fig. 9.3). We make this a more dynamic assessment by asking the athlete to perform five consecutive trials. The examiner notes the patient's overall trunk control and the position of the hip, knee, and foot throughout the test. The test result may be classified according to five categories that are rated as good, fair, or poor (Table 9.9) [72]. The rating may either be done during the test trial or may be recorded in the frontal plane and conducted later when viewing the video. Acceptable inter-rater reliability and intra-rater reliability have been reported in several studies of young adults [72–74].

9.4.8 Single-Leg Hop Test

The single-leg hop test is another simple clinical tool that may be done in arthroplasty patients who desire to return to athletics. This test is one of the most commonly used measures of lower extremity power and dynamic balance [75–81]. Our initial research demonstrated that a limb symmetry index (LSI) of ≥85% was present in the majority (93%) of athletes [75], and this is the goal for the arthroplasty patient that desires to return to more strenuous activities. A tape measure is secured to the ground for a distance of approximately 3 m. The patient stands on the designated leg to be tested with their toe just behind the starting end of the tape. They are instructed to hop as far as possible forward and land on the same leg, holding that position for at least 2 seconds. The patient is allowed to use their arms for balance as required. After a few trials, two single-leg hops are done on each limb. The distance hopped is recorded, and the furthest distance achieved is used to calculate the LSI by dividing the distance hopped of the right leg by the distance hopped of the left leg and multiplying the result by 100. This test has excellent reliability, with ICCs >0.85 [82, 83].

9.5 Physical Activity Guidelines

In the United States, the 2018 Physical Activity Guidelines recommend that adults do at least 150 minutes (2 hours, 30 minutes) to 300 minutes (5 hours) of moderate-intensity aerobic physical activity a week, or 75 (1 hour, 15 minutes) to 150 minutes

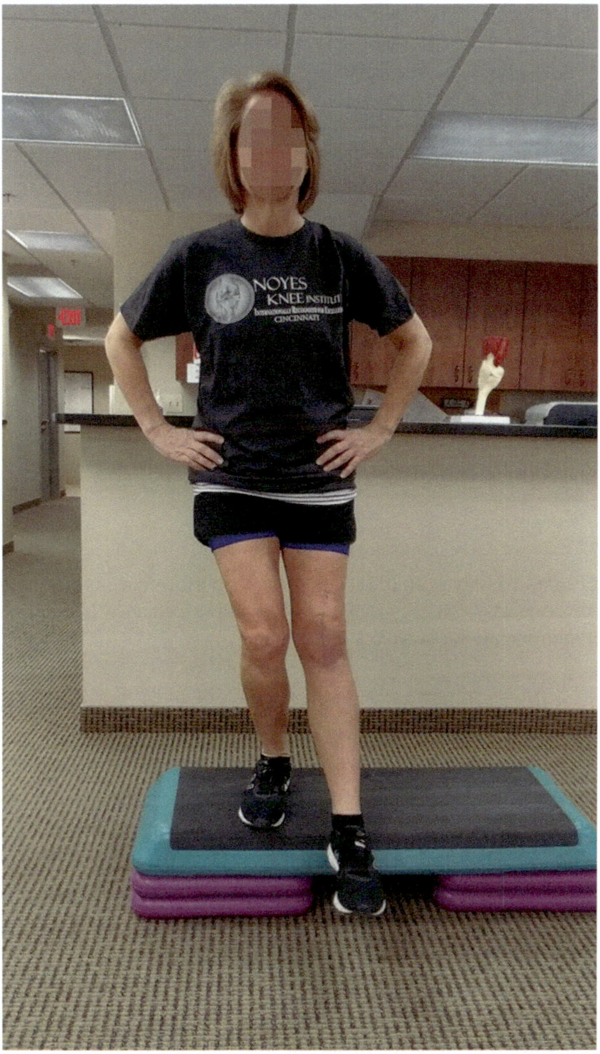

Fig. 9.3 The single-leg squat test

of vigorous-intensity activity [84–86]. During moderate-intensity activity, a person can talk but not sing, and they have noticeable increases in breathing rate and heart rate. During vigorous-intensity activity, a person cannot say more than a few words without pausing for breath, and they have large increases in breathing and heart rate. Aerobic activities may include walking, hiking, dancing, swimming, water aerobics, jogging, bicycling, tennis, and walking while playing golf. In addition, muscle strengthening activities that involve all major muscle groups should be done >2 days a week. These may include exercise bands, weight machines, and body weight exercises.

Table 9.9 Clinical rating criteria for a "good" rating of the single-leg squat test[a]

Overall impression of trial(s)
Athlete does not lose balance
Movement is performed smoothly
Squat goes to at least 60° knee flexion
Squat is performed at a speed of approximately 1 repetition per 2 s
Trunk posture
No trunk/thoracic lateral deviation or shift
No trunk/thoracic rotation
No trunk/thoracic lateral flexion
No trunk/thoracic forward flexion
The pelvis "in space"
No pelvic shunt or lateral deviation
No pelvic rotation
No pelvic tilt
Hip joint
No hip adduction
No hip (femoral) internal rotation
Knee joint
No apparent knee valgus
Center of knee remains over center of foot

[a]From Crossley et al. [72]. The patient's performance is considered good if all of the requirements for at least 4 criteria are achieved. The performance is rated poor if they do not meet all of the requirements for at least 1 criterion

Older adults (ages 65 and older) should do multicomponent physical activity that includes balance training in addition to aerobic and muscle strengthening exercises. If they cannot do 150 minutes of moderate-intensity aerobic activity a week because of chronic conditions, they should be as physically active as possible.

We conducted a systematic review of 19 studies to determine physical activity and recreational sports resumed after primary TKA [87]. There were 5179 knees followed a mean of 4.8 years postoperatively. There was a wide range between studies in the percentage of patients who resumed recreational or sports activities (34–100%). Only two studies used accelerometers to measure physical activity, and both reported a low percentage of patients (0–16.5%) who met physical activity guidelines. See Chap. 10 for further information regarding recommended guidelines for physical activity after TKA.

9.6 Test Batteries

9.6.1 Performance-Based Knee Function Test

Hossain et al. [88] developed a user-friendly performance-based knee outcome test battery for TKA patients. The battery involves (1) timed 10-m walk, (2) stride length, (3) timed single-leg stance, (4) single-leg hop test, (5) triple hop test, (6) kneeling test, (7) timed horizontal leg hold, and (8) ten-step stair climb. The tests are

Objective Function							Subjective Pain
Timed 10-m walk	0	1	2	3	4	5	Pain / No Pain: 0 1 2 3 4 5 6 7 8 9 10
	16.8	13.8	10.8	7.9	4.9	sec	
Stride length	0	1	2	3	4	5	
	82.0	106.4	130.8	155.1	179.5	sec	
Timed single-leg stance	0	1	2	3	4	5	Pain / No Pain: 0 1 2 3 4 5 6 7 8 9 10
	4.5	21.4	38.2	55.1	72.0	sec	
Single-leg hop	0	1	2	3	4	5	Pain / No Pain: 0 1 2 3 4 5 6 7 8 9 10
	12.0	54.3	96.7	139.0	181.3	sec	
Triple hop	0	1	2	3	4	5	Pain / No Pain: 0 1 2 3 4 5 6 7 8 9 10
	25.0	154.8	284.5	414.3	544.0	sec	
Kneeling test	0	1	2	3			Pain / No Pain: 0 1 2 3 4 5 6 7 8 9 10
	Unable	90° on chair	90° on floor	Sit on heels			
Timed horizontal leg hold	0	1	2	3	4	5	Pain / No Pain: 0 1 2 3 4 5 6 7 8 9 10
	10.3	45.2	80.1	115.1	150.0	sec	
10-Step stair climb	0	1	2	3	4	5	Pain / No Pain: 0 1 2 3 4 5 6 7 8 9 10
	39.1	30.2	21.2	12.2	3.2	sec	

Fig. 9.4 The performance test battery includes eight function scores. A 10-point pain score is completed for each test except stride length, which is measured simultaneously during the timed 10-m walk. (Revised from Hossain et al. [88])

scored as shown in Fig. 9.4. In a population of 50 TKA patients and 50 normal controls, the overall score had adequate reliability (ICC, 0.89), internal consistency, construct validity, and responsiveness.

9.6.2 Performance Batteries by Stratford

Stratford and Kennedy [89] described a performance-based test battery for TKA or total hip arthroplasty patients that includes (1) self-paced walk (40 m), (2) stair test (ten steps), (3) TUG, and (4) 6-minute walk test. Patients also complete the 20-item Lower Extremity Functional Scale (LEFS) and the Western Ontario and McMaster Universities Osteoarthritis Index (WOMAC), of which the physical function scale was included in the battery. Later, Stratford et al. [90] reduced the battery to items #1–3 above, along with the LEFS and the WOMAC. The authors reported that the performance battery tests were more sensitive to change (from before surgery to 1 month after surgery) than the WOMAC or LEFS.

9.6.3 Aggregated Locomotor Function Score

McCarthy and Oldham [91] combined three functions of (1) self-paced walk (8 m), (2) stair test (seven steps), and (3) walk-to-sit test (three repetitions) in their aggregated locomotor function (ALF) score. Patients with knee arthritis also completed the WOMAC and Short Form 36 health survey (SF-36). The ALF had excellent ICC (0.99), took 10 minutes to administer, and had higher SEM (more responsive to change) 1 year post TKA than the WOMAC and SF-36.

9.6.4 Short Physical Performance Battery

The Short Physical Performance Battery (SPPB) involves (1) standing tandem balance test, (2) timed 2.4-m walk, and (3) timed five chair-stand repetitions. All times are measured to the nearest 0.01 second with a stopwatch. Each test is scored between 0 and 4 and summed for a maximum score of 12 [92]. For the walk and chair stands, a score of 0 is given if the patient is unable to complete the test. For the walk test, a score of 1 is given for ≥5.7 sec, 2 for 4.1–5.6 sec, 3 for 3.2–4.0 sec, and 4 for ≤3.1 sec. For the chair-stand test, a score of 1 is given for ≥16.7 sec, 2 for 13.7–16.6 sec, 3 for 11.2–13.6 sec, and 4 for ≤11.1 sec. For the balance test, a score of 2 is assigned for ≤2 secs, 2 for 3–9 secs, and 4 for 10 secs. The SPPB is a reliable and valid measure of lower-extremity performance, with ICCs reported from 0.73 to 0.97 [93].

9.6.5 Authors' Return to Activity Test Battery

We developed a test battery to determine readiness of arthroplasty patients to return to recreational sports. The battery includes (1) a comprehensive knee examination, (2) patient and physician rating of pain and swelling according to our Cincinnati knee rating system [94], (3) the Star Excursion Balance Test, (4) the single-leg squat test, (5) the single-leg hop test, (6) a core endurance test, (7) muscle strength tests,

(8) a 6-minute walk test, (9) a stair-climbing test (ten steps), and (10) a fitness guideline test, walking for 20 minutes at a brisk rate. The goals for each test and details are shown in Fig. 9.5. This test is done upon completion of our postoperative rehabilitation program in motivated patients prior to release to activities such as racquet sports (tennis, racquetball, squash, pickleball) and skiing.

Cincinnati Sportsmedicine and Orthopaedic Center and the Noyes knee Institute
Total or Partial Knee Replacement: Return to Recreational Sports/Fitness Test Battery

Patient Name: ______________________ Today's Date: ____________ Age: ______

Date Surgery: ____________ Physician: ____________________

This test battery measures several important factors about your knee condition. The goal is to determine your readiness to return to recreational sports as approved by your physician and identify area of weakness that need further attention.

Knee Examination **Physician:** **Needs Attention** ☐

ROM: ________ Knee swelling? ____ Patellar mobility normal? ______ Patellar pain? ______

Medial tibiofemoral pain? _____ Lateral tibiofemoral pain? _____ Medial/lateral stability _________

Alignment ___________ Symmetrical gait? ____ Joint crepitus with motion? ______ Iliotibial band pain?______

Physician Notes:

Cincinnati Knee Rating Scores **Examiner:** **Needs Attention** ☐

Pain score (**Goal:** ≥ 6) ______ Swelling score (**Goal:** ≥ 6) _______

Star Excursion Balance Test **Examiner:** **Needs Attention** ☐

Measures su=ingle-leg balance in three different directions. Normalize accoring to leg length (reach distance/leg length x 100 = percentage of leg length). Take average of 3 trials.

Goal: < 10% deficit compared with contralateral side.

leg length (from most distal end of anterior superior iliac spine to most distal end of lateral malleolus):

Right ____ cm Left ______ cm

Results Operated Side: Anterior _____ Posterlateral _____ Posteromedial _____
Results Contralateral Side: Anterior _____ Posterlateral _____ Posteromedial _____

Anterior % deficit ______ Posterolateral % deficit _____ Posteromedial % deficit _____

Single-Leg Squat Test **Examiner:** **Needs Attention** ☐

Patient stands on a box with hands on hip and performs 5 squats on each leg. Rating is based on position of hip and knee joints. Measures core, hip, and leg muscle strength.

Goal: no knee valgus, medial-lateral movements, or pelvic tilt.

Results (good, fair, poor): Operated leg ______________ Contralateral leg ______________

Single-Leg Hop Test **Examiner:** **Needs Attention** ☐

Patient stands on one leg, hops forward as far as possible, and lands on the same leg. The landing must be held for 3 seconds for the test to be valid. Complete 2 single-leg hops on each side, calculate mean of each side and the calculate limb symmetry: operated leg mean/contralateral leg mean x 100

Goal: ≤ 15% deficit compared with contralateral side.

Results: Operated leg mean ____in Contralateral leg mean ______in Limb symmetery _____%

Core Endurance Test **Examiner:** **Needs Attention** ☐

Number of partial curl-ups in 1 minute.

Goal: 90% rank for men < 50 y.o. = 75 and > 50 y.o = 74 90% rank for women < 50 y.o. = 50 and > 50 y.o = 48

Result: ________

Fig. 9.5 The authors' test battery includes (**a**) knee examination, rating of pain and swelling, single-leg balance and functional and core endurance tests, and (**b**) muscle strength and fitness tests

Quadriceps, Hamstrings, Hip Abductors Muscle Strength Tests **Examiner:** **Needs Attention** ☐

Option #1: Manual muscle test, **Gold:** 5/5

Result: quadriceps ____ % deficit hamstrings ____ % deficit

Option #2: Isometric max torque Biodex, Goal: < 30% deficit oppoite side

Result: quadriceps ____ % deficit hamstrings ____ % deficit

Option #3: Isometric using handheld dynamometer, quadriceps 60° flaxion, hamstrings 60-90° flaxion, average of 3 reps; **Goal:** < 20% deficit opposite side

Result: quadriceps ____ % deficit hamstrings ____ % deficit hip abductors ____ % deficit

6-Minute Walk Test **Examiner:** **Needs Attention** ☐

Distance a patient can walk in 6 minutes going as fast as comfortable on a treadmill.

Goal: > 0.30 mile (497 meters)

Result: ______ Heart rate before test: ______ Heart rate on completion of test: ______

AHA Firness Guidline Test **Examiner:** **Needs Attention** ☐

Determine if a patient can walk for 20 minutes at a brisk rate that elevates the heart rate

Result:

Completed test: Yes/NO Knee pain: Yes/NO Knee instability: Yes/NO

Cannot do because of knee: Yes/NO Cannot do for reasons other than knee: Yes/NO

Heart rate upon completion of test _______ # steps (pedometer) _______

Stair Climbing Test **Examiner:** **Needs Attention** ☐

Time for a patient to go up 10 steps and back down, may use handrail for support if required.

Goal: < 13 seconds (men and women)

Result: ____ secs

Recommendations (check all that apply)

- ☐ OK return AHA fitness guidelines
- ☐ OK return physical fitness program (10 min flexibility, 20min strength, 30 min aerobic)
- ☐ OK gradual return to recreational sports (will need repeat exam)
- ☐ OK return recreational sports
- ☐ OK return work activities
- ☐ Continue strength, flexibility, aerobic programs

Fig. 9.5 (continued)

CoM, center of mass; ROM, range of motion; CTSIB, Clinical Test of Sensory Integration for Balance; EO, eyes open; EC, eyes closed; TUG, timed up and go. All items are scored from 0 (not able or absent) to 3 (normal), and the scores are summed for each subscale. The sum of the six subscales is the total score. The subscale and total scales are reported as a percentage of the maximum score.

References

1. Aalund PK, Larsen K, Hansen TB, Bandholm T. Normalized knee-extension strength or leg-press power after fast-track total knee arthroplasty: which measure is most closely associated with performance-based and self-reported function? Arch Phys Med Rehabil. 2013;94(2):384–90. https://doi.org/10.1016/j.apmr.2012.09.031.
2. Almeida GJ, Schroeder CA, Gil AB, Fitzgerald GK, Piva SR. Interrater reliability and validity of the stair ascend/descend test in subjects with total knee arthroplasty. Arch Phys Med Rehabil. 2010;91(6):932–8. https://doi.org/10.1016/j.apmr.2010.02.003.
3. Alnahdi AH, Zeni JA, Snyder-Mackler L. Hip abductor strength reliability and association with physical function after unilateral total knee arthroplasty: a cross-sectional study. Phys Ther. 2014;94(8):1154–62. https://doi.org/10.2522/ptj.20130335.
4. Alnahdi AH, Zeni JA, Snyder-Mackler L. Quadriceps strength asymmetry predicts loading asymmetry during sit-to-stand task in patients with unilateral total knee arthroplasty. Knee Surg Sports Traumatol Arthrosc. 2016;24(8):2587–94. https://doi.org/10.1007/s00167-015-3827-x.
5. Farquhar S, Snyder-Mackler L. The Chitranjan Ranawat Award: the nonoperated knee predicts function 3 years after unilateral total knee arthroplasty. Clin Orthop Relat Res. 2010;468(1):37–44. https://doi.org/10.1007/s11999-009-0892-9.
6. Lienhard K, Lauermann SP, Schneider D, Item-Glatthorn JF, Casartelli NC, Maffiuletti NA. Validity and reliability of isometric, isokinetic and isoinertial modalities for the assessment of quadriceps muscle strength in patients with total knee arthroplasty. J Electromyogr Kinesiol. 2013;23(6):1283–8. https://doi.org/10.1016/j.jelekin.2013.09.004.
7. Mizner RL, Petterson SC, Stevens JE, Axe MJ, Snyder-Mackler L. Preoperative quadriceps strength predicts functional ability one year after total knee arthroplasty. J Rheumatol. 2005;32(8):1533–9.
8. Petterson SC, Mizner RL, Stevens JE, Raisis L, Bodenstab A, Newcomb W, Snyder-Mackler L. Improved function from progressive strengthening interventions after total knee arthroplasty: a randomized clinical trial with an imbedded prospective cohort. Arthritis Rheum. 2009;61(2):174–83. https://doi.org/10.1002/art.24167.
9. Mizner RL, Petterson SC, Snyder-Mackler L. Quadriceps strength and the time course of functional recovery after total knee arthroplasty. J Orthop Sports Phys Ther. 2005;35(7):424–36. https://doi.org/10.2519/jospt.2005.35.7.424.
10. Loyd BJ, Stackhouse S, Dayton M, Hogan C, Bade M, Stevens-Lapsley J. The relationship between lower extremity swelling, quadriceps strength, and functional performance following total knee arthroplasty. Knee. 2019;26(2):382–91. https://doi.org/10.1016/j.knee.2019.01.012.
11. Fleeton G, Harmer AR, Nairn L, Crosbie J, March L, Crawford R, van der Esch M, Fransen M. Self-reported knee instability before and after total knee replacement surgery. Arthritis Care Res. 2016;68(4):463–71. https://doi.org/10.1002/acr.22692.
12. Graff C, Hohmann E, Bryant AL, Tetsworth K. Subjective and objective outcome measures after total knee replacement: is there a correlation? ANZ J Surg. 2016;86(11):921–5. https://doi.org/10.1111/ans.13708.
13. Dobson F, Hinman RS, Roos EM, Abbott JH, Stratford P, Davis AM, Buchbinder R, Snyder-Mackler L, Henrotin Y, Thumboo J, Hansen P, Bennell KL. OARSI recommended performance-based tests to assess physical function in people diagnosed with hip or knee osteoarthritis. Osteoarthr Cartil. 2013;21(8):1042–52. https://doi.org/10.1016/j.joca.2013.05.002.
14. Jette DU, Hunter SJ, Burkett L, Langham B, Logerstedt DS, Piuzzi NS, Poirier NM, Radach LJL, Ritter JE, Scalzitti DA, Stevens-Lapsley JE, Tompkins J, Zeni J Jr, American Physical Therapy A. Physical therapist management of total knee arthroplasty. Phys Ther. 2020;100(9):1603–31. https://doi.org/10.1093/ptj/pzaa099.
15. Kean CO, Birmingham TB, Garland SJ, Bryant DM, Giffin JR. Minimal detectable change in quadriceps strength and voluntary muscle activation in patients with knee osteoarthritis. Arch Phys Med Rehabil. 2010;91(9):1447–51. https://doi.org/10.1016/j.apmr.2010.06.002.

16. Staehli S, Glatthorn JF, Casartelli N, Maffiuletti NA. Test-retest reliability of quadriceps muscle function outcomes in patients with knee osteoarthritis. J Electromyogr Kinesiol. 2010;20(6):1058–65. https://doi.org/10.1016/j.jelekin.2010.07.006.
17. Tevald MA, Murray A, Luc BA, Lai K, Sohn D, Pietrosimone B. Hip abductor strength in people with knee osteoarthritis: a cross-sectional study of reliability and association with function. Knee. 2016;23(1):57–62. https://doi.org/10.1016/j.knee.2015.06.006.
18. Schache MB, McClelland JA, Webster KE. Reliability of measuring hip abductor strength following total knee arthroplasty using a hand-held dynamometer. Disabil Rehabil. 2016;38(6):597–600. https://doi.org/10.3109/09638288.2015.1046565.
19. Moon YW, Kim HJ, Ahn HS, Lee DH. Serial changes of quadriceps and hamstring muscle strength following total knee arthroplasty: a meta-analysis. PLoS One. 2016;11(2):e0148193. https://doi.org/10.1371/journal.pone.0148193.
20. Drouin JM, Valovich-mcLeod TC, Shultz SJ, Gansneder BM, Perrin DH. Reliability and validity of the Biodex system 3 pro isokinetic dynamometer velocity, torque and position measurements. Eur J Appl Physiol. 2004;91(1):22–9.
21. Valtonen A, Poyhonen T, Heinonen A, Sipila S. Muscle deficits persist after unilateral knee replacement and have implications for rehabilitation. Phys Ther. 2009;89(10):1072–9. https://doi.org/10.2522/ptj.20070295.
22. Horak FB, Wrisley DM, Frank J. The Balance Evaluation Systems Test (BESTest) to differentiate balance deficits. Phys Ther. 2009;89(5):484–98. https://doi.org/10.2522/ptj.20080071.
23. Opheim A, Jahnsen R, Olsson E, Stanghelle JK. Balance in relation to walking deterioration in adults with spastic bilateral cerebral palsy. Phys Ther. 2012;92(2):279–88. https://doi.org/10.2522/ptj.20100432.
24. Jones KD, Horak FB, Winters-Stone K, Irvine JM, Bennett RM. Fibromyalgia is associated with impaired balance and falls. J Clin Rheumatol. 2009;15(1):16–21. https://doi.org/10.1097/RHU.0b013e318190f991.
25. Beauchamp MK, Sibley KM, Lakhani B, Romano J, Mathur S, Goldstein RS, Brooks D. Impairments in systems underlying control of balance in COPD. Chest. 2012;141(6):1496–503. https://doi.org/10.1378/chest.11-1708.
26. Jacobs JV, Kasser SL. Balance impairment in people with multiple sclerosis: preliminary evidence for the Balance Evaluation Systems Test. Gait Posture. 2012;36(3):414–8. https://doi.org/10.1016/j.gaitpost.2012.03.026.
27. Leddy AL, Crowner BE, Earhart GM. Functional gait assessment and balance evaluation system test: reliability, validity, sensitivity, and specificity for identifying individuals with Parkinson disease who fall. Phys Ther. 2011;91(1):102–13. https://doi.org/10.2522/ptj.20100113.
28. Chan AC, Pang MY. Assessing balance function in patients with total knee arthroplasty. Phys Ther. 2015;95(10):1397–407.
29. Chan ACM, Ouyang XH, Jehu DAM, Chung RCK, Pang MYC. Recovery of balance function among individuals with total knee arthroplasty: comparison of responsiveness among four balance tests. Gait Posture. 2018;59:267–71. https://doi.org/10.1016/j.gaitpost.2017.10.020.
30. Franchignoni F, Horak F, Godi M, Nardone A, Giordano A. Using psychometric techniques to improve the Balance Evaluation Systems Test: the mini-BESTest. J Rehabil Med. 2010;42(4):323–31. https://doi.org/10.2340/16501977-0537.
31. Di Carlo S, Bravini E, Vercelli S, Massazza G, Ferriero G. The Mini-BESTest: a review of psychometric properties. Int J Rehabil Res. 2016;39(2):97–105. https://doi.org/10.1097/MRR.0000000000000153.
32. Padgett PK, Jacobs JV, Kasser SL. Is the BESTest at its best? A suggested brief version based on interrater reliability, validity, internal consistency, and theoretical construct. Phys Ther. 2012;92(9):1197–207. https://doi.org/10.2522/ptj.20120056.
33. Shah Mital B, Thangamani Ramalingam A, Bid Dibyendunarayan D. Intra and inter-rater reliability of brief balance evaluation system test in patients with total knee arthroplasty. Ind J Physiother Occupat Ther. 2018;12(1).

34. Berg KO, Wood-Dauphinee SL, Williams JI, Maki B. Measuring balance in the elderly: validation of an instrument. Can J Public Health. 1992;83 Suppl 2:S7–11.
35. Chou CY, Chien CW, Hsueh IP, Sheu CF, Wang CH, Hsieh CL. Developing a short form of the Berg Balance Scale for people with stroke. Phys Ther. 2006;86(2):195–204.
36. Jogi P, Spaulding SJ, Zecevic AA, Overend TJ, Kramer JF. Comparison of the original and reduced versions of the Berg Balance Scale and the Western Ontario and McMaster Universities Osteoarthritis Index in patients following hip or knee arthroplasty. Physiother Can. 2011;63(1):107–14. https://doi.org/10.3138/ptc.2009-26.
37. Kim D-Y, Kim T-H, Kim J-B. Concurrent validity of the seven-Item BBS-3P with other clinical measures of balance in a sample of stroke patients. J Kor Phys Ther. 2017;29(3):122–7. https://doi.org/10.18857/jkpt.2017.29.3.122.
38. Freund JE, Stetts DM, Oostindie A, Shepherd J, Vallabhajosula S. Lower Quarter Y-Balance Test in healthy women 50-79 years old. J Women Aging. 2019;31(6):475–91. https://doi.org/10.1080/08952841.2018.1510248.
39. Lee DK, Kim GM, Ha SM, Oh JS. Correlation of the Y-balance test with lower-limb strength of adult women. J Phys Ther Sci. 2014;26(5):641–3. https://doi.org/10.1589/jpts.26.641.
40. Lee D-K, Kang M-H, Lee T-S, Oh J-S. Relationships among the Y balance test, Berg Balance Scale, and lower limb strength in middle-aged and older females. Braz J Phys Ther. 2015;19(3):227–34. https://doi.org/10.1590/bjpt-rbf.2014.0096.
41. Robinson RH, Gribble PA. Support for a reduction in the number of trials needed for the star excursion balance test. Arch Phys Med Rehabil. 2008;89(2):364–70. https://doi.org/10.1016/j.apmr.2007.08.139.
42. Sarvestani H, Tabrizi H, Abbasi A, Rahmanpourmoghaddam J. The effect of eight weeks aquatic balance trainingand core stabilization training on dynamic balance in inactive elder males. Middle-East J Sci Res. 2012;11(3):279–86.
43. Shin SS, An DH. Comparison of energy expenditure during the Y-balance test in older adults with different visual acuities. J Phys Ther Sci. 2015;27(3):697–9. https://doi.org/10.1589/jpts.27.697.
44. Sipe CL, Ramey KD, Plisky PP, Taylor JD. Y-balance test: a valid and reliable assessment in older adults. J Aging Phys Act. 2019:1–7. https://doi.org/10.1123/japa.2018-0330.
45. Walaszek R, Chwala W, Walaszek K, Burdacki M, Blaszczuk J. Evaluation of the accuracy of the postural stability measurement with the Y-Balance Test based on the levels of the biomechanical parameters. Acta Bioeng Biomech. 2017;19(2):121–8.
46. Wellman SS, Klement MR, Queen RM. Performance comparison of single-radius versus multiple-curve femoral component in total knee arthroplasty: a prospective, randomized study using the lower quarter Y-balance test. Orthopedics. 2017;40(6):e1074–80. https://doi.org/10.3928/01477447-20171020-02.
47. Gstoettner M, Raschner C, Dirnberger E, Leimser H, Krismer M. Preoperative proprioceptive training in patients with total knee arthroplasty. Knee. 2011;18(4):265–70. https://doi.org/10.1016/j.knee.2010.05.012.
48. Swanik CB, Lephart SM, Rubash HE. Proprioception, kinesthesia, and balance after total knee arthroplasty with cruciate-retaining and posterior stabilized prostheses. J Bone Joint Surg Am. 2004;86(2):328–34. https://doi.org/10.2106/00004623-200402000-00016.
49. Hinman MR. Factors affecting reliability of the Biodex Balance System: a summary of four studies. J Sport Rehabil. 2000;9:240–52.
50. Baldwin SL, VanArnam TW, Ploutz-Snyder LL. Reliability of dynamic bilateral postural stability on the Biodex Stability System in older adults. Med Sci Sports Exerc. 2004;36(5):S30.
51. Parraca JA, Olivares Sánchez-Toledo PR, Carbonell Baeza A, Aparicio García-Molina VA, Adsuar Sala JC, Gusi Fuertes N. Test-Retest reliability of Biodex Balance SD on physically active old people; 2011.
52. Enright PL. The six-minute walk test. Respir Care. 2003;48(8):783–5.
53. Curb JD, Ceria-Ulep CD, Rodriguez BL, Grove J, Guralnik J, Willcox BJ, Donlon TA, Masaki KH, Chen R. Performance-based measures of physical function for high-function populations. J Am Geriatr Soc. 2006;54(5):737–42. https://doi.org/10.1111/j.1532-5415.2006.00700.x.

54. Kennedy DM, Stratford PW, Wessel J, Gollish JD, Penney D. Assessing stability and change of four performance measures: a longitudinal study evaluating outcome following total hip and knee arthroplasty. BMC Musculoskelet Disord. 2005;6:3. https://doi.org/10.1186/1471-2474-6-3.
55. Jakobsen TL, Kehlet H, Bandholm T. Reliability of the 6-min walk test after total knee arthroplasty. Knee Surg Sports Traumatol Arthrosc. 2013;21(11):2625–8. https://doi.org/10.1007/s00167-012-2054-y.
56. Rejeski WJ, Ettinger WH Jr, Schumaker S, James P, Burns R, Elam JT. Assessing performance-related disability in patients with knee osteoarthritis. Osteoarthr Cartil. 1995;3(3):157–67.
57. Steffen TM, Hacker TA, Mollinger L. Age- and gender-related test performance in community-dwelling elderly people: Six-Minute Walk Test, Berg Balance Scale, Timed Up & Go Test, and gait speeds. Phys Ther. 2002;82(2):128–37.
58. Kennedy DM, Stratford PW, Riddle DL, Hanna SE, Gollish JD. Assessing recovery and establishing prognosis following total knee arthroplasty. Phys Ther. 2008;88(1):22–32. https://doi.org/10.2522/ptj.20070051.
59. Moffet H, Collet JP, Shapiro SH, Paradis G, Marquis F, Roy L. Effectiveness of intensive rehabilitation on functional ability and quality of life after first total knee arthroplasty: a single-blind randomized controlled trial. Arch Phys Med Rehabil. 2004;85(4):546–56.
60. Ko V, Naylor JM, Harris IA, Crosbie J, Yeo AE. The six-minute walk test is an excellent predictor of functional ambulation after total knee arthroplasty. BMC Musculoskelet Disord. 2013;14:145. https://doi.org/10.1186/1471-2474-14-145.
61. Sarac D, Unver B, Cekmece S, Karatosun V. FRI0736-HPR validity and reliability of performance tests assessing balance and fall risk in patients with total knee arthroplasty. BMJ Publishing Group Ltd; 2017.
62. Watson MJ. Refining the ten-metre walking test for use with neurologically impaired people. Physiotherapy. 2002;88(7):386–97.
63. Podsiadlo D, Richardson S. The timed "Up & Go": a test of basic functional mobility for frail elderly persons. J Am Geriatr Soc. 1991;39(2):142–8. https://doi.org/10.1111/j.1532-5415.1991.tb01616.x.
64. Boonstra MC, De Waal Malefijt MC, Verdonschot N. How to quantify knee function after total knee arthroplasty? Knee. 2008;15(5):390–5. https://doi.org/10.1016/j.knee.2008.05.006.
65. Doll H, Gentile B, Bush EN, Ballinger R. Evaluation of the measurement properties of four performance outcome measures in patients with elective hip replacements, elective knee replacements, or hip fractures. Value Health. 2018;21(9):1104–14. https://doi.org/10.1016/j.jval.2018.02.006.
66. Piva SR, Fitzgerald GK, Irrgang JJ, Bouzubar F, Starz TW. Get up and go test in patients with knee osteoarthritis. Arch Phys Med Rehabil. 2004;85(2):284–9. https://doi.org/10.1016/j.apmr.2003.05.001.
67. Unnanuntana A, Ruangsomboon P, Keesukpunt W. Validity and responsiveness of the two-minute walk test for measuring functional recovery after total knee arthroplasty. J Arthroplasty. 2018;33(6):1737–44. https://doi.org/10.1016/j.arth.2018.01.015.
68. Jones CJ, Rikli RE, Beam WC. A 30-s chair-stand test as a measure of lower body strength in community-residing older adults. Res Q Exerc Sport. 1999;70(2):113–9. https://doi.org/10.1080/02701367.1999.10608028.
69. Gill S, McBurney H. Reliability of performance-based measures in people awaiting joint replacement surgery of the hip or knee. Physiother Res Int. 2008;13(3):141–52. https://doi.org/10.1002/pri.411.
70. Nightingale EJ, Pourkazemi F, Hiller CE. Systematic review of timed stair tests. J Rehabil Res Dev. 2014;51(3):335–50. https://doi.org/10.1682/JRRD.2013.06.0148.
71. Newcomer KL, Krug HE, Mahowald ML. Validity and reliability of the timed-stands test for patients with rheumatoid arthritis and other chronic diseases. J Rheumatol. 1993;20(1):21–7.
72. Crossley KM, Zhang WJ, Schache AG, Bryant A, Cowan SM. Performance on the single-leg squat task indicates hip abductor muscle function. Am J Sports Med. 2011;39(4):866–73. https://doi.org/10.1177/0363546510395456.

73. Ageberg E, Bennell KL, Hunt MA, Simic M, Roos EM, Creaby MW. Validity and inter-rater reliability of medio-lateral knee motion observed during a single-limb mini squat. BMC Musculoskelet Disord. 2010;11:265. https://doi.org/10.1186/1471-2474-11-265.
74. Alenezi F, Herrington L, Jones P, Jones R. The reliability of biomechanical variables collected during single leg squat and landing tasks. J Electromyogr Kinesiol. 2014;24(5):718–21. https://doi.org/10.1016/j.jelekin.2014.07.007.
75. Barber SD, Noyes FR, Mangine RE, McCloskey JW, Hartman W. Quantitative assessment of functional limitations in normal and anterior cruciate ligament-deficient knees. Clin Orthop Relat Res. 1990;255:204–14.
76. Engelen-van Melick N, van Cingel RE, Tijssen MP, Nijhuis-van der Sanden MW. Assessment of functional performance after anterior cruciate ligament reconstruction: a systematic review of measurement procedures. Knee Surg Sports Traumatol Arthrosc. 2013;21(4):869–79. https://doi.org/10.1007/s00167-012-2030-6.
77. Hegedus EJ, McDonough SM, Bleakley C, Baxter D, Cook CE. Clinician-friendly lower extremity physical performance tests in athletes: a systematic review of measurement properties and correlation with injury. Part 2-the tests for the hip, thigh, foot and ankle including the star excursion balance test. Br J Sports Med. 2015;49(10):649–56. https://doi.org/10.1136/bjsports-2014-094341.
78. Kroman SL, Roos EM, Bennell KL, Hinman RS, Dobson F. Measurement properties of performance-based outcome measures to assess physical function in young and middle-aged people known to be at high risk of hip and/or knee osteoarthritis: a systematic review. Osteoarthr Cartil. 2014;22(1):26–39. https://doi.org/10.1016/j.joca.2013.10.021.
79. Logerstedt D, Grindem H, Lynch A, Eitzen I, Engebretsen L, Risberg MA, Axe MJ, Snyder-Mackler L. Single-legged hop tests as predictors of self-reported knee function after anterior cruciate ligament reconstruction: the Delaware-Oslo ACL cohort study. Am J Sports Med. 2012;40(10):2348–56. https://doi.org/10.1177/0363546512457551.
80. Meierbachtol A, Rohman E, Paur E, Bottoms J, Tompkins M. Quantitative improvements in Hop Test scores after a 6-week neuromuscular training program. Sports Health. 2016;9(1):22–9. https://doi.org/10.1177/1941738116667933.
81. Noyes FR, Barber SD, Mangine RE. Abnormal lower limb symmetry determined by function hop tests after anterior cruciate ligament rupture. Am J Sports Med. 1991;19(5):513–8.
82. Gustavsson A, Neeter C, Thomee P, Silbernagel KG, Augustsson J, Thomee R, Karlsson J. A test battery for evaluating hop performance in patients with an ACL injury and patients who have undergone ACL reconstruction. Knee Surg Sports Traumatol Arthrosc. 2006;14(8):778–88. https://doi.org/10.1007/s00167-006-0045-6.
83. Reid A, Birmingham TB, Stratford PW, Alcock GK, Giffin JR. Hop testing provides a reliable and valid outcome measure during rehabilitation after anterior cruciate ligament reconstruction. Phys Ther. 2007;87(3):337–49.
84. Piercy KL, Troiano RP. Physical activity guidelines for Americans from the US department of health and human services: cardiovascular benefits and recommendations. Circ Cardiovasc Qual Outcomes. 2018;11(11):e005263.
85. Piercy KL, Troiano RP, Ballard RM, Carlson SA, Fulton JE, Galuska DA, George SM, Olson RD. The physical activity guidelines for Americans. JAMA. 2018;320(19):2020–8.
86. Powell KE, King AC, Buchner DM, Campbell WW, DiPietro L, Erickson KI, Hillman CH, Jakicic JM, Janz KF, Katzmarzyk PT. The scientific foundation for the physical activity guidelines for Americans. J Phys Act Health. 2018;16(1):1–11.
87. Barber-Westin SD, Noyes FR. Aerobic physical fitness and recreational sports participation after total knee arthroplasty. Sports Health. 2016;8(6):553–60. https://doi.org/10.1177/1941738116670090.
88. Hossain F, Patel S, Fernandez M, Konan S, Haddad F. A performance based patient outcome score for active patients following total knee arthroplasty. Osteoarthr Cartil. 2013;21(1):51–9.
89. Stratford PW, Kennedy DM. Performance measures were necessary to obtain a complete picture of osteoarthritic patients. J Clin Epidemiol. 2006;59(2):160–7. https://doi.org/10.1016/j.jclinepi.2005.07.012.

90. Stratford PW, Kennedy DM, Riddle DL. New study design evaluated the validity of measures to assess change after hip or knee arthroplasty. J Clin Epidemiol. 2009;62(3):347–52. https://doi.org/10.1016/j.jclinepi.2008.06.008.
91. McCarthy CJ, Oldham JA. The reliability, validity and responsiveness of an aggregated locomotor function (ALF) score in patients with osteoarthritis of the knee. Rheumatology (Oxford). 2004;43(4):514–7. https://doi.org/10.1093/rheumatology/keh081.
92. Guralnik JM, Simonsick EM, Ferrucci L, Glynn RJ, Berkman LF, Blazer DG, Scherr PA, Wallace RB. A short physical performance battery assessing lower extremity function: association with self-reported disability and prediction of mortality and nursing home admission. J Gerontol. 1994;49(2):M85–94. https://doi.org/10.1093/geronj/49.2.m85.
93. Guralnik JM, Ferrucci L, Simonsick EM, Salive ME, Wallace RB. Lower-extremity function in persons over the age of 70 years as a predictor of subsequent disability. N Engl J Med. 1995;332(9):556–61. https://doi.org/10.1056/NEJM199503023320902.
94. Barber-Westin SD, Noyes FR, McCloskey JW. Rigorous statistical reliability, validity, and responsiveness testing of the Cincinnati knee rating system in 350 subjects with uninjured, injured, or anterior cruciate ligament-reconstructed knees. Am J Sports Med. 1999;27(4):402–16.
95. Yoshida Y, Mizner RL, Ramsey DK, Snyder-Mackler L. Examining outcomes from total knee arthroplasty and the relationship between quadriceps strength and knee function over time. Clin Biomech (Bristol, Avon). 2008;23(3):320–8. https://doi.org/10.1016/j.clinbiomech.2007.10.008.
96. Mizner RL, Petterson SC, Clements KE, Zeni JA Jr, Irrgang JJ, Snyder-Mackler L. Measuring functional improvement after total knee arthroplasty requires both performance-based and patient-report assessments: a longitudinal analysis of outcomes. J Arthroplasty. 2011;26(5):728–37. https://doi.org/10.1016/j.arth.2010.06.004.
97. Berg K, Wood-Dauphine S, Williams J, Gayton D. Measuring balance in the elderly: preliminary development of an instrument. Physiother Can. 1989;41(6):304–11.
98. Parent E, Moffet H. Comparative responsiveness of locomotor tests and questionnaires used to follow early recovery after total knee arthroplasty. Arch Phys Med Rehabil. 2002;83(1):70–80.
99. Harada ND, Chiu V, Stewart AL. Mobility-related function in older adults: assessment with a 6-minute walk test. Arch Phys Med Rehabil. 1999;80(7):837–41.

Recommended Guidelines for Physical Activity and Athletics After Knee Arthroplasty

10

Sue Barber-Westin and Frank R. Noyes

10.1 Introduction

In 2013, Weinstein et al. [1] calculated that 655,800 total knee arthroplasty (TKA) recipients in the USA were 50–59 years old and 984,700 patients were 60–69 years old, indicating a large number of individuals that were expected to be active in fitness and recreational activities. Subsequent studies showed a disproportionate increase in the percentage of younger individuals (under the age of 60 years) requiring TKA [2, 3]. This appears to be especially true in individuals that participate in recreational activities over their lifetime who developed knee osteoarthritis (OA) [4–6] and in patients who sustain athletic injuries such as anterior cruciate ligament (ACL) ruptures that underwent meniscectomy [7–12].

TKA is performed in many athletes, as well as individuals who wish to resume a physically active lifestyle after surgery. These patients have high preoperative expectations [13–15] that correlate strongly with postoperative patient satisfaction [14, 16, 17], as detailed in Chap. 12. Therefore, the assessment of which recreational activities are resumed postoperatively is important to determine for preoperative patient counseling and a goal-oriented rehabilitation program to accomplish patient expectations. In addition, objective measurement of the level of physical activity (PA) using validated activity monitors provides realistic data regarding changes in parameters such as percent of time spent in sedentary behaviors compared with light, moderate, or vigorous activities; step counts; time spent walking; distance achieved; and so on. Finally, the determination of whether symptoms of

S. Barber-Westin (✉)
Noyes Knee Institute, Cincinnati, OH, USA
e-mail: sbwestin@csmref.org

F. R. Noyes
Cincinnati SportsMedicine and Orthopaedic Center, The Noyes Knee Institute, Cincinnati, OH, USA

F. R. Noyes, S. Barber-Westin (eds.), *Critical Rehabilitation for Partial and Total Knee Arthroplasty*, https://doi.org/10.1007/978-3-030-87003-4_10

pain and/or swelling occur with recreational activities is also important to assess the ability of TKA to return patients to an active lifestyle, including aerobic fitness, and achieve high levels of satisfaction. This chapter represents an update of the authors' previous systematic review [18] of this topic in published literature through October 2020.

10.2 Current Physical Activity Guidelines for Healthy Adults

In 2018, the American Heart Association (AHA) updated its guidelines for OA for healthy individuals (Table 10.1) [19, 20]. The guidelines were based on the work of a 17-member advisory committee that extensively reviewed the literature on PA and health [21]. Evidence was rated as strong, moderate, limited, or not assignable and was based on risk factors for cardiovascular disease that can be modified by PA, including blood pressure, blood glucose, blood lipids, and body weight.

Recommendations for substantial health benefits for all healthy adults (aged ≥18) were at least 150–300 minutes of moderate-intensity PA a week, or 75–150 minutes of vigorous-intensity activity, or an equivalent combination of moderate- and vigorous-intensity activity. During moderate-intensity activity, a person can talk but not sing. During vigorous-intensity activity, a person cannot say more than a few words without pausing to catch their breath. In addition, muscle-strengthening exercises of moderate or greater intensity that involve all major muscle groups should be performed at least 2 days a week. Adults aged ≥65 years were also encouraged to do multicomponent PA that includes balance training. They were advised to determine their level of effort for PA according to their level of fitness and whether any chronic conditions were present.

The guidelines allow for a cumulative effect of PA throughout the week. Therefore, the first recommendation was that "adults should move more and sit less throughout the day. Some physical activity is better than none." Therefore, sedentary patients who begin to perform some PA, such as taking the stairs or parking further from a store, could be expected to achieve some benefits.

The 2018 CDC Physical Activity Guidelines [22] further defined activity in terms of metabolic equivalents (METs), which is the most commonly used unit to measure PA. One MET is the rate of energy expenditure while sitting at rest, 1.3 for sitting and reading, 2.0 for walking slowly, 3.3 for walking at 3 miles per hour, and 8.3 for running at 5 miles per hour. Vigorous-intensity activity requires >6.0 METs; moderate-intensity activity, 3.0 to <6.0; light-intensity activity, 1.6 to <3.0; and sedentary activity ≤1.5. PA is also reported in terms of frequency (sessions of moderate-to-vigorous PA per day or week), duration (length of each session), and intensity (in METs). Volume is calculated in MET minutes or MET hours per day or week. The use of personal devices (pedometers and accelerometers) to measure PA allows for volume to be expressed as activity counts or step counts during a period of time.

Table 10.1 Examples of aerobic physical activities and intensities for adults[a]

Adults aged 18–64	
Moderate intensity (person can talk, but not sing, during activity)	Walking briskly (≥2.5 miles per hour) Recreational swimming Bicycling on level terrain (<10 miles per hour) Doubles tennis Active yoga Ballroom or line dancing General yard work and home repair work Exercise classes such as water aerobics
Vigorous intensity (person cannot say more than a few words without pausing for a breath)	Jogging or running Swimming laps Singles tennis Vigorous dancing Bicycling (>10 miles per hour) Jumping rope Heavy yard work (digging or shoveling, with heart rate increases) Hiking uphill or with a heavy backpack High-intensity interval training Exercise classes such as step aerobics or kickboxing
Adults aged ≥65	
Either moderate or vigorous intensity (depending upon the level of fitness and chronic conditions) Moderate intensity: On a scale of 0–10 (0 = sitting, 10 = greatest effort possible), levels 5–6 and produces noticeable increases in breathing and heart rate Vigorous intensity: levels ≥7 and produces large increases in breathing and heart rate	Walking or hiking Dancing Swimming Water aerobics Jogging or running Aerobic exercise classes Some forms of yoga Bicycle riding Some yard work (raking, pushing a lawn mower) Tennis or basketball Walking as part of golf

[a]From Physical Activity Guidelines for Americans, 2nd edition, 2018; U.S. Department of Health and Human Services

10.3 Sports and Recreational Activities After TKA

We assessed data from 21 studies that detailed recreational and sports activities patients participated in postoperatively (Table 10.2) [23–43]. The studies reported a wide range of patients that returned to recreational activities (25–100%, Fig. 10.1). The mean percentages of patients that participated in the most common activities

Table 10.2 Studies that determined sports and recreational activity after TKA

Study	No. of knees	Age mean	F.U. yr mean	Activity monitor	Sports/physical activity rating instruments
Naylor et al. [23]	718	67.8	3	None	Authors' own questionnaire
Rocha Da Silva et al. [24]	59	69.5	>0.5	None	IPAQ
Hepperger et al. [25]	200	72.2	2.0	None	Tegner
Vielgut et al. [26]	260	62.7	14.9	None	Tegner, authors' own questionnaire
Bercovy et al. [27]	494	70.6	7.5	None	UCLA Activity Score
Mayr et al. [28]	81	71.8	6.4	None	Authors' own questionnaire
Chang et al. [29]	369	68.8	2	None	UCLA Activity Score, authors' own questionnaire
Long et al. [30]	108	All ≤55	25.1	None	Tegner
Argenson et al. [31]	104	69.0	10.6	None	UCLA Activity Score
Jones et al. [32]	83	66.5	1	None	Self-Efficacy for Exercise, Historical Leisure Activity
Kersten et al. [33]	830	72.0	3	None	SQUASH
Meding et al. [34]	98	NA	21.1	None	UCLA Activity Score
Bonnin et al. [35]	141	66.4	3.7	None	Knee Function Survey
Jackson et al. [36]	93	66.0	8.7	None	UCLA Activity Score, authors' own questionnaire
Dahm et al. [37]	1206	67.0	5.7	None	UCLA Activity Score, authors' own questionnaire
Hopper et al. [38]	76	62.1	1.8	None	Authors' own questionnaire
Mont et al. [39]	33	66.0	4.1	None	Authors' own questionnaire
Mont et al. [40]	114	70.0	7	None	Authors' own questionnaire
Walton et al. [41]	122	71.5	1	None	Grimby, authors' own questionnaire
Chatterji et al. [42]	144	70.8	1.5	None	Authors' own questionnaire
Huch et al. [43]	312	66.0	5	None	Authors' own questionnaire

F.U. follow-up, *IPAQ* International Physical Activity Questionnaire, *SQUASH* Short Questionnaire to Assess Health-Enhancing Physical Activity, *UCLA* University of California at Los Angeles

including walking, bicycling (stationary or road), hiking, swimming, dancing, fitness training or classes such as aerobic or aquatic, and golf are shown in Fig. 10.2. Evidence was not routinely available regarding the number of sports patients participated in on a weekly basis, although some studies indicated patients took part in more than one sports activity [27, 38, 40]. Frequency of participation was highly variable due to the differing methods reported that included the number of days/week [25, 38], number of days/month [36], mean hours/week [28, 32, 43], mean minutes/week [33], and mean number of times per week any activity was performed [39, 40] (Table 10.3).

Only a few studies described symptoms or limitations that occurred with activity [36, 38, 43, 44]. A "major limitation" during participation was found in 14% in one study [44]. Pain in the knee was reported during activity in 16% in one study [43] and in 17% in another (while golfing) [36]. One investigation [38] reported that 26% of patients had pain in their knee and 26% had a feeling of instability during

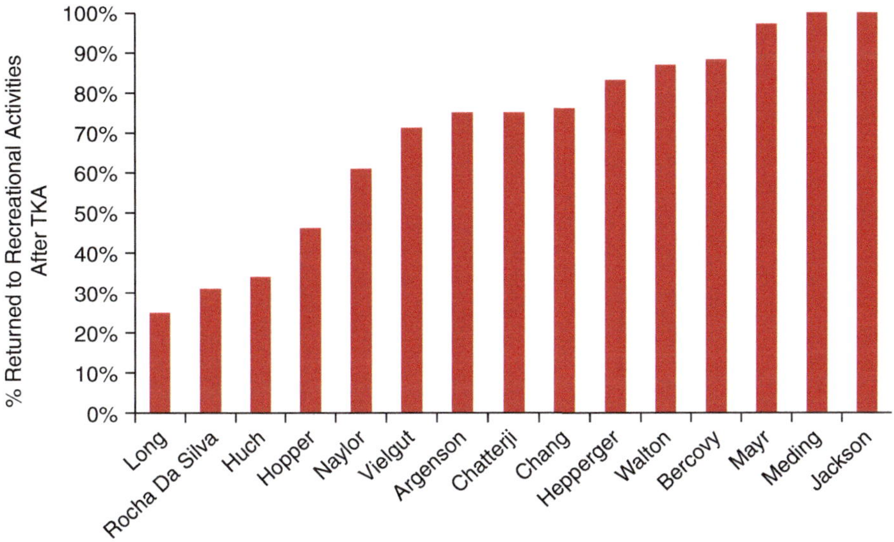

Fig. 10.1 The overall percent of TKA patients that returned to sports and recreational activities per study. These data were not available for five of the 20 studies

Fig. 10.2 The most common sports and recreational activities reported after TKA. Only studies that reported multiple activities were included. The number of studies for each activity was: walking 8, bicycling 13, hiking 8, swimming 13, dancing 7, fitness/classes 8, and golf 9

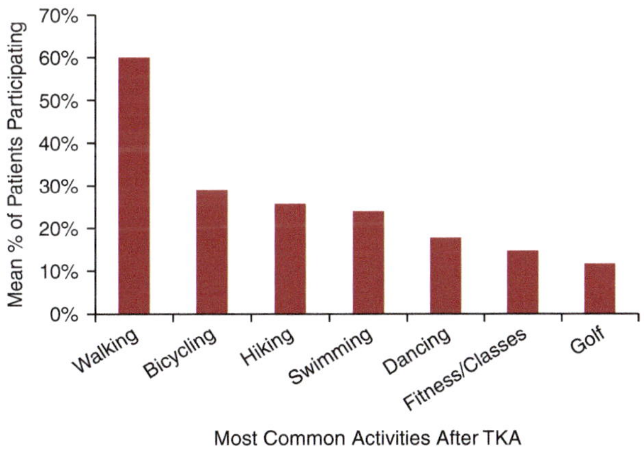

participation. Factors responsible for the inability to return to PA were usually other musculoskeletal problems or persistent pain in the TKA joint [23, 31, 37, 38, 43].

Factors that influenced return to recreational activities included higher preoperative levels of activity [23, 26, 27], higher educational level [24], male gender [37], and body mass index less than 30 [37]. Most studies found that younger patient age at TKA led to higher postoperative activity levels (<70 years [37], <65 years [33], or "younger" age [26]). There were significant correlations found between University of California at Los Angeles (UCLA) activity scores and SF-36 and Western Ontario and McMaster Universities Osteoarthritis Index (WOMAC) scores in one study

Table 10.3 Sports and recreational activities after TKA

Study	% Postoperative participation in sports and recreational activities	Sports and recreational activities	Other results
Naylor et al. [23]	61%	Walking 46%, swimming 9%, fitness exercise 8%, cycling 6%, golf 5%, lawn bowling 4%, tai chi 2%, tennis 1%	Significant factors return to PA: regular PA 1 year preop ($P < 0.001$). Main reasons not able to participate in PA: other musculoskeletal problems 10%, problem with TKA 5%, other medical problem 5%
Rocha Da Silva et al. [24]	34%	Low impact (water aerobics, walking, cycling, weight lifting, pilates) 26%, gymnastics 5%	Significant factors return to PA: older age ($P < 0.001$), lower pain VAS ($P < 0.001$), educational level ($P < 0.05$)
Hepperger et al. [25]	83%	Hiking 74%, skiing 70%, cycling 55%, swimming 38%, cross-country skiing 17%	Frequency of PA (all sports combined): 13% >5 days/week, 57% 2–3 x/week, 13% occasionally
Vielgut et al. [26]	71%	Cycling 26%, hiking 26%, nordic walking 22%, gymnastics 22%, swimming 20%, dancing 9%, fitness training 3%, bowling 3%, badminton 3%, golf 2%, jogging 2%, soccer 2%	Significant factors return to PA: preop Tegner score ($P < 0.001$), younger age ($P < 0.05$)
Bercovy et al. [27]	88%	88% had UCLA score ≥ 7 points 30% had UCLA score ≥ 8 points 21% participated in more than 1 activity	Significant factors UCLA score: pre-disease UCLA score, age (unknown older or younger age; $P = 0.001$)
Mayr et al. [28]	97%	Cycling 94%, swimming 76%, hiking 70%, fitness training 33%, nordic walking 31%, cross-country skiing 27%, water aerobics 26%, dancing 26%, alpine skiing 25%, tennis 20%, golf 11%, rock climbing 9%	All patients >60 years age. Mean frequency participation (all sports combined): 5.3 hours/week. Significant correlation level PA activity and KOOS sports score ($P = 0.02$), KOOS quality of life score ($P = 0.04$), WOMAC score ($P = 0.03$)
Chang et al. [29]	76%	Walking 60%, swimming 23%, cycling 22%, hiking 6%, gymnastics 5%, <2% badminton, running, golf, table tennis	Regular PA associated higher satisfaction. Postop UCLA scores significantly correlated with SF-36 and WOMAC function scores. No effects in sociodemographic factors, pain relief, postoperative range of motion on PA levels

Study	% Postoperative participation in sports and recreational activities	Sports and recreational activities	Other results
Long et al. [30]	25%	Tegner scores: 4 (8%), 5 (3%), 6 (11%), 7 (3%)	NA
Argenson et al. [31]	75%	75% involved in sports or recreation; most frequent walking, hiking, gardening, swimming, exercising, cycling, and golfing	Mean time to return to PA 6 ± 3 mos. Limitations with PA: 71% none, 23% mild, 6% major. No PA: reasons not related to TKA 19%
Jones et al. [32]	NA	Walking 64%, fitness exercising 32%, weight lifting 31%, gardening 30%, bicycling 24%, swimming 7%, hiking 4%, golfing 4%	Mean frequency of PA: 19.6 hours/week (range, 0–125.6)
Kersten et al. [33]	NA	NA 51% met PA guidelines (≥30 min. moderate-intensity aerobic PA ≥5 days/week or ≥20 min. vigorous-intensity PA ≥3 days/week)	Mean frequency of PA: 1347 minutes/week; 167 ± 135 minutes/week for walking, 122 ± 242 minutes/week for cycling, 52 ± 140 minutes/week for sports. Patients < 65 years of age had greater mean PA per week than those > 65 years ($P < 0.001$)
Meding et al. [34]	100%	36% impact activities such as jogging, volleyball, and singles tennis	All patients participated in moderate activity (UCLA scores ≥5)
Bonnin et al. [35]	NA	Gardening 52%, hiking 35%, stationary cycling 31%, swimming 31%, gymnastics 16%, downhill skiing 8%, dancing 6%, cross-country skiing 5%	Correlation between participation in PA and patient motivation ($P = 0.0001$)
Jackson et al. [36]	100%	Studied only patients who returned to golf	Frequency: 33% 1 x/mo, 36% 2–7 x/mo, 31% >7 x/mo. Time to return: 3 mos in 13%, 4–6 mos in 44%, 7–9 mos in 20%, 10–12 mos in 8%, >12 mos in 15% Pain while golfing: 17%
Dahm et al. [37]	NA	Walking 67%, stationary cycling 45%, swimming 29%, dancing 25%, hiking 24%, golfing 21%, low-impact aerobics 17%, road cycling 15%, weight lifting 15%, speed walking 10%, croquet 7%, canoeing 6%, bowling 6%	Significant factors higher UCLA score: age < 70 years ($P < 0.001$), male gender ($P < 0.0001$)
Hopper and Leach [38]	46%	1 sport 28%, 2 sports 17%, >2 sports 3%. Swimming 30%, dancing 14%, cycling 9%, bowling 9%, golfing 6%	Mean frequency of PA 2 x/wk, minimum 37.5 mins/session; mean time to return to PA 4.1 mos.

(continued)

Table 10.3 (continued)

Study	% Postoperative participation in sports and recreational activities	Sports and recreational activities	Other results
Mont et al. [39]	100%	All high-impact sports such as jogging, tennis (singles), racquetball, and high-impact aerobics	Mean frequency 4 x/week, 3.5 hours
Mont et al. [40]	NA	High activity group: walking 89%, swimming 53%, weight training 46%, gardening 44%	Mean frequency of PA: high activity group 11 x/week, low activity group 4 x/week
Walton et al. [41]	87%	Walking 66%, swimming 11%, green bowls 11%, fishing 6%, gym work 6%, golfing 5%, cycling 4%	NA
Chatterji et al. [42]	75%	Walking 72%, swimming 15%, bowling 12%, water aerobics 8%, fishing 8%, golfing 6%, exercise class 6%	Mean time to return: 5–6 weeks aqua aerobics, 8 weeks exercise walking, 12–13 weeks exercise class, cycling, golf, 18 weeks bowling
Huch et al. [43]	34%	Swimming ~35%, cycling ~31%, hiking 29%, gymnastics ~8%, dancing ~4%	Frequencies of all PA: 15% <1 hour/week, 15% 1–2 hours/week, 5% >2 hours/week, 65% none

KOOS Knee Injury and Osteoarthritis Outcome Score, *NA* not available, *PA* physical activity, *UCLA* University of California at Los Angeles, *VAS* visual analogue scale, *WOMAC* Western Ontario and McMaster Universities Osteoarthritis Index

[29], and between patient activity levels (high, medium, and low impact) and Knee Injury and Osteoarthritis Outcome Score (KOOS) sports, KOOS quality of life, and WOMAC scores in another study [28].

Although the majority of studies that reported return to activity data following TKA found the majority participated in low-impact activities [45], a few described patients who returned to high-impact sports. However, an analysis of symptoms or limitations with these activities has not been rigorously conducted to our knowledge. For instance, Mont et al. [39] followed a cohort of 31 patients (who represented 4% of their TKA population) that returned to sports that involved running and other high-impact activities a mean of 4 years postoperatively. All but one had excellent clinical outcomes and were satisfied with the result of the operation. The authors stressed their opinion that these types of activities were not appropriate for the majority of patients. However, with a small percentage choosing to return, surgeons should work closely to individualize recommendations. Mayr et al. [28] found that 25% of 81 patients who lived in an Alpine area returned to high-impact activities such as downhill skiing and tennis, and 47% returned to medium-impact sports such as mountain hiking and cross-country skiing. All but one patient had been involved in sports during their lifetime. While most patients were participating in low-impact activities at the 1-year evaluation, the evaluation at 6 years showed increased involvement in higher-impact sports. Hepperger et al. [25] reported that 74% of 200 patients from Austria returned to hiking and 70% returned to downhill skiing 2 years postoperatively. These authors attributed the results to living in the Alpine region and noted that the home geographic environment plays an important role in activities resumed postoperatively.

10.4 Objective Measured Physical Activity After TKA

Eight studies measured movement-related activity, three of which determined the percent of patients who achieved AHA recommended PA guidelines (Table 10.4) [46–53]. At 6 months postoperatively, two studies reported that 0% [47] to 18% [46] met the guidelines, and at 12 months postoperatively, one study [48] found that 16.5% met the guidelines. There was wide variability in study conclusions regarding time spent in sedentary behavior compared with preoperative data, as four studies reported no change [47–49, 51] and three studies reporting a significant decrease [46, 50, 52]. Postoperative PA levels were considerably lower than those of healthy controls in one study [48] and were lower than previously published data in another study [50].

It is important to note that in normal adult populations, investigators have shown that only a small percentage of adults meet AHA guidelines. Whether the data from TKA studies and those from control populations regarding problems achieving PA guidelines are strictly related to aging or are due to other factors such as socioeconomic status and motivation is unclear and worthy of future study. One investigation that measured PA in 2450 healthy adults aged 70–93 years reported that only 15% of men and 10% of women achieved >150 minutes a week of PA [54]. Another

Table 10.4 Studies that determined physical activity after TKA

Study	No. of knees, age mean	Activity monitor, time measured	% Met PA guidelines[a]	Results
Frimpong et al. [46]	45, 63.8	ActiGraph Preoperative, 6 months postop	18%	Sedentary behavior: decreased from 70% preop to 64% at 6 mos postop (~56 mins/day; $P = 0.009$). Proportion time spent in light PA increased from 29% preop to 35% at 6 mos postop (~50 min/day; $P = 0.008$). No change in time spent in moderate to vigorous PA. Significant improvements in UCLA activity scores ($P < 0.001$)
Harding et al. [47]	25, 69.0	ActiGraph Preoperative, 6 months postop	0%	No patient met American PA guidelines. No change in measured PA. Proportion of time in sedentary behavior: 82% preop, 83% postop. Significant improvements in UCLA activity scores ($P < 0.001$)
Lutzner et al. [48]	97, 68.9	activPAL Preoperative, 12 months postop	16.5%	16.5% met PA guidelines. Moderate to vigorous steps/day increased from 1150 ± 982 to 1935 ± 1728 ($P < 0.001$). Time spent in sedentary behavior did not change. Patients took significantly fewer steps/day than age-matched controls
Vissers et al. [49]	21[b], NA	Activity Monitor Preoperative, 6 months, 4 years postop	NA	No significant improvement in either time period: all movement-related activity/24 hour period, % time walking/24 hour period, % time standing/24 hour period, number of sit-to-stand movements/24 hour period. No significant improvement in KOOS Sport and Recreation score
Brandes et al. [50]	44, 65.8	SAM Preoperative, 2, 6, 12 months postop	NA	Gait cycles: significant increase 6 ($P < 0.05$) and 12 ($P = 0.003$) mos postop Significant increase in time spent in moderate and high-intensity walking (>50 gait cycles/ minute) 12 mos postop ($P = 0.01$)
de Groot et al. [51]	42, 62.1	Activity Monitor Preoperative, 3, 6 months postop	NA	No significant improvement in all movement-related activity/24 hour period, % time walking/24 hour period, % time standing/24 hour period, number of sit-to-stand movements/24 hour period
Walker et al. [52]	19, 69.0	Numact Preoperative, 1, 3, 6 months postop	NA	Significant increase in total overall ambulatory activity (79%, $P = 0.02$, effect size 1.66), total time standing/24 hour period (64 min. longer, $P = 0.01$), energy expenditure in longest continuous walk ($P = 0.03$). No change in mean amplitude steps/24 hour period

(continued)

Table 10.4 (continued)

Study	No. of knees, age mean	Activity monitor, time measured	% Met PA guidelines[a]	Results
Hoorntge et al. [53]	52 58.4	Activ8 Preoperative, 6 months postop	NA	Small improvement in total waking active time (0.7 ± 0.6%), standing time (1.0 ± 0.9%), and sedentary time (−2.5 ± 1.3%). No improvement with use of an individualized rehabilitation program based on preoperative goal setting

[a]≥150 minutes of moderate to vigorous PA per week
[b]21/42 patients from de Groot et al.'s [51] study

study of 3459 US adults aged 49–85 years measured PA for 7 days and reported that only 2.5% achieved adherence of PA guidelines of ≥30 min/day of moderate-to-vigorous movement intensity [55].

In a systematic review of 26 studies that measured PA levels after total joint (hip and knee) arthroplasty (using either objective instruments or recall questionnaires), Naal and Impellizzeri [56] reported noteworthy heterogeneity and provided recommendations to standardize future studies. They noted patients undergoing total joint arthroplasty were less active than recommended AHA levels. Accelerometers provide realistic data of all types of activity (light, moderate, and vigorous) and give feedback and motivation to patients [57]. Total daily step count is a beneficial motivator, and Garber et al. [58] recommended ≥7000 steps/day, which could be achieved by increasing step counts by ≥2000 as necessary to achieve this level. In 2018, Hammett et al. [59] systematically reviewed the literature for studies that only used accelerometers from preoperative to postoperative from inception of the PubMed database to January 2016 for TKA and total hip arthroscopy. Seven studies were included, four of which focused on TKA, and the authors found no significant increase in PA at 6 months (compared with preoperative) and only a small to moderate effect at 12 months.

Clinical studies usually employ patient self-reporting of activity levels with questionnaires such as the UCLA activity scale [60]. These data are not always reliable, may be subject to recall bias [51, 61], and may overestimate PA compared with objective activity measurements [47, 50, 51]. For example, Harding et al. [47] reported no change in PA parameters 6 months after TKA measured with an accelerometer in 25 patients. However, there was a significant increase in the UCLA activity scores between the preoperative and follow-up evaluations (3 ± 1 and 5 ± 3, respectively; $P < 0.001$). Brandes et al. [50] also reported no correlation between PA and clinical outcomes as measured with the Knee Society Score and SF-36.

10.5 Recommended Sports and Recreational Activities

At the time of writing, the most recent activity recommendations following TKA by the American Association of Hip and Knee Surgeons were published in 2009 (Table 10.5) [62]. Based on the results of 139 completed surveys from the 2007 annual meeting, consensus was reached for low-impact activities such as walking, climbing stairs, bicycling on level surfaces, swimming, doubles tennis, and golfing. Activities that were consistently discouraged included jogging, sprinting, skiing on difficult terrain, and singles tennis. A survey of 94 surgeons from the Netherland Orthopaedic Association included 40 sports, of which the surgeons indicated whether they were allowed, allowed with experience, discouraged, or no opinion [63]. The results for patients <65 years of age are shown in Table 10.5. For patients >65 years of age, the same activities achieved consensus for allowed and not allowed as the younger group. Two additional activities reached consensus for allowed with

Table 10.5 Survey activity recommendations after TKA

Society, study	Activities allowed all patients	Activities allowed with experience	Activities not allowed
American Association of Hip and Knee Surgeons, 2009 [62]	Walking Climbing Bicycling on level surfaces Swimming Doubles tennis Golfing	NA	Jogging Sprinting Skiing on difficult terrain Singles tennis
Netherland Orthopaedic Association, 2018 [63]	*For patients < 65 years:* Aqua fitness Bicycling Dancing Fitness/fysiofitness Golf Game of bowls Nordic walking Swimming Walking	*For patients < 65 years:* Aerobics Canoeing Cross-country skiing Cycling Ice skating Horseback riding Sailing Surfing Table tennis Doubles tennis Yoga	Basketball Football Handball Hockey Korfball Martial arts Running Snowboarding Volleyball
Systematic review 21 studies [64]	Low-impact aerobics Bowling Golf Dancing Walking Swimming	Cycling Hiking Rowing Cross-country skiing Stationary skiing Speed walking Doubles tennis Ice skating	Racquetball/squash Contact sports (football, hockey, soccer) Rock climbing Jogging/running Singles tennis Waterskiing Baseball/softball Handball Martial arts

experience (cross-walking and rowing). A systematic review of 21 studies published from 1986 through 2010 by Vogel et al. [64] provided advice regarding the most appropriate activities after TKA. These authors stressed the avoidance of sports that create high-impact loads and noted that rehabilitation may take at least 3 months to allow low-impact activities.

10.6 Authors' Discussion

Important goals of TKA in younger active patients include maintaining a healthy lifestyle and returning to desired realistic recreational or sports activities. However, in patients who wish to resume moderate- or high-intensity recreational and sports activities after TKA, the high loads placed on the knee joint may result in chronic effusions and muscle dysfunction.

There was a wide range of patients that resumed mostly light, low-impact recreational activities after TKA (25–100%). There are many potential reasons for lack of postoperative participation in recreational activities or PA, including lingering effects of the operation (pain or swelling), the natural aging process, income, educational status, area of residency, personal barriers and beliefs, self-efficacy, and social support [65–68]. The reasons patients elect not to participate in recreational activities after TKA are important to determine, especially in studies in which return to PA is a main focus. Five studies reported that the factors most commonly responsible for the inability to return to PA were other musculoskeletal problems or persistent pain in the TKA joint [23, 31, 37, 38, 43].

Few studies provided data regarding symptoms or functional limitations that occurred during recreational or sports activities. For patient counseling purposes, future studies should provide these data to ensure that preoperative patient expectations are realistic in terms of activities that are resumed after surgery. Finally, no study provided detail regarding the postoperative rehabilitation program. This book describes in detail the role of the physical therapist in guiding a patient back to recreational or fitness activities. Rehabilitation programs that incorporate strength, balance, flexibility, and neuromuscular function have been recommended to safely resume PA [69–71]. Objective assessment of muscular and neuromuscular function prior to release to activities is also recommended [72–75]. A careful balance of joint loads must be managed to reduce chronic knee joint effusions (which is an indicator of the need to reduce activities) and chronic muscle weakness.

References

1. Weinstein AM, Rome BN, Reichmann WM, Collins JE, Burbine SA, Thornhill TS, Wright J, Katz JN, Losina E. Estimating the burden of total knee replacement in the United States. J Bone Joint Surg Am. 2013;95(5):385–92. https://doi.org/10.2106/JBJS.L.00206.
2. Sloan M, Premkumar A, Sheth NP. Projected volume of primary total joint arthroplasty in the U.S., 2014 to 2030. J Bone Joint Surg Am. 2018;100(17):1455–60. https://doi.org/10.2106/JBJS.17.01617.

3. Maradit Kremers H, Larson DR, Crowson CS, Kremers WK, Washington RE, Steiner CA, Jiranek WA, Berry DJ. Prevalence of total hip and knee replacement in the United States. J Bone Joint Surg Am. 2015;97(17):1386–97. https://doi.org/10.2106/JBJS.N.01141.
4. Elleuch MH, Guermazi M, Mezghanni M, Ghroubi S, Fki H, Mefteh S, Baklouti S, Sellami S. Knee osteoarthritis in 50 former top-level soccer players: a comparative study. Ann Readapt Med Phys. 2008;51(3):174–8. https://doi.org/10.1016/j.annrmp.2008.01.003.
5. Spector TD, Harris PA, Hart DJ, Cicuttini FM, Nandra D, Etherington J, Wolman RL, Doyle DV. Risk of osteoarthritis associated with long-term weight-bearing sports: a radiologic survey of the hips and knees in female ex-athletes and population controls. Arthritis Rheum. 1996;39(6):988–95.
6. Tveit M, Rosengren BE, Nilsson JA, Karlsson MK. Former male elite athletes have a higher prevalence of osteoarthritis and arthroplasty in the hip and knee than expected. Am J Sports Med. 2012;40(3):527–33. https://doi.org/10.1177/0363546511429278.
7. Granan LP, Bahr R, Lie SA, Engebretsen L. Timing of anterior cruciate ligament reconstructive surgery and risk of cartilage lesions and meniscal tears: a cohort study based on the Norwegian National Knee Ligament Registry. Am J Sports Med. 2009;37(5):955–61. 0363546508330136 [pii]. https://doi.org/10.1177/0363546508330136.
8. Brophy RH, Rai MF, Zhang Z, Torgomyan A, Sandell LJ. Molecular analysis of age and sex-related gene expression in meniscal tears with and without a concomitant anterior cruciate ligament tear. J Bone Joint Surg Am. 2012;94(5):385–93. https://doi.org/10.2106/JBJS.K.00919.
9. Mihelic R, Jurdana H, Jotanovic Z, Madjarevic T, Tudor A. Long-term results of anterior cruciate ligament reconstruction: a comparison with non-operative treatment with a follow-up of 17–20 years. Int Orthop. 2011;35(7):1093–7. https://doi.org/10.1007/s00264-011-1206-x.
10. Gerhard P, Bolt R, Duck K, Mayer R, Friederich NF, Hirschmann MT. Long-term results of arthroscopically assisted anatomical single-bundle anterior cruciate ligament reconstruction using patellar tendon autograft: are there any predictors for the development of osteoarthritis? Knee Surg Sports Traumatol Arthrosc. 2013;21(4):957–64. https://doi.org/10.1007/s00167-012-2001-y.
11. Ahn JH, Kim JG, Wang JH, Jung CH, Lim HC. Long-term results of anterior cruciate ligament reconstruction using bone-patellar tendon-bone: an analysis of the factors affecting the development of osteoarthritis. Arthroscopy. 2012;28(8):1114–23. https://doi.org/10.1016/j.arthro.2011.12.019.
12. Janssen RP, du Mee AW, van Valkenburg J, Sala HA, Tseng CM. Anterior cruciate ligament reconstruction with 4-strand hamstring autograft and accelerated rehabilitation: a 10-year prospective study on clinical results, knee osteoarthritis and its predictors. Knee Surg Sports Traumatol Arthrosc. 2013;21(9):1977–88. https://doi.org/10.1007/s00167-012-2234-9.
13. Deakin AH, Smith MA, Wallace DT, Smith EJ, Sarungi M. Fulfilment of preoperative expectations and postoperative patient satisfaction after total knee replacement. A prospective analysis of 200 patients. Knee. 2019;26(6):1403–12. https://doi.org/10.1016/j.knee.2019.07.018.
14. Jain D, Nguyen LL, Bendich I, Nguyen LL, Lewis CG, Huddleston JI, Duwelius PJ, Feeley BT, Bozic KJ. Higher patient expectations predict higher patient-reported outcomes, but not satisfaction, in total knee arthroplasty patients: a prospective multicenter study. J Arthroplasty. 2017;32(9S):S166–70. https://doi.org/10.1016/j.arth.2017.01.008.
15. Jassim SS, Douglas SL, Haddad FS. Athletic activity after lower limb arthroplasty: a systematic review of current evidence. Bone Joint J. 2014;96-B(7):923–7. https://doi.org/10.1302/0301-620X.96B7.31585.
16. Lützner C, Postler A, Beyer F, Kirschner S, Lützner J. Fulfillment of expectations influence patient satisfaction 5 years after total knee arthroplasty. Knee Surg Sports Traumatol Arthrosc. 2019;27(7):2061–70. https://doi.org/10.1007/s00167-018-5320-9.
17. Husain A, Lee GC. Establishing realistic patient expectations following total knee arthroplasty. J Am Acad Orthop Surg. 2015;23(12):707–13. https://doi.org/10.5435/JAAOS-D-14-00049.
18. Barber-Westin SD, Noyes FR. Aerobic physical fitness and recreational sports participation after total knee arthroplasty. Sports Health. 2016;8(6):553–60. https://doi.org/10.1177/1941738116670090.

19. Piercy KL, Troiano RP, Ballard RM, Carlson SA, Fulton JE, Galuska DA, George SM, Olson RD. The physical activity guidelines for Americans. JAMA. 2018;320(19):2020–8.
20. Piercy KL, Troiano RP. Physical activity guidelines for Americans from the US department of health and human services: cardiovascular benefits and recommendations. Circ Cardiovasc Qual Outcomes. 2018;11(11):e005263.
21. DiPietro L, Buchner DM, Marquez DX, Pate RR, Pescatello LS, Whitt-Glover MC. New scientific basis for the 2018 US Physical Activity Guidelines. J Sport Health Sci. 2019;8(3):197.
22. U.S. Department of Health and Human Services. 2018 physical activity guidelines advisory committee scientific report. Washington, DC; 2018.
23. Naylor JM, Pocovi N, Descallar J, Mills KA. Participation in regular physical activity after total knee or hip arthroplasty for osteoarthritis: prevalence, associated factors, and type. Arthritis Care Res. 2019;71(2):207–17. https://doi.org/10.1002/acr.23604.
24. Rocha Da Silva R, Filardi De Oliveira P, Almeida Matos M. Sports activity after total knee arthroplasty. Ortop Traumatol Rehabil. 2018;20(2):133–8. https://doi.org/10.5604/01.3001.0012.0423.
25. Hepperger C, Gfoller P, Abermann E, Hoser C, Ulmer H, Herbst E, Fink C. Sports activity is maintained or increased following total knee arthroplasty. Knee Surg Sports Traumatol Arthrosc. 2018;26(5):1515–23. https://doi.org/10.1007/s00167-017-4529-3.
26. Vielgut I, Leitner L, Kastner N, Radl R, Leithner A, Sadoghi P. Sports activity after low-contact-stress total knee arthroplasty - a long term follow-up study. Sci Rep. 2016;6:24630. https://doi.org/10.1038/srep24630.
27. Bercovy M, Langlois J, Beldame J, Lefebvre B. Functional results of the ROCC(R) mobile bearing knee. 602 cases at midterm follow-up (5 to 14 years). J Arthroplasty. 2015;30(6):973–9. https://doi.org/10.1016/j.arth.2015.01.003.
28. Mayr HO, Reinhold M, Bernstein A, Suedkamp NP, Stoehr A. Sports activity following total knee arthroplasty in patients older than 60 years. J Arthroplasty. 2015;30(1):46–9. https://doi.org/10.1016/j.arth.2014.08.021.
29. Chang MJ, Kim SH, Kang YG, Chang CB, Kim TK. Activity levels and participation in physical activities by Korean patients following total knee arthroplasty. BMC Musculoskelet Disord. 2014;15:240. https://doi.org/10.1186/1471-2474-15-240.
30. Long WJ, Bryce CD, Hollenbeak CS, Benner RW, Scott WN. Total knee replacement in young, active patients: long-term follow-up and functional outcome: a concise follow-up of a previous report. J Bone Joint Surg Am. 2014;96(18):e159. https://doi.org/10.2106/JBJS.M.01259.
31. Argenson JN, Parratte S, Ashour A, Saintmard B, Aubaniac JM. The outcome of rotating-platform total knee arthroplasty with cement at a minimum of ten years of follow-up. J Bone Joint Surg Am. 2012;94(7):638–44. https://doi.org/10.2106/JBJS.K.00263.
32. Jones DL, Bhanegaonkar AJ, Billings AA, Kriska AM, Irrgang JJ, Crossett LS, Kwoh CK. Differences between actual and expected leisure activities after total knee arthroplasty for osteoarthritis. J Arthroplasty. 2012;27(7):1289–96. https://doi.org/10.1016/j.arth.2011.10.030.
33. Kersten RF, Stevens M, van Raay JJ, Bulstra SK, van den Akker-Scheek I. Habitual physical activity after total knee replacement. Phys Ther. 2012;92(9):1109–16. https://doi.org/10.2522/ptj.20110273.
34. Meding JB, Meding LK, Ritter MA, Keating EM. Pain relief and functional improvement remain 20 years after knee arthroplasty. Clin Orthop Relat Res. 2012;470(1):144–9. https://doi.org/10.1007/s11999-011-2123-4.
35. Bonnin M, Laurent JR, Parratte S, Zadegan F, Badet R, Bissery A. Can patients really do sport after TKA? Knee Surg Sports Traumatol Arthrosc. 2010;18(7):853–62. https://doi.org/10.1007/s00167-009-1009-4.
36. Jackson JD, Smith J, Shah JP, Wisniewski SJ, Dahm DL. Golf after total knee arthroplasty: do patients return to walking the course? Am J Sports Med. 2009;37(11):2201–4. https://doi.org/10.1177/0363546509339009.
37. Dahm DL, Barnes SA, Harrington JR, Sayeed SA, Berry DJ. Patient-reported activity level after total knee arthroplasty. J Arthroplasty. 2008;23(3):401–7. https://doi.org/10.1016/j.arth.2007.05.051.

38. Hopper GP, Leach WJ. Participation in sporting activities following knee replacement: total versus unicompartmental. Knee Surg Sports Traumatol Arthrosc. 2008;16(10):973–9. https://doi.org/10.1007/s00167-008-0596-9.
39. Mont MA, Marker DR, Seyler TM, Jones LC, Kolisek FR, Hungerford DS. High-impact sports after total knee arthroplasty. J Arthroplasty. 2008;23(6 Suppl 1):80–4. https://doi.org/10.1016/j.arth.2008.04.018.
40. Mont MA, Marker DR, Seyler TM, Gordon N, Hungerford DS, Jones LC. Knee arthroplasties have similar results in high- and low-activity patients. Clin Orthop Relat Res. 2007;460:165–73. https://doi.org/10.1097/BLO.0b013e318042b5e7.
41. Walton NP, Jahromi I, Lewis PL, Dobson PJ, Angel KR, Campbell DG. Patient-perceived outcomes and return to sport and work: TKA versus mini-incision unicompartmental knee arthroplasty. J Knee Surg. 2006;19(2):112–6.
42. Chatterji U, Ashworth MJ, Lewis PL, Dobson PJ. Effect of total knee arthroplasty on recreational and sporting activity. ANZ J Surg. 2005;75(6):405–8. https://doi.org/10.1111/j.1445-2197.2005.03400.x.
43. Huch K, Muller KA, Sturmer T, Brenner H, Puhl W, Gunther KP. Sports activities 5 years after total knee or hip arthroplasty: the Ulm Osteoarthritis Study. Ann Rheum Dis. 2005;64(12):1715–20. https://doi.org/10.1136/ard.2004.033266.
44. Argenson JN, Parratte S, Ashour A, Komistek RD, Scuderi GR. Patient-reported outcome correlates with knee function after a single-design mobile-bearing TKA. Clin Orthop Relat Res. 2008;466(11):2669–76. https://doi.org/10.1007/s11999-008-0418-x.
45. Hanreich C, Martelanz L, Koller U, Windhager R, Waldstein W. Sport and physical activity following primary total knee arthroplasty: a systematic review and meta-analysis. J Arthroplasty. 2020;35(8):2274–2285.e2271. https://doi.org/10.1016/J.ARTH.2020.04.013.
46. Frimpong E, McVeigh JA, van der Jagt D, Mokete L, Kaoje YS, Tikly M, Meiring RM. Light intensity physical activity increases and sedentary behavior decreases following total knee arthroplasty in patients with osteoarthritis. Knee Surg Sports Traumatol Arthrosc. 2019;27(7):2196–205. https://doi.org/10.1007/s00167-018-4987-2.
47. Harding P, Holland AE, Delany C, Hinman RS. Do activity levels increase after total hip and knee arthroplasty? Clin Orthop Relat Res. 2014;472(5):1502–11. https://doi.org/10.1007/s11999-013-3427-3.
48. Lutzner C, Kirschner S, Lutzner J. Patient activity after TKA depends on patient-specific parameters. Clin Orthop Relat Res. 2014;472(12):3933–40. https://doi.org/10.1007/s11999-014-3813-5.
49. Vissers MM, Bussmann JB, de Groot IB, Verhaar JA, Reijman M. Physical functioning four years after total hip and knee arthroplasty. Gait Posture. 2013;38(2):310–5. https://doi.org/10.1016/j.gaitpost.2012.12.007.
50. Brandes M, Ringling M, Winter C, Hillmann A, Rosenbaum D. Changes in physical activity and health-related quality of life during the first year after total knee arthroplasty. Arthritis Care Res. 2011;63(3):328–34. https://doi.org/10.1002/acr.20384.
51. de Groot IB, Bussmann HJ, Stam HJ, Verhaar JA. Small increase of actual physical activity 6 months after total hip or knee arthroplasty. Clin Orthop Relat Res. 2008;466(9):2201–8. https://doi.org/10.1007/s11999-008-0315-3.
52. Walker DJ, Heslop PS, Chandler C, Pinder IM. Measured ambulation and self-reported health status following total joint replacement for the osteoarthritic knee. Rheumatology (Oxford). 2002;41(7):755–8. https://doi.org/10.1093/rheumatology/41.7.755.
53. Hoorntje A, Witjes S, Kuijer P, Bussmann JBJ, Horemans HLD, Kerkhoffs G, van Geenen RCI, Koenraadt KLM. Does activity-based rehabilitation with goal attainment scaling increase physical activity among younger knee arthroplasty patients? Results from the randomized controlled ACTION trial. J Arthroplasty. 2020;35(3):706–11. https://doi.org/10.1016/j.arth.2019.10.028.
54. Jefferis BJ, Sartini C, Lee IM, Choi M, Amuzu A, Gutierrez C, Casas JP, Ash S, Lennnon LT, Wannamethee SG, Whincup PH. Adherence to physical activity guidelines in older adults,

using objectively measured physical activity in a population-based study. BMC Public Health. 2014;14:382. https://doi.org/10.1186/1471-2458-14-382.
55. Berkemeyer K, Wijndaele K, White T, Cooper A, Luben R, Westgate K, Griffin S, Khaw K-T, Wareham N, Brage S. The descriptive epidemiology of accelerometer-measured physical activity in older adults. Int J Behav Nutr Phys Act. 2016;13(1):2.
56. Naal FD, Impellizzeri FM. How active are patients undergoing total joint arthroplasty?: a systematic review. Clin Orthop Relat Res. 2010;468(7):1891–904. https://doi.org/10.1007/s11999-009-1135-9.
57. Sparling PB, Howard BJ, Dunstan DW, Owen N. Recommendations for physical activity in older adults. BMJ (Clinical research ed). 2015;350:h100. https://doi.org/10.1136/bmj.h100.
58. Garber CE, Blissmer B, Deschenes MR, Franklin BA, Lamonte MJ, Lee IM, Nieman DC, Swain DP. American College of Sports Medicine position stand. Quantity and quality of exercise for developing and maintaining cardiorespiratory, musculoskeletal, and neuromotor fitness in apparently healthy adults: guidance for prescribing exercise. Med Sci Sports Exerc. 2011;43(7):1334–59. https://doi.org/10.1249/MSS.0b013e318213fefb.
59. Hammett T, Simonian A, Austin M, Butler R, Allen KD, Ledbetter L, Goode AP. Changes in physical activity after total hip or knee arthroplasty: a systematic review and meta-analysis of six- and twelve-month outcomes. Arthritis Care Res. 2018;70(6):892–901. https://doi.org/10.1002/acr.23415.
60. Zahiri CA, Schmalzried TP, Szuszczewicz ES, Amstutz HC. Assessing activity in joint replacement patients. J Arthroplasty. 1998;13(8):890–5.
61. Welk GJ, Kim Y, Stanfill B, Osthus DA, Calabro MA, Nusser SM, Carriquiry A. Validity of 24-h physical activity recall: physical activity measurement survey. Med Sci Sports Exerc. 2014;46(10):2014–24. https://doi.org/10.1249/MSS.0000000000000314.
62. Swanson EA, Schmalzried TP, Dorey FJ. Activity recommendations after total hip and knee arthroplasty: a survey of the American Association for Hip and Knee Surgeons. J Arthroplasty. 2009;24(6 Suppl):120–6. https://doi.org/10.1016/j.arth.2009.05.014.
63. Meester SB, Wagenmakers R, van den Akker-Scheek I, Stevens M. Sport advice given by Dutch orthopaedic surgeons to patients after a total hip arthroplasty or total knee arthroplasty. PLoS One. 2018;13(8):e0202494. https://doi.org/10.1371/journal.pone.0202494.
64. Vogel LA, Carotenuto G, Basti JJ, Levine WN. Physical activity after total joint arthroplasty. Sports Health. 2011;3(5):441–50. https://doi.org/10.1177/1941738111415826.
65. Crombie IK, Irvine L, Williams B, McGinnis AR, Slane PW, Alder EM, McMurdo ME. Why older people do not participate in leisure time physical activity: a survey of activity levels, beliefs and deterrents. Age Ageing. 2004;33(3):287–92. https://doi.org/10.1093/ageing/afh089.
66. Li F, Harmer PA, Cardinal BJ, Bosworth M, Acock A, Johnson-Shelton D, Moore JM. Built environment, adiposity, and physical activity in adults aged 50–75. Am J Prev Med. 2008;35(1):38–46. https://doi.org/10.1016/j.amepre.2008.03.021.
67. Parks SE, Housemann RA, Brownson RC. Differential correlates of physical activity in urban and rural adults of various socioeconomic backgrounds in the United States. J Epidemiol Community Health. 2003;57(1):29–35.
68. Trost SG, Owen N, Bauman AE, Sallis JF, Brown W. Correlates of adults' participation in physical activity: review and update. Med Sci Sports Exerc. 2002;34(12):1996–2001. https://doi.org/10.1249/01.MSS.0000038974.76900.92.
69. Meier W, Mizner RL, Marcus RL, Dibble LE, Peters C, Lastayo PC. Total knee arthroplasty: muscle impairments, functional limitations, and recommended rehabilitation approaches. J Orthop Sports Phys Ther. 2008;38(5):246–56. https://doi.org/10.2519/jospt.2008.2715.
70. Mistry JB, Elmallah RD, Bhave A, Chughtai M, Cherian JJ, McGinn T, Harwin SF, Mont MA. Rehabilitative guidelines after total knee arthroplasty: a review. J Knee Surg. 2016;29(3):201–17. https://doi.org/10.1055/s-0036-1579670.
71. Piva SR, Teixeira PE, Almeida GJ, Gil AB, DiGioia AM 3rd, Levison TJ, Fitzgerald GK. Contribution of hip abductor strength to physical function in patients with total knee arthroplasty. Phys Ther. 2011;91(2):225–33. https://doi.org/10.2522/ptj.20100122.

72. Marmon AR, McClelland JA, Stevens-Lapsley J, Snyder-Mackler L. Single-step test for unilateral limb ability following total knee arthroplasty. J Orthop Sports Phys Ther. 2013;43(2):66–73. https://doi.org/10.2519/jospt.2013.4372.
73. Marmon AR, Milcarek BI, Snyder-Mackler L. Associations between knee extensor power and functional performance in patients after total knee arthroplasty and normal controls without knee pain. Int J Sports Phys Ther. 2014;9(2):168–78.
74. Ko V, Naylor JM, Harris IA, Crosbie J, Yeo AE. The six-minute walk test is an excellent predictor of functional ambulation after total knee arthroplasty. BMC Musculoskelet Disord. 2013;14:145. https://doi.org/10.1186/1471-2474-14-145.
75. Boonstra MC, De Waal Malefijt MC, Verdonschot N. How to quantify knee function after total knee arthroplasty? Knee. 2008;15(5):390–5. https://doi.org/10.1016/j.knee.2008.05.006.

Return to Work Following Knee Arthroplasty

11

A. J. Kievit, M. U. Schafroth, and P. P. F. M. Kuijer

Take-Home Messages

- On average one in three patients do not return to work after knee arthroplasty
- Patients return to work around 12 weeks post-surgery, although large differences exist between patients and full return to work may take more than 6 months.
- The cause for not returning to work is multifactorial, but known prognostic factors are preoperative sick leave of more than 2 weeks, female sex, high body mass index (BMI), patient-reported work-relatedness of knee symptoms, and physically demanding jobs. Age and Knee Injury and Osteoarthritis Outcome Scores (KOOS) were not associated with no return to work.
- At present, no studies are available that evaluated the effect of exercise-based rehabilitation, active referral to an occupational physician or therapist, or other forms of multidisciplinary care for knee arthroplasty on return to work.
- Promising interventions for return to work are better expectation management by setting preoperative patient-centered realistic work-related activity goals, preoperative referral to an occupational physician or therapist to actively address prognostic factors hindering return to work, and the use of personalized e/mHealth including activity trackers to support KA patients on a daily basis in return to work.

A. J. Kievit (✉) · M. U. Schafroth
Department of Orthopedic Surgery, Amsterdam Movement Sciences, Amsterdam Centre for European Studies, Amsterdam University Medical Centers, Amsterdam, Netherlands
e-mail: a.j.kievit@amsterdamumc.nl; m.u.schafroth@amsterdamumc.nl

P. P. F. M. Kuijer
Department of Public and Occupational Health, Amsterdam Public Health Research Institute, Amsterdam Movement Sciences, Amsterdam University Medical Centers, Amsterdam, Netherlands
e-mail: p.p.kuijer@amsterdamumc.nl

F. R. Noyes, S. Barber-Westin (eds.), *Critical Rehabilitation for Partial and Total Knee Arthroplasty*, https://doi.org/10.1007/978-3-030-87003-4_11

11.1 Introduction

If knee arthroplasty (KA) surgery has been successful and patients' pain is reduced and mobility returns, it becomes vital for both patients' health and society that patients return to normal daily life activities. For many patients, returning to work will require them to accept the fact that their "new" KA knee will not function as their healthy knee. The largest increase in primary KA demands is namely not among the classic knee arthroplasty population of patients aged 70 years and older but among patients of working age [1]. For instance, the number of patients aged 45–65 years who undergo total knee arthroplasty (TKA) has tripled (Swedish knee arthroplasty register) in the past 30 years. Germany – one of the leading countries in the prevalence of knee arthroplasty – foresees the highest increase in patients aged 50–65 years until 2050, and in a similar study using the same database, even among patients aged 40–49 years until 2040 [2, 3]. In several countries, the current proportion of knee arthroplasty patients under 65 years is already substantial at 30–40%. It is expected in 2030 that the USA will be the first country where the majority of these patients will be younger than 65 years, followed by the UK in 2035 [4, 5]. In addition, it was found that the combined loss of productivity plus medical costs for conservatively treated symptomatic knee osteoarthritis for those in paid employment in the Netherlands amounts to €871 per patient per month, with loss of productivity accounting for 83% and medical costs for 17% [6].

Previously little was known about return to work in either employed or self-employed patients undergoing TKA. Because the numbers of working patients undergoing TKA are increasing, it is important to find out which factors will help or hinder patients in returning to work following surgery in a swift and also effective manner. What is the impact of surrounding medical as well as social support, the type of work a patient performs, and the general health of the patient? How do these factors interact with one another?

There is sparsity although increasing data about the variety of outcomes regarding this working population. It seems that patients have varying expectations about returning to work after TKA surgery. Remarkably, it was found that only 72% of the patients expected that TKA would improve their ability to work prior to surgery. Six months after TKA, this was even further reduced to 28%. With respect to knee-demanding activities, only 34% expected severe difficulty in kneeling, 30% in crouching, and 17% in clambering at 6 months after TKA [7].

Rehabilitation with Goal Attainment Scaling (GAS) could be a useful tool to manage expectations of functional postoperative outcome. When preoperative goals are set as studied in unicompartmental knee arthroplasty (UKA) patients for postoperative daily life activity, work, and leisure time, it was found that 100% met these goals, compared to 82% of TKA patients [8]. When realistic goals are set and expectations are adjusted, this might improve perceived outcome.

More detailed knowledge about the impact of KA on ability to return to work can help in making better informed decisions about whether KA is the appropriate treatment for the patient's problem. Furthermore, no randomized or appropriately adjusted comparison has yet been made to find out whether UKA patients return to work sooner or perform better than patients with TKA. UKA surgery is less invasive, and patients seem to function better and be more active and are even able to return to sport sooner despite reported higher revision rates, but the role of bias is unclear [9, 10].

There is increasing interest in the development of health care toward more outcome-oriented care in a broad sense, in which the choice of treatment looks at what best fits the specific situation of the patient instead of population-based objective group outcomes.

Outcome-oriented care can be defined as the outcome that really matters for the health and well-being of a specific patient. The goal is to focus care better on what matters to the patient which in turn can lead to better decision-making choices and more timely work-directed care. This is of importance given that the first prospective cohort study among working age TKA patients showed that even after 1 year, only 71% of workers had fully returned to work [11].

11.2 Patient-Reported Outcome Measures in Working KA Patients

To study patients' physical difficulty experienced in work before or following KA, the Work, Osteoarthritis or joint-Replacement Questionnaire (WORQ) was developed [6]. The WORQ (range 0–100, with a minimal clinically important difference of 13) assesses the experienced difficulty for 13 work-related activities, like kneeling, working with the hands below knee height, and walking on rough terrain. This 13-item questionnaire was tested for internal consistency by factor analysis, internal reliability (Cronbach's α), and construct validity. A test-retest reproducibility was performed for analyzing standard error of measurement (SEM agreement), reliability (ICC), and smallest detectable change (SDC) in individuals and groups. Lastly, responsiveness (standardized response means [SRM]), floor and ceiling effects, and interpretability (minimal important change [MIC]) were analyzed. It was shown that the WORQ is a reliable, valid, and responsive questionnaire following TKA that can be used to evaluate the impact of knee complaints on patients' ability to work [12].

Other patient-reported outcome measures (PROMs) commonly applied to TKA patients are the KOOS, Oxford, and the new Knee Society Scoring System questionnaires. These mainly assess home-life activities and do not look at specific activities that are necessary to return to the work. Gagnier et al. performed a review on PROMs for TKA to critically appraise, compare, and summarize their psychometric properties using accepted methods. Although not all psychometric properties were studied, they concluded that the WORQ had the highest overall ratings and thus could be a useful PROM for evaluating patients undergoing TKA [13, 14].

In an early cross-sectional survey, it was found that approximately one-third of TKA patients worked within 2 years prior to surgery [15]. When looking at these working patients, activities that most improved were operating foot pedals,

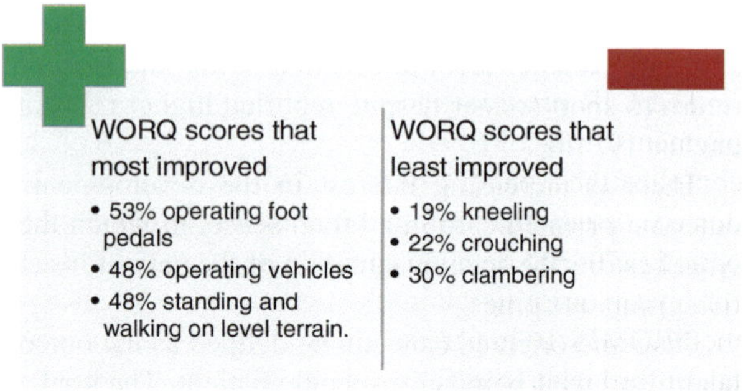

Fig. 11.1 WORQ score improvements in % performing work-related activities following knee arthroplasty between T0 (before the knee problems arose) and T2 (at 2 years after TKA) [15]

operating vehicles, and standing and walking on level terrain. Activities that least improved were kneeling, crouching, and clambering (Fig. 11.1).

Fifty patients scored 5 or less on the Work Ability Index (WAI), an index from 0 to 10 in which a patient can report how well they are able to perform their work with a TKA. TKA significantly, but unequally, reduces difficulties in carrying out knee-burdening work activities [15]. When UKA patients (median 60 years, 51% male) were compared to TKA patients (median 60 years, 49% male) (n.s.), it was found that WORQ scores improved similarly in both groups. The WAI score was also comparable between the groups. Dissatisfaction with work ability was comparable (UKA 15% versus TKA 18%) (n.s.). TKA and UKA patients have similar WORQ, WAI, and satisfaction scores [16].

11.3 Return to Work Timing Following TKA and UKA

Return to work between TKA and UKA patients has been reported to be around 70–80% (Table 11.1 [16]). In the same multi-center retrospective cohort study as mentioned above, the time period between stopping work and returning to work was assessed [10]. UKA patients ($n = 157$, median 60 years, 51% male) were compared to TKA patients ($n = 167$, median 60 years, 49% male) (n.s.). Of the 157 UKA patients, 115 (73%) returned to work within 2 years compared to 121 (72%) of TKA patients (n.s.). More UKA patients returned to work within 3 months (73% versus 48%) ($p < 0.01$) (Fig. 11.2) [16]. UKA patients return to work significantly sooner after surgery than TKA patients, which might improve their quality of life and allow them to re-participate more actively in society at an earlier time.

11.4 Prognostic Factors for Not Returning to Work

In the Netherlands, it has been studied what patient characteristics are associated with no return to work (RTW) [38]. Backward stepwise logistic regression analyses were performed to predict no RTW. One hundred and sixty-seven patients met the inclusion criteria, and 46 did not RTW. Preoperative sick leave of more than 2 weeks

Table 11.1 Summary of timing of return to work reported in a KSSTA study in 2020 [16]

Author	Journal	PubMed ID	Year	Total patients with TKA	Total patients with UKA	Age at operation of study group	Patients working pre-op	Patients returning to work post-op	% Returned	Interval return to work in median weeks	Definition
Kievit et al. [16]	KSSTA	31471724	2020		315	60	157	117	75	27% at 1 month, 73% at 3 months	Assessed at mean 3.1 years post-surgery
Jinnah et al. [17]	Surg Technol Int	29611158	2018		30		30			6.4 (mean)	Assessed at 2, 4, 6, and 12 weeks
Scott et al. [18]	Bone Joint J	28768780	2017	289		59.0	261	105	40	13.5 (mean)	Assessed at 2–4 years post-surgery
Stigmar et al. [19]	Acta Orthop.	27996342	2017	4421		55.0	996	857	86	15	Assessed until 24 months post-surgery (calculated from median sick leave of F:M 117:96 days)
Leichtenberg et al. [20]	Ann R Coll Surg Engl	27138849	2016	120		56.0	56	50	89	–	Assessed at 12 months post-surgery
Bardgett et al. [21]	BMJ Open	26832426	2016	10		54.0	10	10	100	9.4 (mean)	Assessed at 8–35 months post-surgery
Tilbury et al. [22]	Rheumatol Int.	26119221	2015	322		57.4	64	56	83	12.9 (mean)	Assessed at 12 months post-surgery

(continued)

Table 11.1 (continued)

Author	Journal	PubMed ID	Year	Total patients with TKA	Total patients with UKA	Age at operation of study group	Patients working pre-op	Patients returning to work post-op	% Returned	Interval return to work in median weeks	Definition
Kleim et al. [23]	Knee Surg Sports Traumatol Arthrosc	25193567	2015	127		54.0	50	41	82	13	Assessed at mean 21 months
Belmont et al. [24]	J Arthroplasty	25677939	2015	159		45.7	159	130	82		Assessed at 24 months post-surgery
Kievit et al. [15]	J Arthroplasty	24524779	2013	480		66	173	121	70	50.4% within 12 weeks	Assessed at 24–86 months
Glebus et al. [25]	J Arthroplasty	23830502	2013	20	2	45.0	22	?	86		Assessed at 4.5 years post-surgery
Sankar et al. [26]	Osteoarthritis Cartilage	23774473	2013	494		57.5	170	144	85	24% at 1 month. 57% at 3 months	Assessed until 1 year post-surgery
Lombardi et al. [27]	Clin Orthop Relat Res.	23761175	2013	661		54.0	494	482	98	8.9	Assessed at 12–36 months post-surgery
Clyde et al. [28]	J Arthroplasty	23583541	2013	98		55.0	98	64	65	15.5 (mean)	Assessed at 17–125 months
Husted et al. [29]	J Bone Joint Surg Br.	21357957	2011	421		68.3	82	46	56	–	Assessed at 24 months
Styron et al. [30]	J Bone Joint Surg Am.	21209263	2011	162		57.0	162	122	75	8.9	Assessed at 3 months

Author	Journal	PubMed ID	Year	Total patients with TKA	Total patients with UKA	Age at operation of study group	Patients working pre-op	Patients returning to work post-op	% Returned	Interval return to work in median weeks	Definition
Lyall et al. [31]	Ann R Coll Surg Engl	19344550	2009	56		57.9	41	40	98	10 (mean)	Assessed at 47–112 months post-surgery
Foote et al. [32]	Knee	19632120	2009	41		54.1	27	22	82	12	Assessed at 14–61 months
Foote et al. [32]	Knee	19632120	2009		31	52.6	22	18	82	11	Assessed at 14–61 months
Lombardi et al. [33]	Clin Orthop Relat Res.	19225852	2009	113	113	62	–	–	–	8	Assessed at 2–52 months post-surgery
Walton et al. [34]	J Knee Surg.	16642887	2006	120		71.5	21	17	81	–	
Jorn et al. [35]	Acta Orthop Scand.	10569263	1999	102	60	56.0	88	52	59	(54% within 26 weeks)	Assessed at 2 years post-surgery
Nielsen et al. [36]	Ugeskr Laeger	10434787	1999	926		–	51	40	78	–	Assessed at 1 year post-surgery
Weingarten et al. [37]	Am J Med.	9688019	1998	287		69.7	56	41	81	–	Assessed at 3–5 months
Sumarized				9429	551	58	3285	2575	78		

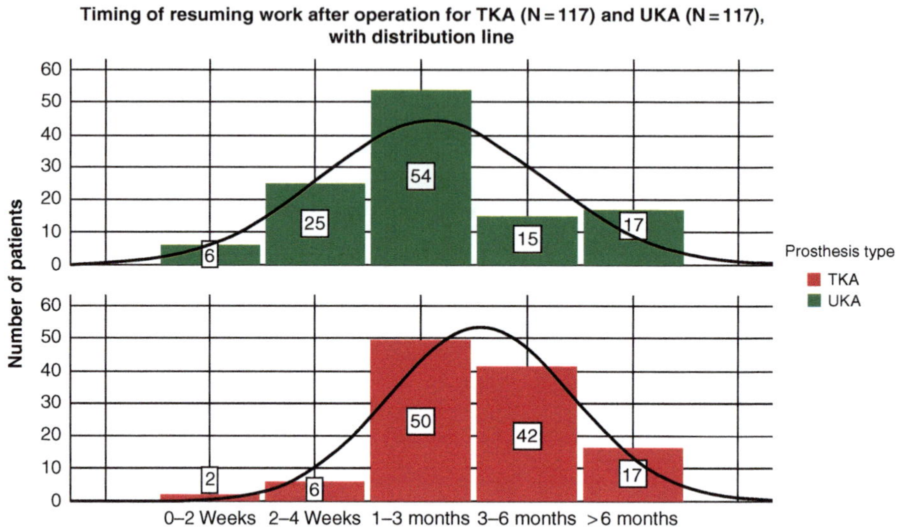

Fig. 11.2 Time when patients resumed work after unicompartmental (UKA, N = 117) and total knee arthroplasty (TKA, N = 117) in absolute numbers, with distribution line [16]

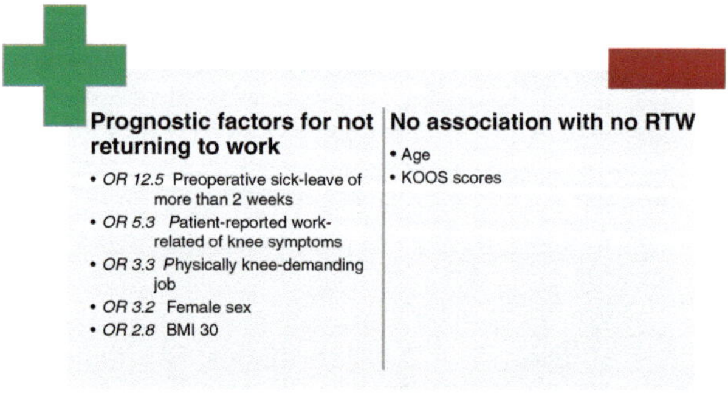

Fig. 11.3 Prognostic factors for not returning to work – stepwise logistic regression analyses [38]

(OR, 12.5; 90% CI 5.0–31.5) was most strongly associated with no RTW. Other associations found were female sex (OR, 3.2; 90% CI 1.3–8.2), BMI 30 (OR, 2.8; 90% CI 1.1–7.1), patient-reported work-relatedness of knee symptoms (OR, 5.3; 90% CI 2.0–14.1), and physically knee-demanding job (OR, 3.3; 90% CI 1.2–8.9). Age and KOOS scores were not associated with no RTW (Fig. 11.3). Especially obese female workers, with a preoperative sick leave duration >2 weeks who performed knee-demanding work and indicated that their knee symptoms were work related, had a high chance for no RTW after TKA. These results stress the importance of a timelier referral for work-directed care of patients at risk for no RTW after TKA.

In a qualitative study performed in 50 TKA patients by Bardgett et al., three key factors were identified that influenced RTW from the patients' perspective [39]. These patients reported an improved physical and psychological performance at work after surgery in comparison to preoperative functioning. The three factors reported were that (1) patients did not receive specific advice to facilitate their RTW following surgery, (2) patients perceived that the current provision of information for joint replacement patients is focused on the needs of elderly patients and reported that more clarity and consistency are required regarding RTW advice, and (3) these patients reported a lack of support and adaptation in the workplace and described a negative influence on their experience of RTW although this was not reflected in increased duration of sickness absence [39].

Furthermore, patients who had a slower return to work often reported that comorbidities, especially musculoskeletal like low back pain or OA affecting other joints, prevented their RTW even when the surgical outcome was positive [40]. However, the most recent review on prognostic factors for return to work concluded that based on 14 studies and 3073 patients, the most important prognostic factors associated with a slower or no RTW were a more physically demanding job and preoperative absence from work [41].

11.5 Interventions Aimed at Improving Return to Work After KA

Remarkably, little to no evidence is available for effective return-to-work interventions for KA patients. Although the provision of exercise-based rehabilitation after KA is almost universal, a systematic literature review performed in Ovid Medline and EMBASE concluded that "no studies were found evaluating the effect of rehabilitation programmes for knee arthroplasty on return to work" [42]. To come to this conclusion, a detailed search was performed with the support of a clinical librarian specialized in the outcome work participation, and despite that, 3788 studies were independently assessed by two reviewers. If the search was broadened and also included integrated multidisciplinary care, like active referral to an occupational physician or an occupational therapist or including e/mHealth interventions, again no studies were found for KA patients and RTW [43]. Therefore, to develop an occupational advice intervention to support early recovery to usual activities including work that is tailored to the requirements of KA patients, Baker and colleagues performed an intervention mapping approach, including 110 stakeholder interviews and a survey of 152 practices [44]. The intervention included information resources, a personalized return-to-work plan, and coordination from the health-care team. To support delivery, a range of tools (e.g., occupational checklists, patient workbooks, and employer information), roles (e.g., return-to-work coordinator), and training resources were created. The intervention was assessed in 26 patients and staff and showed high rates of adherence to the defined performance objectives. The overall results demonstrated that the occupational advice intervention developed for KA patients is deliverable. However, the intervention warrants a randomized controlled trial to assess its clinical effectiveness and cost-effectiveness to improve rates and timing of return to work. Two other promising return-to-work interventions for KA patients and using limited health-care resources are Goal Attainment Scaling (GAS) and the use of a personalized e-Health application, iRecover (in Dutch: ikHerstel) [45, 46]. GAS personalizes exercise-based rehabilitation by setting patient-specific, activity-oriented rehabilitation goals in close collaboration between the patient and the physical therapist, thereby setting realistic patient expectations and securing close monitoring of these goals during the rehabilitation period. A randomized controlled trial (RCT) among 120 working-age KA patients showed that GAS resulted in higher patient satisfaction with work activities compared to care as usual in the control group: an increase of 11 points on a scale from 0 to 100 with a 98% confidence interval of 2–19 points [45]. For the iRecover application, multidisciplinary consensus on recommendations regarding the resumption of 27 activities of daily life, including work, has been reached among a multidisciplinary expert panel of six orthopedic surgeons, three physical therapists, five occupational physicians, and one physician assistant for fast, average, and slow recovery [46]. These consensus recommendations are integrated into the algorithm of the iRecover application (Fig. 11.4) [47]. In combination with the use of an activity tracker and GAS for work-related activities, this intervention is currently evaluated in the so-called Active RCT among 368 patients (https://www.trialregister.nl/trial/8525).

11.6 Discussion

11.6.1 Cost-Effectiveness of KA From a Personal and Societal Perspective

Despite good results with respect to return to work for most of the KA patients, a large proportion of these patients do not return to work. Also within this population, when patients return to work, not all aspects of functional recovery improve, but patients' overall satisfaction can still be high. Information regarding time to return to work including what work-related activities will improve most after KA is of primary importance for patients and care providers, as meeting preoperative expectations is key for satisfaction [48, 49]. This is especially true for patients approaching their retirement age. As, on average, patients return to work 3 months after KA, it is still unclear if the cost of the 3-month sick leave in addition to the cost of KA weighs up to the potential improvement of productivity from a societal economical perspective. This may be relatively easy in patients who are already on full sick leave and unable to perform their job because of OA-related knee complaints as they can only improve. Such a simple cost-benefit analysis is less straightforward in patients who are still able to perform their work, but in a less productive manner. Will they improve sufficiently from surgery? As shown earlier, activities like kneeling and crouching only improved marginally. Therefore, KA will probably improve general quality of life but not necessary productivity for most plumbers, gardeners, and builders getting close to pension age as the "return of investment" time is too short. On the other hand, if a patient's work mainly consists of driving a vehicle, such as is the case in taxi drivers or lorry drivers, it might be advantageous to perform arthroplasty surgery earlier on as these activities do seem to improve. It needs

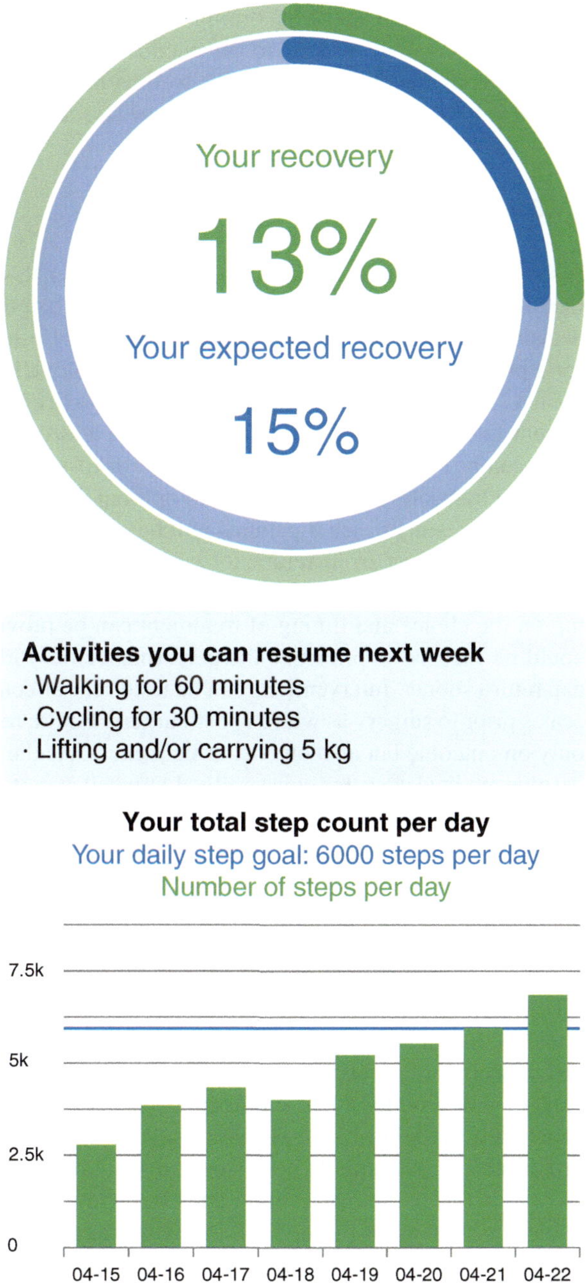

Fig. 11.4 An example of a dashboard of the iRecover app, providing knee arthroplasty patients tailored guidance on resumption of activities of daily life, including work. Guidance on the resumption of activities and the recovery status of these activities (upper two panels) can be provided, while wearable devices can be used to provide patients with feedback on their physical activities, helping them to work toward self-chosen (work-directed) goals [47]

to be further investigated what timings are advantageous for specific working groups and whether active referral to an occupational physician or therapist might be advantageous for return to work, as well as for professions in order to find work-related solutions for activities that improve less after KA.

11.6.2 UKA or TKA?

It seems that UKA patients return to work sooner than TKA patients. Despite the fact that prosthetic survival of a UKA is shorter than that of TKA, a well-informed decision can be made in the case of anteromedial osteoarthritis. If it is paramount for a patient to return to work as soon as possible, UKA could be the prosthesis of choice. This can be the case for patients who are self-employed. However, if a patient finds it most important to receive an arthroplasty which will last longer, a TKA can be chosen despite the longer return-to-work interval. Future research will focus on translating research data into optimal decision-making in the workplace. It will be interesting to see if patients will be more satisfied if they are better informed on what to expect from return to work after TKA or UKA surgery. With better insight into what a specific patient needs to be able to return to work, better coaching on the choice and timing of treatment can be provided. Specific physiotherapy could be focused to prioritize the performance of work activities to see if patients can return sooner. Interventions can be tested for effectiveness by assessing WORQ scales prior to surgery as well as post-surgery. Future research will need to focus not only on outcome but also on cost-effectiveness. As the combined loss of productivity plus medical costs for conservatively treated symptomatic knee osteoarthritis for those in paid employment in the Netherlands amounts to €871 per patient per month (with loss of productivity accounting for 83% and medical costs for 17% [6]), better assessment of cost-benefit and cost-effectiveness will become possible. One might expect that arthroplasty surgery may reduce these costs. If arthroplasty surgery would reduce the loss of productivity to zero at the moment of return to work at 3 months, and the total cost of arthroplasty surgery is on average around €10.000 [50], surgery would accrue positive cost-benefit outcome if absence from work could be shortened by 12 months (=10.000/871) or more. However, these rough estimates ignore the fact that three out of ten patients do not return to work and that surgery will produce adverse outcomes in others. To make an accurate assessment of when is the best time to perform surgery for specific patients, new comparative prospective studies should be performed. Challenges for future research are the difference between the intervention and the control arm, not only with respect to the choice and timing of surgery but also with respect to other covariates such as management of expectations, quantification of medical and societal costs (such as loss of productivity), and adequate as well as feasible follow-up. The results of one study demonstrated that the total economic cost to society for treatment of severe knee osteoarthritis in a relatively young working person is markedly lower with TKA than it is with non-operative treatment [51]. As furthermore stated by the authors of this paper:

The results of this model illustrate the need to account for the implications of treatment choices, not only at the individual patient level, but also for society at large. When deciding among available treatment options, patients, physicians, payers, and policymakers must consider individual treatment cost and effectiveness but also should account for future potential earnings generated when a treatment may restore a patient's ability to contribute to society [51].

11.7 Conclusion

Knee arthroplasty is becoming more and more important to keep patients active as members of the workforce. Therefore, not only in clinical practice and in research but also in guideline development, this important outcome should be more often addressed, especially regarding effective multidisciplinary care.

References

1. Kuijer PPF, Burdorf A. Prevention at work needed to curb the worldwide strong increase in knee replacement surgery for working-age osteoarthritis patients. Scand J Work Environ Health. 2020;46(5):457–60.
2. Klug A, Gramlich Y, Rudert M, Drees P, Hoffmann R, Weißenberger M, et al. The projected volume of primary and revision total knee arthroplasty will place an immense burden on future health care systems over the next 30 years. Knee Surg Sports Traumatol Arthrosc. 2020:1–12.
3. Rupp M, Lau E, Kurtz SM, Alt V. Projections of primary TKA and THA in Germany from 2016 through 2040. Clin Orthop Relat Res. 2020;478(7):1622–33.
4. Kurtz S, Ong K, Lau E, Mowat F, Halpern M. Projections of primary and revision hip and knee arthroplasty in the United States from 2005 to 2030. J Bone Joint Surg Am. 2007;89(4):780–5.
5. Culliford D, Maskell J, Judge A, Cooper C, Prieto-Alhambra D, Arden NK. Future projections of total hip and knee arthroplasty in the UK: results from the UK Clinical Practice Research Datalink. Osteoarthr Cartil. 2015;23(4):594–600.
6. Hermans J, Koopmanschap MA, Bierma-Zeinstra SM, van Linge JH, Verhaar JA, Reijman M, et al. Productivity costs and medical costs among working patients with knee osteoarthritis. Arthritis Care Res (Hoboken). 2012;64(6):853–61.
7. van Zaanen Y, van Geenen RCI, Pahlplatz TMJ, Kievit AJ, Hoozemans MJM, Bakker EWP, et al. Three out of ten working patients expect no clinical improvement of their ability to perform work-related knee-demanding activities after total knee arthroplasty: a multicenter study. J Occup Rehabil. 2019;29(3):585–94.
8. Witjes S, Hoorntje A, Kuijer PP, Koenraadt KL, Blankevoort L, Kerkhoffs GM, et al. Goal setting and achievement in individualized rehabilitation of younger total and unicondylar knee arthroplasty patients: a cohort study. Arch Phys Med Rehabil. 2019;100(8):1434–41.
9. Kleeblad LJ, van der List JP, Zuiderbaan HA, Pearle AD. Larger range of motion and increased return to activity, but higher revision rates following unicompartmental versus total knee arthroplasty in patients under 65: a systematic review. Knee Surg Sports Traumatol Arthrosc. 2018;26(6):1811–22.
10. Witjes S, Gouttebarge V, Kuijer PP, van Geenen RC, Poolman RW, Kerkhoffs GM. Return to sports and physical activity after total and unicondylar knee arthroplasty: a systematic review and meta-analysis. Sports Med (Auckland, NZ). 2016;46(2):269–92.
11. Hylkema TH, Stevens M, van Beveren J, Rijk PC, Brouwer RW, Bulstra SK, et al. Recovery courses of patients who return to work by 3, 6 or 12 months after total knee arthroplasty. J Occup Rehabil. 2021.

12. Kievit AJ, Kuijer PPFM, Kievit RA, Sierevelt IN, Blankevoort L, Frings-Dresen MHW. A reliable, valid and responsive questionnaire to score the impact of knee complaints on work following total knee arthroplasty: the WORQ. J Arthroplasty. 2014;29(6):1169–75.
13. Terwee CB, Bot SD, de Boer MR, van der Windt DA, Knol DL, Dekker J, et al. Quality criteria were proposed for measurement properties of health status questionnaires. J Clin Epidemiol. 2007;60(1):34–42.
14. Gagnier JJ, Mullins M, Huang H, Marinac-Dabic D, Ghambaryan A, Eloff B, et al. A systematic review of measurement properties of patient-reported outcome measures used in patients undergoing total knee arthroplasty. J Arthroplasty. 2017;32(5):1688–97.e7.
15. Kievit AJ, van Geenen RCI, Kuijer PPFM, Pahlplatz TMJ, Blankevoort L, Schafroth MU. Total knee arthroplasty and the unforeseen impact on return to work: a cross-sectional multicenter survey. J Arthroplasty. 2014;29(6):1163–8.
16. Kievit AJ, Kuijer P, de Haan LJ, Koenraadt KLM, Kerkhoffs G, Schafroth MU, et al. Patients return to work sooner after unicompartmental knee arthroplasty than after total knee arthroplasty. Knee Surg Sports Traumatol Arthrosc. 2020;28(9):2905–16.
17. Jinnah AH, Augart MA, Lara DL, Jinnah RH, Poehling GG, Gwam CU, et al. Decreased time to return to work using robotic-assisted unicompartmental knee arthroplasty compared to conventional techniques. Surg Technol Int. 2018;32:279–83.
18. Scott CEH, Turnbull GS, MacDonald D, Breusch SJ. Activity levels and return to work following total knee arthroplasty in patients under 65 years of age. Bone Joint J. 2017;99-b(8):1037–46.
19. Stigmar K, Dahlberg LE, Zhou C, Jacobson Lidgren H, Petersson IF, Englund M. Sick leave in Sweden before and after total joint replacement in hip and knee osteoarthritis patients. Acta Orthop. 2017;88(2):152–7.
20. Leichtenberg CS, Tilbury C, Kuijer P, Verdegaal S, Wolterbeek R, Nelissen R, et al. Determinants of return to work 12 months after total hip and knee arthroplasty. Ann R Coll Surg Engl. 2016;98(6):387–95.
21. Bardgett M, Lally J, Malviya A, Deehan D. Return to work after knee replacement: a qualitative study of patient experiences. BMJ Open. 2016;6(2):e007912.
22. Tilbury C, Leichtenberg CS, Tordoir RL, Holtslag MJ, Verdegaal SH, Kroon HM, et al. Return to work after total hip and knee arthroplasty: results from a clinical study. Rheumatol Int. 2015;35(12):2059–67.
23. Kleim BD, Malviya A, Rushton S, Bardgett M, Deehan DJ. Understanding the patient-reported factors determining time taken to return to work after hip and knee arthroplasty. Knee Surg Sports Traumatol Arthrosc. 2015;23(12):3646–52.
24. Belmont PJ Jr, Heida K, Keeney JA, Hamilton W, Burks R, Waterman BR. Return to work and functional outcomes following primary total knee arthroplasty in U.S. Military Servicemembers. J Arthroplasty. 2015;30(6):968–72.
25. Glebus GP, Feather TW, Hsu JR, Gerlinger TL. Return to duty and deployment after major joint arthroplasty. J Arthroplasty. 2013;28(8):1270–3.
26. Sankar A, Davis AM, Palaganas MP, Beaton DE, Badley EM, Gignac MA. Return to work and workplace activity limitations following total hip or knee replacement. Osteoarthr Cartil. 2013;21(10):1485–93.
27. Lombardi AV Jr, Nunley RM, Berend KR, Ruh EL, Clohisy JC, Hamilton WG, et al. Do patients return to work after total knee arthroplasty? Clin Orthop Relat Res. 2014;472(1):138–46.
28. Clyde CT, Goyal N, Matar WY, Witmer D, Restrepo C, Hozack WJ. Workers' compensation patients after total joint arthroplasty: do they return to work? J Arthroplasty. 2013;28(6):883–7.
29. Husted H, Troelsen A, Otte KS, Kristensen BB, Holm G, Kehlet H. Fast-track surgery for bilateral total knee replacement. J Bone Joint Surg Br. 2011;93(3):351–6.
30. Styron JF, Barsoum WK, Smyth KA, Singer ME. Preoperative predictors of returning to work following primary total knee arthroplasty. J Bone Joint Surg Am. 2011;93(1):2–10.
31. Lyall H, Ireland J, El-Zebdeh MY. The effect of total knee replacement on employment in patients under 60 years of age. Ann R Coll Surg Engl. 2009;91(5):410–3.
32. Foote JA, Smith HK, Jonas SC, Greenwood R, Weale AE. Return to work following knee arthroplasty. Knee. 2010;17(1):19–22.

33. Lombardi AV Jr, Berend KR, Walter CA, Aziz-Jacobo J, Cheney NA. Is recovery faster for mobile-bearing unicompartmental than total knee arthroplasty? Clin Orthop Relat Res. 2009;467(6):1450–7.
34. Walton NP, Jahromi I, Lewis PL, Dobson PJ, Angel KR, Campbell DG. Patient-perceived outcomes and return to sport and work: TKA versus mini-incision unicompartmental knee arthroplasty. J Knee Surg. 2006;19(2):112–6.
35. Jorn LP, Johnsson R, Toksvig-Larsen S. Patient satisfaction, function and return to work after knee arthroplasty. Acta Orthop Scand. 1999;70(4):343–7.
36. Nielsen MB, Kristensen PW, Lamm M, Schroder HM. Knee alloplasty and working ability. The significance of knee alloplasty for working ability of patients who were working prior to surgery. Ugeskr Laeger. 1999;161(18):2666–9.
37. Weingarten S, Riedinger MS, Sandhu M, Bowers C, Ellrodt AG, Nunn C, et al. Can practice guidelines safely reduce hospital length of stay? Results from a multicenter interventional study. Am J Med. 1998;105(1):33–40.
38. Kuijer PP, Kievit AJ, Pahlplatz TM, Hooiveld T, Hoozemans MJ, Blankevoort L, et al. Which patients do not return to work after total knee arthroplasty? Rheumatol Int. 2016;36(9):1249–54.
39. Bardgett M, Lally J, Malviya A, Kleim B, Deehan D. Patient-reported factors influencing return to work after joint replacement. Occup Med (Oxford, England). 2016;66(3):215–21.
40. Hylkema TH, Brouwer S, Stewart RE, van Beveren J, Rijk PC, Brouwer RW, et al. Two-year recovery courses of physical and mental impairments, activity limitations, and participation restrictions after total knee arthroplasty among working-age patients. Disabil Rehabil. 2020:1–10.
41. Van Leemput D, Neirynck J, Berger P, Vandenneucker H. Return to work after primary total knee arthroplasty under the age of 65 years: a systematic review. J Knee Surg. 2021.
42. Kuijer P, van Haeren MM, Daams JG, Frings-Dresen MHW. Better return to work and sports after knee arthroplasty rehabilitation? Occup Med (Oxford, England). 2018;68(9): 626–30.
43. Coenen P, Hulsegge G, Daams JG, van Geenen RC, Kerkhoffs GM, van Tulder MW, et al. Integrated care programmes for sport and work participation, performance of physical activities and quality of life among orthopaedic surgery patients: a systematic review with meta-analysis. BMJ Open Sport Exerc Med. 2020;6(1):e000664.
44. Baker P, Coole C, Drummond A, Khan S, McDaid C, Hewitt C, et al. Occupational advice to help people return to work following lower limb arthroplasty: the OPAL intervention mapping study. Health Technol Assess (Winchester, England). 2020;24(45):1–408.
45. Hoorntje A, Waterval-Witjes S, Koenraadt KLM, Kuijer P, Blankevoort L, Kerkhoffs G, et al. Goal attainment scaling rehabilitation improves satisfaction with work activities for younger working patients after knee arthroplasty: results from the randomized controlled ACTION trial. J Bone Joint Surg Am. 2020;102(16):1445–53.
46. Straat AC, Coenen P, Smit DJM, Hulsegge G, Bouwsma EVA, Huirne JAF, et al. Development of a personalized m/ehealth algorithm for the resumption of activities of daily life including work and sport after total and unicompartmental knee arthroplasty: a multidisciplinary delphi study. Int J Environ Res Public Health. 2020;17(14):4952.
47. Coenen P, Straat C, Kuijer PP. Knee arthroplasty: a window of opportunity to improve physical activity in daily life, sports and work. BMJ Open Sport Exerc Med. 2020;6(1):e000822.
48. Swarup I, Henn CM, Gulotta LV, Henn RF 3rd. Patient expectations and satisfaction in orthopaedic surgery: a review of the literature. J Clin Orthop Trauma. 2019;10(4):755–60.
49. Deakin AH, Smith MA, Wallace DT, Smith EJ, Sarungi M. Fulfilment of preoperative expectations and postoperative patient satisfaction after total knee replacement. A prospective analysis of 200 patients. Knee. 2019.
50. ZorgkaartNederlandR. Wat kost een totale knieprothese? 2015. Available from: https://www.zorgkaartnederland.nl/aandoeningen/knievervanging/artikelen/wat-kost-een-totale-knieprothese.
51. Bedair H, Cha TD, Hansen VJ. Economic benefit to society at large of total knee arthroplasty in younger patients: a Markov analysis. J Bone Joint Surg Am. 2014;96(2):119–26.

12 Key Factors for Achieving Expectations in Patient Satisfaction and Quality of Life After Knee Arthroplasty

Sue Barber-Westin and Frank R. Noyes

12.1 Introduction

In order to determine the most important factors for achieving patient satisfaction and improving quality of life (QOL) following total knee arthroplasty (TKA), validated scales must be used and influences of compounding factors must be accounted for such as mental and emotional problems and pain in other joints. Although a variety of scales and questions have been used to rate patient satisfaction, few have been validated and there is tremendous variation in recent literature regarding this topic. Conversely, QOL instruments have well-documented psychometric properties and historically have been used throughout the orthopedic literature. Many preoperative and postoperative factors have been shown to be predictive of patient satisfaction. Validated scales such as the Medical Outcomes Short Form 12 scores (mental and physical component scores), the Western Ontario and McMaster Universities Osteoarthritis Index, and the Knee Society Score have been the most commonly used instruments to identify relationships with both patient satisfaction and dissatisfaction postoperatively. This chapter summarizes the current knowledge regarding methods for determining patient satisfaction and quality of life as well as significant predictors of postoperative satisfaction and dissatisfaction following primary TKA.

S. Barber-Westin (✉)
Noyes Knee Institute, Cincinnati, OH, USA
e-mail: sbwestin@csmref.org

F. R. Noyes
Cincinnati SportsMedicine and Orthopaedic Center, The Noyes Knee Institute, Cincinnati, OH, USA

F. R. Noyes, S. Barber-Westin (eds.), *Critical Rehabilitation for Partial and Total Knee Arthroplasty*, https://doi.org/10.1007/978-3-030-87003-4_12

12.2 Validated Patient Satisfaction and Quality of Life Scales

A variety of scales and questions have been used to rate patient satisfaction; however, few have been validated and there is tremendous variation in recent literature regarding this topic. In a systematic review of patient satisfaction after TKA encompassing 208 studies published between 2007 and 2017, Kahlenberg et al. [1] reported that only 27 (13%) used a validated scale. Of these, 15 used the 2011 Knee Society Score (KSS) system, which evaluates satisfaction for five activities (Table 12.1). The most commonly used method for determining satisfaction (127 studies, 61%) was the use of a single (nonvalidated) question (such as how satisfied are you with the outcome of your TKA?) that could be answered on an ordinal or Likert scale (such as 1 = very satisfied, 2 = somewhat satisfied, 3 = barely satisfied, 4 = dissatisfied, and 5 = very dissatisfied). Other methods included a simple binary scale (satisfied: yes or no), willingness to undergo surgery again (yes or no), and use of a numeric or visual analogue scale (VAS). Our internal review of more recent literature found similar single-question methods used in many studies [2–12].

Clement et al. [13] conducted a study of 2512 patients to determine whether the focus of questions regarding satisfaction significantly influenced the rate and predictors after TKA. This study used a questionnaire previously published that has adequate reliability, internal consistency, and modest correlations with the Medical Outcomes Short Form 36 (SF-36) Physical Component Score (PCS) and Western Ontario and McMaster Universities Osteoarthritis Index (WOMAC) scores after TKA [14]. The questions focused on overall outcome, activity, work, and pain (Table 12.2). Using overall outcome as the standard (89.8% satisfied), there was no difference in the rate of satisfaction for pain relief (odds ratio [OR], 0.5); however, patients were more likely to be dissatisfied with activities (OR, 2.22; $P < 0.001$) and work (OR, 1.47; $P < 0.001$). The authors concluded that the focus of the question influences the rate of satisfaction and, in agreement with Kahlenberg et al. [1], recommended standardizing patient satisfaction reporting for future studies.

Table 12.1 2011 Knee Society Score patient satisfaction subscale[a]

Question
1. Currently, how satisfied are you with the pain level of your knee while sitting?
2. Currently, how satisfied are you with the pain level of your knee while lying in bed?
3. Currently, how satisfied are you with your knee function while getting out of bed?
4. Currently, how satisfied are you with your knee function while performing light household duties?
5. Currently, how satisfied are you with your knee function while performing leisure recreational activities?
Scale (same for each question)
Very satisfied (8 points)
Satisfied (6 points)
Neutral (4 points)
Dissatisfied (2 points)
Very dissatisfied (0 points)
Maximum total 40 points

[a]From Scuderi et al. [53]

Table 12.2 The Self-Administered Patient Satisfaction Scale[a]

Question
1. How satisfied are you with the results of your surgery?
2. How satisfied are you with the results of your surgery for improving your pain?
3. How satisfied are you with the results of your surgery for improving your ability to do home or yard work?
4. How satisfied are you with the results of your surgery for improving your ability to do recreational activities?
Scale (same for each question)
Very satisfied
Somewhat satisfied
Somewhat dissatisfied
Very dissatisfied

[a]From Mahomed et al. [14]

The use of a general health score, such as the SF-36, to indicate patient satisfaction was investigated by Teo et al. [11] in 6659 TKA patients. Two years postoperatively, 25% rated their satisfaction as excellent; 39%, very good; 28%, good; 6%, fair; 1%, poor; and < 1%, terrible. Combining the first three categories, the authors reported that overall satisfaction was achieved in 92%. The minimal clinically important difference in the SF-36 PCS (increase of ≥10 points) was only met in 68%.

Overall patient satisfaction rates after TKA range from 60% to 100% [1, 13]. The variation may be caused by (1) the type of questions used to determine satisfaction as just discussed, (2) the use of a validated satisfaction instrument versus non-validated single questions, (3) the interpretation of responses to questions (for instance, in Table 12.1, the combining of very satisfied and satisfied responses to form a single response versus keeping the two answers separate), (4) the definition of satisfied groups (for instance, grouping together very satisfied and somewhat satisfied patients into one group [3, 15]), and (5) the influence of preoperative comorbidities and psychological issues.

More work has been performed in developing and validating QOL scales. The most commonly used instruments are the SF-36 (available at https://www.rand.org/health-care/surveys_tools/mos/36-item-short-form.html), the SF-12 (available at https://www.rand.org/health-care/surveys_tools/mos/12-item-short-form.html), and the EuroQOL questionnaire (EQ-5D; available at https://euroqol.org/support/how-to-obtain-eq-5d/). Reliability, validity, and responsiveness of these scales are well-established [16–21]. Lan et al. [22] determined trends from 2005 through 2019 in outcomes reporting and usage of the most common PROM (patient-reported outcome measures) instruments. This review of 4616 articles found only seven articles in 2005 that used QOL instruments compared with 82 in 2019. In 2005, only one published article used the EQ-5D and six used the SF-36, while in 2019, 23 reported EQ-5D and 30 reported SF-36 outcomes. The change represented a significant increase in EQ-5D and a significant decrease in SF-36 utilization rates ($P < 0.001$ for both comparisons).

More recently, disease-specific PROMs such as the OsteoArthritis Knee and Hip Quality of Life (OAKHQOL) [23, 24] and the Knee Quality of Life-26 (KQoL-26)

[25, 26] have been introduced in an effort to specifically assess QOL outcome after TKA. However, few studies to date have employed usage of these instruments.

12.3 Predictors of Satisfaction

A multitude of studies have investigated the ability of various factors to predict or correlate with patient satisfaction after TKA [3, 9, 10, 27–35]. Walker et al. [12] found that the WOMAC score 1 year postoperatively could be used to predict patient satisfaction in 2578 patients. Categories of excellent, good, fair, and poor were developed for WOMAC scores for pain, function, stiffness, and total. Patient satisfaction was determined with one question (how satisfied are you with the results of your knee replacement surgery?) with a four-point Likert scale (very satisfied, somewhat satisfied, somewhat dissatisfied, and very dissatisfied). Receiver operating characteristic (ROC) curve analysis was used to identify point total thresholds in the WOMAC scores that were predictive of each of the satisfaction groups. The threshold values predictive of very satisfied versus satisfied patients are shown in Table 12.3, and values predictive of satisfied versus dissatisfied patients are shown in Table 12.4.

Bryan et al. [3] used a multivariable model to predict satisfaction at 6 months post-TKA and change in satisfaction from 6 to 12 postoperative months in 515 patients (Table 12.5). Satisfaction at 6 months was predicted by preoperative WOMAC pain score (OR, 2.65; $P < 0.001$), SF-12 mental component score (MCS; OR, 3.25; $P = 0.001$), and SF-12 physical component score (PCS; OR, 3.16; $P = 0.002$) and change in pain level from baseline to 6 months (OR, 2.31; $P < 0.001$). Change in satisfaction from 6 to 12 months was predicted by improvements in

Table 12.3 Threshold values for WOMAC scores that predict very satisfied from satisfied patients[a]

WOMAC	Threshold value	Sensitivity, specificity	AUC	95% CI	*P* value
Pain	>78	80, 76	80.6	78.0–82.2	<0.001
Function	>72	76, 77	80.1	78.1–82.0	<0.001
Stiffness	>69	77, 71	75.9	73.7–78.2	<0.001
Total	>75	75, 75	81.7	83.5–79.8	<0.001

AUC area under receiver operating characteristic curve, *CI* confidence interval
[a]From Walker et al. [12]

Table 12.4 Threshold values for WOMAC scores that predict satisfied from dissatisfied patients[a]

WOMAC	Threshold value	Sensitivity, specificity	AUC	95% CI	*P* value
Pain	>58	75, 60	71.8	67.5–76.0	<0.001
Function	>54	68, 65	71.1	67.1–75.1	<0.001
Stiffness	>56	54, 72	65.5	61.2–69.9	<0.001
Total	>56	68, 67	72.3	68.3–76.2	<0.001

[a]From Walker et al. [12]

Table 12.5 Factors that influence patient satisfaction

Study	Type analysis	Factor	Odds ratio	95% C.I.	*P* value
Bryan et al. [3]	Multivariate model	Preoperative WOMAC pain	2.65	1.76–4.01	<0.001
		Preoperative SF-12 MCS	3.25	1.67–6.34	0.001
		Preoperative SF-12 PCS	3.16	1.50–6.65	0.002
		Change WOMAC pain baseline to 6 months postop	2.31	1.49–3.56	<0.001
Rooks [10]	Univariate	Moderate-severe preoperative radiographic severity OA	0.17	0.04–0.88	0.03
	Univariate	Male gender	NA	NA	0.05
	Univariate	Can kneel postoperatively	0.10	0.01–0.80	0.005
	Univariate	Patient would have surgery again	NA	NA	<0.0001
Lutzner [9]	Multivariate model	Postoperative KSS (5 years)	NA	0.02–0.07	<0.001
		Fulfillment expectations HSS-KRES	NA	0.01–0.05	0.005
Clement [27]	Univariate	Age < 55 years: independent variable (note: not a predictor when adjusted for confounding variables)	0.54	0.37–0.79	0.001
Jain [28]	Univariate	Postoperative HSS-KRFES (6 months)	NA	NA	<0.001
	Univariate	Postoperative HSS-KRFES (12 months)	NA	NA	<0.001
Hamilton [29]	Multivariate model	Meeting preoperative expectations	2.62	2.24–3.07	<0.001
		Achieving pain relief	2.40	2.00–2.87	<0.001
		Satisfied with hospital experience	1.67	1.45–1.91	<0.001
		Postoperative OKS (12 months)	1.08	1.05–1.10	<0.001
		Preoperative OKS	0.95	0.93–0.97	<0.001
Matsuda [30]	Linear regression	Younger patient age (years NA)	NA	NA	0.02
	Linear regression	Valgus alignment postoperatively	NA	NA	0.04
Merle-Vincent [31]	Multivariate model	No complications	6.6	1.8–24.7	0.004
		Age ≥ 70 years	3.9	1.1–14.3	0.04
		Preoperative BMI <27 kg/m^2	0.1	0.03–0.7	0.02
		Joint space narrowing score > 3	3.9	1.1–14.3	0.04

(continued)

Table 12.5 (continued)

Study	Type analysis	Factor	Odds ratio	95% C.I.	P value
Furu [32]	Stepwise regression	Postoperative KSS function score (12 months)	NA	NA	<0.01
	Stepwise regression	Postoperative KSS symptom score (12 months)	NA	NA	<0.01
	Stepwise regression	Postoperative knee extensor isometric strength (12 months)	NA	NA	<0.01
Nakahara [33]	Multivariate model	Postoperative walking and standing (KSS score 5 years)	NA	NA	0.02
		Postoperative climbing up or down 1 flight of stairs (KSS score 5 years)	NA	NA	<0.01
		Postoperative getting into or out of a car (KSS score 5 years)	NA	NA	<0.01
		Postoperative moving laterally (KSS score 5 years)	NA	NA	<0.01
Baker [34]	Multivariate model	Postoperative OKS pain elements (follow-up NA)	0.77	0.74–0.79	<0.001
		Postoperative OKS function elements (follow-up NA)	0.88	0.87–0.90	<0.001
		Age 70–80	1.23	1.01–1.49	<0.05
		Male gender	1.19	1.01–1.39	<0.05

HSS-KRFES Hospital for Special Surgery Knee Replacement Fulfillment of Expectations Survey, *KSS* Knee Society Score, *MCS* mental component score, *NA* not available, *OA* osteoarthritis, *OKS* Oxford Knee Score, *PCS* physical component score, *WOMAC* Western Ontario and McMaster Universities Osteoarthritis Index

WOMAC pain (OR, 1.24; $P = 0.001$), SF-12 PCS (OR, 1.55; $P = 0.005$), and SF-12 MCS (OR, 1.30; $P = 0.01$).

Rooks et al. [10] examined the relationship between preoperative radiographic severity of OA (Kellgren-Lawrence [K-L] scale) and patient satisfaction in 420 TKA patients 2–3 years postoperatively. Satisfaction was determined by selecting either very satisfied, no concerns with knee; partially satisfied, few concerns; or not satisfied. Overall, 76% were satisfied, 20% were partially satisfied, and 4% were not satisfied. Satisfaction was greater in males (OR, 0.29; $P = 0.05$), patients who could kneel postoperatively (OR, 0.10; $P = 0.005$), and patients with preoperative K-L grades 3–4 (OR, 0.17; $P = 0.03$). Patients with mild preoperative radiographic OA had lower satisfaction rates (64% very satisfied) than those with moderate to severe (76% very satisfied).

Lutzner et al. [9] reported two variables predicted patient satisfaction in their model 5 years postoperatively: the KSS ($P < 0.001$) and fulfillment of expectations using the HSS-KRES ($P = 0.005$). Only 59% of the patient expectations were fulfilled. Factors not associated on multivariate analysis were gender, age, American Society of Anesthesiologists physical status classification, body mass index (BMI), re-interventions, implant design, and SF-36.

Clement et al. [27] followed 2589 patients for 1 year post-TKA and reported that patient age less than 55 years was not an independent predictor of patient satisfaction. Although patients in this age group were less likely to be satisfied than those ≥55 years of age, logistic regression analysis used to adjust for confounding variables showed that age group was not an independent predictor with overall outcome, pain relief, return to work, or return to recreation.

Jain et al. [28] reported that the Hospital for Special Surgery Knee Replacement Expectations Survey (HSS-KRES) score at 6 and 12 months postoperatively predicted patients satisfaction in 83 patients ($P < 0.001$). Satisfaction was assessed with the four-question instrument published by Clement et al. [13] discussed previously (Table 12.2). Higher fulfillment of expectations predicting patient satisfaction has also been reported by others [29, 36–38]. Preoperative expectations predicted patient satisfaction at 12 months postoperatively in the series reported by Deakin et al. [4]. Thirteen of the 17 HSS-KRES items were significantly correlated with overall satisfaction.

Hamilton et al. [29] in a cohort of 4709 TKA patients reported that overall patient satisfaction was predicted by meeting preoperative expectations (OR, 2.62; $P < 0.001$), achieving pain relief (OR, 2.40; $P < 0.001$), and being satisfied with the hospital experience (OR, 1.67; $P < 0.001$). These three factors predicted 97% of the variation in overall patient satisfaction response. The preoperative and 12-month postoperative Oxford Scores were also significant predictors (OR, 0.95 and 1.08, respectively; $P < 0.001$); however, these scores carried little weight in the algorithm. Factors such as age, gender, comorbidities, and length of hospital stay did not predict satisfaction. Matsuda et al. [30] reported that in 375 patients followed an average of 5 years postoperatively, no relationship existed between satisfaction and gender, BMI, primary diagnosis, and postoperative range of motion. Negative correlations were found (worse results) for older age ($P = 0.02$) and varus alignment ($P < 0.05$).

Merle-Vincent et al. [31] reported four factors predicted patient satisfaction 2 years after TKA (237 patients): absence of complications (OR, 6.6; $P = 0.004$), age ≥ 70 years (OR, 3.9; $P < 0.05$), preoperative BMI <27 kg/m^2 (OR, 0.1; $P < 0.05$), and joint space narrowing score > 3 ($P < 0.05$).

Furu et al. [32] reported in a small group of 28 patients that the 1-year KSS function score, KSS symptom score, and knee extensor isometric strength were significant predictors of patients satisfaction ($P < 0.01$).

Perez-Prieto et al. [39] compared satisfaction between 200 depressed patients (according to the preoperative Geriatric Depression Scale) and 516 non-depressed patients 1 year postoperatively and found no significant differences with those who felt pleased or very pleased with the results (79% and 85%, respectively)

Ponzio et al. [40] reported no associations between preoperative patient expectations as determined by the HSS-KRES and patient satisfaction at 2 years postoperatively. These authors matched 1008 active patients with 1008 inactive patients and reported that overall satisfaction was equivalent between the groups for pain relief, ability to do daily activities, and overall opinion. A higher percentage of the active group was satisfied with their ability to participate in recreation (72% versus 63%, $P = 0.0003$).

Kunze et al. [7] reported the sensitivity and negative predictive value of an 11-item knee survey for identifying patient satisfaction after primary TKA. The survey (0–100 points) was developed by two fellowship trained senior surgeons and included location and number of osteophytes, flexion contracture, patella thickness to soft tissue shadow, previous knee surgeries, obesity, diabetes, number and type of comorbidities, drug allergies, chronic opioid use before surgery, etiology of arthritis, and smoking (Table 12.6). Patient satisfaction was determined using a binary (yes or no) question and a continuous scale (1–10) in 484 patients in a mean of 1.5 years postoperatively. Patients with a higher survey score had greater odds of being satisfied (OR, 1.03; $P = 0.003$); BMI and age were not significant predictors of satisfaction. ROC analysis determined that a survey score of 96.5 was associated with a 97.5% sensitivity and a 93.0% specificity rate. In other words, 97.5% of patients who were dissatisfied had a survey score < 96.5. A score of <96.5 predicted dissatisfied patients.

Van Onsem et al. [41] developed a ten-item questionnaire prediction model to predict patient satisfaction (as determined by the 2011 KSS). The questions, selected from commonly used PROMs, were completed in 113 patients preoperatively. At 3 months postoperatively, 88% were rated as satisfied, and the authors reported the instrument could accurately be used to predict this factor. However, the model only explained 36% of the variability in satisfaction. Later studies of this same instrument [5, 42] failed to validate its predictive value. Calkins et al. [42] reported that in 145 patients examined 3 months postoperatively, the model did not predict any of the dissatisfied patients. Halawi et al. [5] analyzed data from 203 patients and concluded this model failed to predict either satisfaction or dissatisfaction after TKA.

12.4 Predictors of Dissatisfaction

There have been a wide variety of preoperative and postoperative factors associated with patient dissatisfaction (Table 12.7) [15, 27, 40, 43–51]. In a study of 3324 TKA patients, Clement et al. [44] reported that older age, increasing BMI, and absence of hypertension were independent predictors of dissatisfaction with recreational activities 1 year postoperatively. In another study, Clement et al. [27] followed 2589 patients for 1 year post-TKA and reported an increased risk of dissatisfaction with diabetes (OR, 0.63; $P = 0.02$), liver disease (OR, 0.36; $P = 0.01$), depression (OR, 0.58; $P = 0.008$), and back pain (OR, 0.42; $P < 0.0001$) and worse preoperative scores on the SF-12 PCS (OR, 1.04; $P = 0.009$) and SF-12 MCS (OR, 1.01; $P = 0.04$).

Ponzio et al. [40] reported significant associations between patient comorbidities (Charlson Comorbidity Index of 1–2) and dissatisfaction with the overall results of the TKA (OR, 1.0; $P = 0.01$) and pain relief (OR, 2.3; $P = 0.001$). Female patients were more likely to be dissatisfied with pain relief compared with male patients

Table 12.6 Knee survey used in prediction model for satisfaction after TKA[a]

Factor	Scale	Points
Body mass index (kg/m^2)	20–30	10
	35–35	8
	35–40	5
	40–50	0
	>50	−5
Drug allergies	0	10
	1–2	8
	3–4	0
	>4	−5
Osteophytes	Medial, lateral, patellofemoral, and posterior	10
	Medial, patellofemoral, and posterior	8
	Medial and patellofemoral	5
	Medial only	0
	None	−5
Patella thickness to soft tissue shadow skin thickness	Ratio > 1	10
	Ratio 0.8–1	5
	Ratio 0.5–0.79	0
	Ratio < 0.5	−5
Flexion contracture (°)	0–5	10
	5–10	8
	10–20	5
	20–30	0
	>30 or recurvatum	−5
Diabetes	Non-diabetic	10
	NIDDM with HgbAlc <7.5	8
	NIDDM with HgbAlc 7.5–8.5	5
	NIDDM with HgbAlc 8.5–9.5	0
	IDDM or NIDDM with HgbAlc >9.5	−5
Opioid use	None	10
	Taken for <3 months preoperatively	0
	Taken for >3 months preoperatively	−5
Comorbidity score (based on #). If patient has >5 comorbidities that include fibromyalgia or depression, score is −5	0	10
	1–2	8
	3–4	5
	5	0
	>5	−5
	Any report of fibromyalgia or depression	−5
Previous knee surgery	None	10
	1 scope >1 year prior to TKA	8
	>1 scope or 1 scope within a year prior to TKA	5
	Open prior surgery without hardware	0
	Open prior surgery with hardware	−5
Surgical indication	Primary OA	10
	Secondary OA	8
	Inflammatory DJD	5
	Post-traumatic DJD/osteonecrosis	0
Smoking	Never	10
	Quit >10 years ago	5
	Quit <10 years ago	0
	Current smoker	−5

DJD degenerative joint disease, *IDDM* insulin-dependent diabetes mellitus. *NIDDM* non-insulin-dependent diabetes mellitus, *OA* osteoarthritis

[a]From Kunze et al. [7]

Table 12.7 Factors that influence patient dissatisfaction

Study	Type analysis	Factor	Odds ratio	95% C.I.	*P* value
Clement [44]	Bivariate regression (dissatisfied with recreational activity)	Older age	1.03	1.01–1.04	0.008
		Increasing BMI	1.05	1.01–1.08	0.01
		Absence of hypertension	0.66	0.47–0.94	0.02
Clement [27]	Bivariate regression	Diabetes	0.63	0.42–0.93	0.02
		Liver disease	0.36	0.16–0.80	0.01
		Depression	0.58	0.39–0.87	0.008
		Back pain	0.42	0.30–0.59	<0.001
		Low preoperative SF-12 PCS	1.04	1.01–1.06	0.009
		Low preoperative SF-12 MCS	1.01	1.00–1.03	0.04
Ponzio [40]	Multivariate regression	Charlson Comorbidity Index 1–2 (dissatisfied with overall results)	1.90	NA	0.01
		Charlson Comorbidity Index 1–2 (dissatisfied with pain relief)	2.3	NA	0.001
		Female gender (dissatisfied with pain relief)	1.7	NA	0.03
		Lower preoperative SF-12 PCS (dissatisfied ability to do recreational activities)	1.04	NA	0.005
		Lower preoperative SF-12 PCS (dissatisfied ability to do housework or yard work)	1.03	NA	0.04
		Lower preoperative SF-12 PCS (dissatisfied overall results)	1.03	NA	0.04
		Lower preoperative SF-12 MCS (dissatisfied quality of life)	1.02	NA	0.03
Ali [47]	Multiple regression (compared with satisfied patients)	Poorer postoperative VAS pain score	NA	NA	<0.001
		Anxiety or depression	NA	NA	0.001
		Poorer range of motion	NA	NA	<0.001
Nazzai [45]	T test (compared with satisfied patients)	Shorter postoperative walking distance and magnitude of improvement compared with preoperative	NA	NA	<0.05
		Poorer postoperative number of stairs climbed and magnitude of improvement compared with preoperative	NA	NA	<0.05
		Poorer VAS pain scores and magnitude of improvement compared with preoperative	NA	NA	<0.05

(continued)

Table 12.7 (continued)

Study	Type analysis	Factor	Odds ratio	95% C.I.	*P* value
Schnurr [46]	Logistic regression	Kellgren-Lawrence grade II arthritis (compared with grade IV)	2.96	1.61–5.44	<0.001
		Kellgren-Lawrence grade III arthritis (compared with grade IV)	2.55	1.70–3.84	<0.001
Barrack [48]	Multivariate	Income <25,000 USD, overall knee function	2.29	1.13–4.64	0.02
		Income <25,000 USD, ability to perform daily activities	2.01	1.03–3.83	<0.05
		Income <25,000 USD, pain relief	2.49	1.23–5.04	0.01
		Female gender, overall knee function	3.13	1.54–6.35	0.002
		Female gender, ability to perform daily activities	1.76	1.01–3.07	<0.05
		Female gender, pain relief	2.03	1.06–3.07	<0.05
Bourne [15]	Logistic regression	Expectations not met	10.66	NA	<0.05
		Preoperative pain at rest	2.36	NA	<0.05
		Complication requiring readmission	1.86	NA	<0.05
		Older age	1.03	NA	<0.05
		Low preoperative WOMAC function score	1.01	NA	<0.05
		Low postoperative WOMAC pain score	2.45	NA	<0.05
		Low postoperative WOMAC function score	2.46	NA	<0.05
Scott [49]	Multivariate regression	Lower preoperative SF-12 MCS	NA	NA	<0.001
		Depression	NA	NA	<0.001
		Pain in other joints	NA	NA	<0.001
		Low SF-12 postoperative score	NA	NA	<0.001
		Lower improvement OKS pain	NA	NA	<0.001
Kim [50]	Multivariate regression	Low preoperative WOMAC pain score	7.6	2.3–25.1	0.001
		Decrease in range of motion postoperatively	2.1	1.5–2.9	<0.001
Du [51]	Logistic regression	Low postoperative WOMAC pain score	1.9	NA	<0.001

BMI body mass index, *MCS* mental component score, *PCS* physical component score, *WOMAC* Western Ontario and McMaster Universities Osteoarthritis Index, *VAS* visual analogue scale

(OR, 1.7; $P < 0.05$). Lower baseline SF-12 PCS and SF-12 MCS were associated with dissatisfaction for several variables.

Nazzal et al. [45] reported significant differences between satisfied and unsatisfied patients 3 months after surgery in VAS pain scores (2.69 and 2.9, respectively; $P = 0.01$), maximum walking distance (503 m and 334 m, respectively; $P = 0.03$), and maximum number of stairs climbed (40 and 33, respectively; $P = 0.02$).

Barrack et al. [48] studied the effect of socioeconomic factors on patient dissatisfaction and found that those that had an annual income of less than 25,000 USD (year 2014) had greater odds of being dissatisfied with overall knee function, ability to perform daily activities, and degree of pain relief. There was no effect of minority status or employment 3 months before surgery.

Scott et al. [49] in a study of 1217 TKA patients reported five factors related to dissatisfaction at 1 year postoperatively: lower preoperative SF-12 MCS score, depression, pain in other joints, low SF-12 postoperative score, and lower improvement in the OKS pain score.

Lizaur-Utrilla et al. [52] analyzed factors that resulted in clinical failure of TKA (defined as KSS score < 70 points) a mean of 5.8 years postoperatively in a cohort of 412 knees. Predictors of clinical failure in the multivariate regression analysis included a high Charlson index of more than two comorbidities (OR, 2.11; $P = 0.03$), lower KSS function score (OR, 0.76; $P = 0.006$), and worse preoperative WOMAC pain score (OR, 0.3; $P = 0.01$).

12.5 Conclusions

In order to determine the most important factors for achieving patient satisfaction and improving quality of life (QOL) following total knee arthroplasty (TKA), validated scales must be used and influences of compounding factors must be accounted for such as mental and emotional problems and pain in other joints. Although a variety of scales and questions have been used to rate patient satisfaction, few have been validated and there is tremendous variation in recent literature regarding this topic. Many factors have been shown to be predictive of patient satisfaction, including meeting patient preoperative expectations and postoperative function and pain relief as shown by scores on the Knee Society and Oxford Knee Society scales. Factors predictive of patient dissatisfaction include the presence of two or more comorbidities, female gender, depression, and low preoperative scores on the Medical Outcomes Short Form 12 and Western Ontario and McMaster Universities Osteoarthritis Index instruments. Preoperative patient counseling should include discussion of these factors to provide realistic expectations regarding outcomes. Further work is required on the research front to devise standardized and validated measures for satisfaction. In addition, work is required to determine strategies and interventions appropriate to modify expectations when required in order to improve postoperative outcomes and satisfaction [35].

References

1. Kahlenberg CA, Nwachukwu BU, McLawhorn AS, Cross MB, Cornell CN, Padgett DE. Patient satisfaction after total knee replacement: a systematic review. HSS J. 2018;14(2):192–201. https://doi.org/10.1007/s11420-018-9614-8.

2. Bierke S, Häner M, Karpinski K, Hees T, Petersen W. Midterm effect of mental factors on pain, function, and patient satisfaction 5 years after uncomplicated total knee arthroplasty. J Arthroplasty. 2020;35(1):105–11. https://doi.org/10.1016/j.arth.2019.08.008.
3. Bryan S, Goldsmith LJ, Davis JC, Hejazi S, MacDonald V, McAllister P, Randall E, Suryaprakash N, Wu AD, Sawatzky R. Revisiting patient satisfaction following total knee arthroplasty: a longitudinal observational study. BMC Musculoskelet Disord. 2018;19(1):423. https://doi.org/10.1186/s12891-018-2340-z.
4. Deakin AH, Smith MA, Wallace DT, Smith EJ, Sarungi M. Fulfilment of preoperative expectations and postoperative patient satisfaction after total knee replacement. A prospective analysis of 200 patients. Knee. 2019;26(6):1403–12. https://doi.org/10.1016/j.knee.2019.07.018.
5. Halawi MJ, Jongbloed W, Baron S, Savoy L, Williams VJ, Cote MP. Patient dissatisfaction after primary total joint arthroplasty: the patient perspective. J Arthroplasty. 2019;34(6):1093–6. https://doi.org/10.1016/j.arth.2019.01.075.
6. Hamilton DF, Lane JV, Gaston P, Patton JT, Macdonald DJ, Simpson AH, Howie CR. Assessing treatment outcomes using a single question: the net promoter score. Bone Joint J. 2014;96-B(5):622–8. https://doi.org/10.1302/0301-620X.96B5.32434.
7. Kunze KN, Akram F, Fuller BC, Zabawa L, Sporer SM, Levine BR. Internal validation of a predictive model for satisfaction after primary total knee arthroplasty. J Arthroplasty. 2019;34(4):663–70. https://doi.org/10.1016/j.arth.2018.12.020.
8. Lange JK, Lee YY, Spiro SK, Haas SB. Satisfaction rates and quality of life changes following Total knee arthroplasty in age-differentiated cohorts. J Arthroplasty. 2018;33(5):1373–8. https://doi.org/10.1016/j.arth.2017.12.031.
9. Lützner C, Postler A, Beyer F, Kirschner S, Lützner J. Fulfillment of expectations influence patient satisfaction 5 years after total knee arthroplasty. Knee Surg Sports Traumatol Arthrosc. 2019;27(7):2061–70. https://doi.org/10.1007/s00167-018-5320-9.
10. Rooks K, Houdek D, Obaid H, Dust W. Primary total knee arthroplasty: correlation between preoperative radiographic severity of arthritis and postoperative patient satisfaction. J Knee Surg. 2020. https://doi.org/10.1055/s-0040-1710384.
11. Teo BJX, Koh JSB, Jiang L, Allen JC, Yeo SJ, Howe TS. Association of the 36-item short form health survey physical component summary score with patient satisfaction and improvement 2 years after total knee arthroplasty. JAMA Netw Open. 2019;2(2):e190062. https://doi.org/10.1001/jamanetworkopen.2019.0062.
12. Walker LC, Clement ND, Bardgett M, Weir D, Holland J, Gerrand C, Deehan DJ. The WOMAC score can be reliably used to classify patient satisfaction after total knee arthroplasty. Knee Surg Sports Traumatol Arthrosc. 2018;26(11):3333–41. https://doi.org/10.1007/s00167-018-4879-5.
13. Clement ND, Bardgett M, Weir D, Holland J, Gerrand C, Deehan DJ. The rate and predictors of patient satisfaction after total knee arthroplasty are influenced by the focus of the question: a standard satisfaction question is required. Bone Joint J. 2018;100-b(6):740–8. https://doi.org/10.1302/0301-620x.100b6.Bjj-2017-1292.R1.
14. Mahomed N, Gandhi R, Daltroy L, Katz JN. The self-administered patient satisfaction scale for primary hip and knee arthroplasty. Arthritis. 2011;2011:591253. https://doi.org/10.1155/2011/591253.
15. Bourne RB, Chesworth BM, Davis AM, Mahomed NN, Charron KD. Patient satisfaction after total knee arthroplasty: who is satisfied and who is not? Clin Orthop Relat Res. 2010;468(1):57–63. https://doi.org/10.1007/s11999-009-1119-9.
16. Devlin NJ, Brooks R. EQ-5D and the EuroQol group: past, present and future. Appl Health Econ Health Policy. 2017;15(2):127–37. https://doi.org/10.1007/s40258-017-0310-5.
17. EuroQOL. EuroQol--a new facility for the measurement of health-related quality of life. Health Policy. 1990;16(3):199–208. https://doi.org/10.1016/0168-8510(90)90421-9.
18. Gandhi SK, Salmon JW, Zhao SZ, Lambert BL, Gore PR, Conrad K. Psychometric evaluation of the 12-item short-form health survey (SF-12) in osteoarthritis and rheumatoid arthritis clinical trials. Clin Ther. 2001;23(7):1080–98.

19. McHorney CA, Ware JE, Rachel JF, Sherbourne CD. The MOS 36-item short-form health survey (SF-36): III. Tests of data quality, scaling assumptions, and reliability across diverse patient groups. Med Care. 1994;32(1):40–66.
20. McHorney CA, Ware JE, Raczek AE. The MOS 36-item short-form health survey (SF-36): II. Psychometric and clinical tests of validity in measuring physical and mental health constructs. Med Care. 1993;31(3):247–63.
21. Ware J Jr, Kosinski M, Keller SD. A 12-Item Short-Form Health Survey: construction of scales and preliminary tests of reliability and validity. Med Care. 1996;34(3):220–33.
22. Lan RH, Bell JW, Samuel LT, Kamath AF. Evolving outcome measures in total knee arthroplasty: trends and utilization rates over the past 15 years. J Arthroplasty. 2020. https://doi.org/10.1016/j.arth.2020.06.036.
23. Rat A-C, Coste J, Pouchot J, Baumann M, Spitz E, Retel-Rude N, Le Quintrec J-S, Dumont-Fischer D, Guillemin F. OAKHQOL: a new instrument to measure quality of life in knee and hip osteoarthritis. J Clin Epidemiol. 2005;58(1):47–55.
24. Rat A-C, Pouchot J, Coste J, Baumann C, Spitz E, Retel-Rude N, Baumann M, Le Quintrec J-S, Dumont-Fischer D, Guillemin F. Development and testing of a specific quality-of-life questionnaire for knee and hip osteoarthritis: OAKHQOL (OsteoArthritis of Knee Hip Quality Of Life). Joint Bone Spine revue du rhumatisme. 2006;73(6):697–704.
25. Garratt AM, Brealey S, Robling M, Atwell C, Russell I, Gillespie W, King D, Team DT. Development of the knee quality of life (KQoL-26) 26-item questionnaire: data quality, reliability, validity and responsiveness. Health Qual Life Outcomes. 2008;6:48. https://doi.org/10.1186/1477-7525-6-48.
26. Chuang L-H, Garratt A, Brealey S. Comparative responsiveness and minimal change of the Knee Quality of Life 26-item (KQoL-26) questionnaire. Qual Life Res. 2013;22(9):2461–75.
27. Clement ND, Walker LC, Bardgett M, Weir D, Holland J, Gerrand C, Deehan DJ. Patient age of less than 55 years is not an independent predictor of functional improvement or satisfaction after total knee arthroplasty. Arch Orthop Trauma Surg. 2018;138(12):1755–63. https://doi.org/10.1007/s00402-018-3041-7.
28. Jain D, Nguyen LL, Bendich I, Nguyen LL, Lewis CG, Huddleston JI, Duwelius PJ, Feeley BT, Bozic KJ. Higher patient expectations predict higher patient-reported outcomes, but not satisfaction, in total knee arthroplasty patients: a prospective multicenter study. J Arthroplasty. 2017;32(9S):S166–70. https://doi.org/10.1016/j.arth.2017.01.008.
29. Hamilton DF, Lane JV, Gaston P, Patton JT, Macdonald D, Simpson AH, Howie CR. What determines patient satisfaction with surgery? A prospective cohort study of 4709 patients following total joint replacement. BMJ Open. 2013;3(4). https://doi.org/10.1136/bmjopen-2012-002525.
30. Matsuda S, Kawahara S, Okazaki K, Tashiro Y, Iwamoto Y. Postoperative alignment and ROM affect patient satisfaction after TKA. Clin Orthop Relat Res. 2013;471(1):127–33. https://doi.org/10.1007/s11999-012-2533-y.
31. Merle-Vincent F, Couris CM, Schott AM, Conrozier T, Piperno M, Mathieu P, Vignon E, Osteoarthritis Section of the French Society for R. Factors predicting patient satisfaction 2 years after total knee arthroplasty for osteoarthritis. Joint Bone Spine revue du rhumatisme. 2011;78(4):383–6. https://doi.org/10.1016/j.jbspin.2010.11.013.
32. Furu M, Ito H, Nishikawa T, Nankaku M, Kuriyama S, Ishikawa M, Nakamura S, Azukizawa M, Hamamoto Y, Matsuda S. Quadriceps strength affects patient satisfaction after total knee arthroplasty. J Orthop Sci. 2016;21(1):38–43. https://doi.org/10.1016/j.jos.2015.10.002.
33. Nakahara H, Okazaki K, Mizu-Uchi H, Hamai S, Tashiro Y, Matsuda S, Iwamoto Y. Correlations between patient satisfaction and ability to perform daily activities after total knee arthroplasty: why aren't patients satisfied? J Orthop Sci. 2015;20(1):87–92. https://doi.org/10.1007/s00776-014-0671-7.
34. Baker PN, van der Meulen JH, Lewsey J, Gregg PJ, National Joint Registry for E, Wales. The role of pain and function in determining patient satisfaction after total knee replacement. Data from the National Joint Registry for England and Wales. J Bone Joint Surg. 2007;89(7):893–900. https://doi.org/10.1302/0301-620X.89B7.19091.

35. Swarup I, Henn CM, Gulotta LV, Henn RF 3rd. Patient expectations and satisfaction in orthopaedic surgery: a review of the literature. J Clin Orthop Trauma. 2019;10(4):755–60. https://doi.org/10.1016/j.jcot.2018.08.008.
36. Noble PC, Conditt MA, Cook KF, Mathis KB. The John Insall Award: patient expectations affect satisfaction with total knee arthroplasty. Clin Orthop Relat Res. 2006;452:35–43. https://doi.org/10.1097/01.blo.0000238825.63648.1e.
37. Scott CE, Bugler KE, Clement ND, MacDonald D, Howie CR, Biant LC. Patient expectations of arthroplasty of the hip and knee. J Bone Joint Surg. 2012;94(7):974–81. https://doi.org/10.1302/0301-620X.94B7.28219.
38. Hafkamp FJ, Gosens T, de Vries J, den Oudsten BL. Do dissatisfied patients have unrealistic expectations? A systematic review and best-evidence synthesis in knee and hip arthroplasty patients. EFORT Open Rev. 2020;5(4):226–40. https://doi.org/10.1302/2058-5241.5.190015.
39. Perez-Prieto D, Gil-Gonzalez S, Pelfort X, Leal-Blanquet J, Puig-Verdie L, Hinarejos P. Influence of depression on total knee arthroplasty outcomes. J Arthroplasty. 2014;29(1):44–7. https://doi.org/10.1016/j.arth.2013.04.030.
40. Ponzio DY, Chiu YF, Salvatore A, Lee YY, Lyman S, Windsor RE. An analysis of the influence of physical activity level on total knee arthroplasty expectations, satisfaction, and outcomes: increased revision in active patients at five to ten years. J Bone Joint Surg Am. 2018;100(18):1539–48. https://doi.org/10.2106/jbjs.17.00920.
41. Van Onsem S, Van Der Straeten C, Arnout N, Deprez P, Van Damme G, Victor J. A new prediction model for patient satisfaction after total knee arthroplasty. J Arthroplasty. 2016;31(12):2660–2667 e2661. https://doi.org/10.1016/j.arth.2016.06.004.
42. Calkins TE, Culvern C, Nahhas CR, Della Valle CJ, Gerlinger TL, Levine BR, Nam D. External validity of a new prediction model for patient satisfaction after total knee arthroplasty. J Arthroplasty. 2019;34(8):1677–81. https://doi.org/10.1016/j.arth.2019.04.021.
43. Gunaratne R, Pratt DN, Banda J, Fick DP, Khan RJK, Robertson BW. Patient dissatisfaction following total knee arthroplasty: a systematic review of the literature. J Arthroplasty. 2017;32(12):3854–60. https://doi.org/10.1016/j.arth.2017.07.021.
44. Clement ND, Walker LC, Merrie K, Bardgett M, Weir D, Holland J, Deehan DJ. Which patients are satisfied with their overall outcome but dissatisfied with their return to recreational activities after total knee arthroplasty? Knee. 2019;26(1):258–66. https://doi.org/10.1016/j.knee.2018.09.013.
45. Nazzal MI, Bashaireh KH, Alomari MA, Nazzal MS, Maayah MF, Mesmar M. Relationship between improvements in physical measures and patient satisfaction in rehabilitation after total knee arthroplasty. Int J Rehabil Res. 2012;35(2):94–101. https://doi.org/10.1097/MRR.0b013e32834df63c.
46. Schnurr C, Jarrous M, Gudden I, Eysel P, Konig DP. Pre-operative arthritis severity as a predictor for total knee arthroplasty patients' satisfaction. Int Orthop. 2013;37(7):1257–61. https://doi.org/10.1007/s00264-013-1862-0.
47. Ali A, Sundberg M, Robertsson O, Dahlberg LE, Thorstensson CA, Redlund-Johnell I, Kristiansson I, Lindstrand A. Dissatisfied patients after total knee arthroplasty: a registry study involving 114 patients with 8-13 years of followup. Acta Orthop. 2014;85(3):229–33. https://doi.org/10.3109/17453674.2014.916487.
48. Barrack RL, Ruh EL, Chen J, Lombardi AV Jr, Berend KR, Parvizi J, Della Valle CJ, Hamilton WG, Nunley RM. Impact of socioeconomic factors on outcome of total knee arthroplasty. Clin Orthop Relat Res. 2014;472(1):86–97. https://doi.org/10.1007/s11999-013-3002-y.
49. Scott CE, Howie CR, MacDonald D, Biant LC. Predicting dissatisfaction following total knee replacement: a prospective study of 1217 patients. J Bone Joint Surg. 2010;92(9):1253–8. https://doi.org/10.1302/0301-620X.92B9.24394.
50. Kim TK, Chang CB, Kang YG, Kim SJ, Seong SC. Causes and predictors of patient's dissatisfaction after uncomplicated total knee arthroplasty. J Arthroplasty. 2009;24(2):263–71. https://doi.org/10.1016/j.arth.2007.11.005.

51. Du H, Tang H, Gu JM, Zhou YX. Patient satisfaction after posterior-stabilized total knee arthroplasty: a functional specific analysis. Knee. 2014;21(4):866–70. https://doi.org/10.1016/j.knee.2014.03.007.
52. Lizaur-Utrilla A, Gonzalez-Parreno S, Miralles-Munoz FA, Lopez-Prats FA, Gil-Guillen V. Patient-related predictors of treatment failure after primary total knee arthroplasty for osteoarthritis. J Arthroplasty. 2014;29(11):2095–9. https://doi.org/10.1016/j.arth.2014.07.011.
53. Scuderi GR, Bourne RB, Noble PC, Benjamin JB, Lonner JH, Scott WN. The new knee society knee scoring system. Clin Orthop Relat Res. 2012;470(1):3–19. https://doi.org/10.1007/s11999-011-2135-0.

Index

F. R. Noyes, S. Barber-Westin (eds.), *Critical Rehabilitation for Partial and Total Knee Arthroplasty*, https://doi.org/10.1007/978-3-030-87003-4

GPSR Compliance

The European Union's (EU) General Product Safety Regulation (GPSR) is a set of rules that requires consumer products to be safe and our obligations to ensure this.

If you have any concerns about our products, you can contact us on ProductSafety@springernature.com

In case Publisher is established outside the EU, the EU authorized representative is:

Springer Nature Customer Service Center GmbH
Europaplatz 3
69115 Heidelberg, Germany

Batch number: 10726135

Printed by Printforce, the Netherlands